HYDROCEPHALUS

A Guide for Patients, Families, and Friends

Chuck Toporek and Kellie Robinson

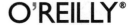

O'REILLY®

Beijing • Cambridge • Köln • Paris • Sebastopol • Taipei • Tokyo

Hydrocephalus: A Guide for Patients, Families, and Friends
by Chuck Toporek and Kellie Robinson

Copyright © 1999 O'Reilly & Associates, Inc. All rights reserved.
Printed in the United States of America.

Published by O'Reilly & Associates, Inc., 101 Morris Street, Sebastopol, CA 95472.

Editor: Linda Lamb

Production Editor: Claire Cloutier LeBlanc

Printing History:

> February 1999: First Edition

Library of Congress Cataloging-in-Publication Data:

Toporek, Chuck, 1965– .
    Hydrocephalus: a guide for patients, families, and friends / Chuck Toporek and
      Kellie Robinson.
       p. cm.—(Patient-centered guides)
      ISBN 1-56592-410-X (pbk.)
      1. Hydrocephalus—Popular works. I. Robinson, Kellie, 1967– .
II. Title. III. Series.
RC391.T66   1999
616.85'8843—dc21

                                98-52974
                                    CIP

For all hydrocephalus patients and their families.
May this book provide you with knowledge, comfort, and hope.

Table of Contents

Foreword

THE NEUROSURGICAL SERVICE at the Brigham and Women's Hospital and Children's Hospital in Boston performs over 2,000 procedures a year. Of these, about 2 percent in children and 5 percent in adult procedures are for hydrocephalus. Hydrocephalus is therefore a major neurosurgical problem, although it is often not accorded the same attention as stroke, brain tumors, epilepsy, or other neurosurgical conditions.

The relative neglect of this important condition and its treatments extends well beyond neurosurgery. It is only briefly covered in most medical textbooks, and there are few resources for families. In this book, Chuck Toporek and Kellie Robinson have provided a wonderful entry into the world of hydrocephalus to begin to remedy this situation. They begin with a very personal account of the problem and its management, and then branch out into a comprehensive and thoughtful discussion of the causes, manifestations, and treatment of hydrocephalus.

In the discussion, it becomes clear that more attention is needed to this condition. Properly treated, it becomes merely an inconvenience in a patient's life. Ignored or misdiagnosed, it can be a source of permanent disability, distress, or even death. For patients with myelomeningoceles, brain tumors, subarachnoid hemorrhage, aqueductal stenosis, and a myriad of other conditions, it is a treatable problem that can be no problem at all. However, for this to be the case, it is important to raise public awareness and to try to improve our present valve systems. This volume is an important contribution to this effort; as physicians dedicated to the care of patients with hydrocephalus, we are immensely grateful to Chuck and Kellie for their groundbreaking efforts.

—Peter M. Black, M.D., Ph.D.
Franc D. Ingraham Professor of Neurosurgery, Harvard Medical School
Neurosurgeon-in-Chief, Brigham and Women's Hospital, Children's Hospital
Boston, Massachusetts

Preface

HYDROCEPHALUS IS A COMPLEX AND UNFORGIVING CONDITION. The more you know about hydrocephalus, its side effects, and how to live with the condition, the more you will be able to prepare yourself for the road ahead.

"Knowledge is power." These words—spoken by the English philosopher Francis Bacon—hold great meaning when it comes to any medical condition, and in particular, hydrocephalus. There is much to know, and very few places for parents to turn when their child is first diagnosed with hydrocephalus. We hope this book fills that much-needed space to provide you with information, resources, and most importantly, support.

Why we wrote this book

It wasn't until Kellie's second shunt revision in 1991, when she was 24 and just after we were married, that we started to learn more about hydrocephalus. Kellie's neurosurgeon told us what a shunt was and how it worked. Remarkably, he explained it all to us in terms that we could both understand and without talking down to us. This was the first time we actually knew what a shunt looked like because he pulled a sample out of his desk drawer and showed it to us.

This began our quest for knowledge about hydrocephalus. We knew that in order for our relationship to survive, we had to know more about the condition, which in a moment's notice turned our world upside down. However, we were quite amazed at how little information there was out there for non-medical laypersons about hydrocephalus. Everything we encountered was highly technical, written by and for neurosurgeons.

It wasn't until 1995 when *The Shunt Book*, by James Drake and Christian Sainte-Rose, was released that more information about hydrocephalus came into the mainstream. Although *The Shunt Book* was useful for finding out more information about the mechanical devices people with hydrocephalus rely on, it lacked the kind of information we craved. We wanted to know what was happening in Kellie's body. We wanted to know what symptoms to be aware of. We wanted to know how to deal with the uncertainty of not knowing when and if her shunt would fail again, where to get support, and how to live with hydrocephalus as normally as possible without being in constant fear. We had a lot of questions and nowhere to turn, except to each other.

Around the same time that *The Shunt Book* was published, we stumbled across a mailing list on the Internet called HYCEPH-L. Compared to the popularity of the Web, mailing lists are kind of the underworld of the Internet, yet most teem with energy. We subscribed to HYCEPH-L and were amazed by some of the email messages people were sending out to the list. People from around the globe shared their feelings and frustrations of living with hydrocephalus and watching their children or loved ones going through shunt revision after shunt revision. People offered caring messages of support, understanding, and love.

But the most common questions to the list were about how to find more information about hydrocephalus. Some people recommended mainstream medical journals like the *New England Journal of Medicine* or the journal *Neurosurgery*. Although these journals offer great insight on the latest treatments and studies about hydrocephalus, they are written for neurosurgeons—using their vocabulary and addressing their concerns.

HYCEPH-L not only brought us closer to others who have hydrocephalus, it was also our first introduction to the Hydrocephalus Association in San Francisco. The fact that there was an organization out there for the condition renewed our hopes of learning more about hydrocephalus.

This book started with our own search for answers, but it could not have come about without the similar search by many others impacted by hydrocephalus. Some of the answers have come from medical doctors and medical texts, some from patient organizations dedicated to finding and sharing information, and much from the shared wisdom of patients and parents living and coping with hydrocephalus.

What this book offers

Our goal was to create a book that contained all the information you need to know about hydrocephalus.

- Medical information. We have included medical background so that you will be informed, able to ask your doctor questions, and participate in care decisions. Where medical terms are used—and they are—we explain to you what they mean; there is also a glossary of terms at the back of the book.

- Practical matters. As every patient and family knows, the medical facts are just one facet of hydrocephalus. We go into some detail on practical matters that can make life less stressful—for example, how to prepare for emergencies or write appeal letters for claims denied under insurance.

- Emotional support and stories. We have tried to let you know that you are not alone. We include many resources for emotional support and patient organizations. Throughout the book you will find stories and suggestions from parents and patients who wanted to share what they learned and what they have been through. The words are their own; some names have been changed to protect the person's privacy.

While researching the material for this book, we were constantly asked to write about the things that doctors don't tell patients. Some doctors feel they are best serving their patients by only giving them information on a need-to-know basis. What some doctors don't understand, however, is that after patients are discharged from the hospital, they may have many questions that still need to be answered.

The audience for this book encompasses a wide range of ages and experience: parents of newborns, parents of children, teens curious about what lies ahead and lifestyle decisions, and adults in charge of their own health and treatment. Other family members, such as spouses of those with hydrocephalus, will also be involved in watching for symptoms (especially neurological side effects such as confusion, mood changes, or lethargy) and seeking treatment. The "you" that this book is for is all of you who need to learn about the condition and make decisions, whether on behalf of your child, your spouse, or yourself.

How this book is organized

We have organized the book in the order that most people need the information.

The first two chapters are about finding out about the condition. Chapter 1, *What Is Hydrocephalus?* describes hydrocephalus, the areas and structures of the brain, and the flow of cerebrospinal fluid through the brain. Chapter 2, *Getting the Diagnosis*, discusses the different types of hydrocephalus, causes of the condition, and how hydrocephalus is diagnosed. You also hear first-hand stories from patients and parents about how they reacted to learning about the diagnosis.

The next four chapters are about treating the condition. Chapter 3, *Selecting a Neurosurgeon*, teaches how to find out more about your neurosurgeon and to choose the best doctor for your situation. Chapter 4, *Treating Hydrocephalus*, explains shunt systems, where they are placed, differences among shunts, sample shunt surgeries, and nonsurgical treatments. Chapter 5, *Hospitalization and Recovery*, describes what to expect during a neurosurgery stay, preparing your family, admissions process, common hospital rules, and the recovery process. Chapter 6, *Shunt Revisions*, looks at some of the reasons why a shunt can fail, what to look for as signs of a possible shunt malfunction, how your neurosurgeon determines the extent of the problem, and what will happen if the shunt needs to be replaced or revised.

The last five chapters talk about living with the condition. Chapter 7, *Side Effects*, describes potential side effects that may follow shunt surgeries and how they are treated. Chapter 8, *Finding Support*, talks about the wide range of support available to families dealing with hydrocephalus, and how to start a local support group if none is available. Chapter 9, *School*, examines issues for school-age children, including absences for hospitalization or recovery, the potential for learning disabilities, and individualized education plans. Chapter 10, *Insurance*, looks at insurance issues of importance to those with hydrocephalus, such as preexisting conditions, lifetime caps, provider networks, billing problems, and appealing denied claims or services. Chapter 11, *The Well-Informed Patient*, describes managing hydrocephalus for the long term. It includes knowing your medical history, planning for emergencies, researching new treatments and findings, and being aware of medical legislation that affects you.

Appendixes A–E include a list of pediatric neurosurgeons, contact information for organizations and associations, medical libraries and medical journals, suggested reading, and additional Internet resources. A glossary of medical terms can also be found at the back of the book, along with a bibliography listing the reference sources used for this book.

How to use this book

Consider this book a personal resource guide. This book does not need to be read from cover to cover. Read only the sections that apply to your present situation and needs. Then, when you get a chance or have some time to spare, go back and check out the rest of the book to answer other questions that may not be as critical. If you still crave more information, there are substantial resources at the end of the book.

The personal stories shared throughout this book are written into each chapter to give you more insight as to what others have been through with hydrocephalus and how they have coped. The stories may or may not reflect your present situation. Every person's situation and experience will be different, although many issues are held in common.

Acknowledgments

We have many people to acknowledge for their efforts in helping this book come together.

First and foremost, we would like to acknowledge Emily Fudge, executive director and founder of the Hydrocephalus Association in San Francisco. Emily, you have been behind us all the way since we first knocked on your door a year ago with a draft of the outline for this book. Your unflagging dedication to the treatment and care of people with hydrocephalus truly inspired us. By giving us complete access to your wealth of knowledge, as well as your medical advisory board, you helped mold this book into its present form. You were our guiding light, and we are forever in your debt.

To our technical reviewers, we also owe you many thanks. Knowing that we are not medical professionals, you gave valuable input that not only made the book technically correct, but also helped set the benchmark for future editions and other books on hydrocephalus. Our reviewers included: Dr. Peter Black, Dr. Alexa Canady, Dr. Samuel Ciricillo, Dr. Michael Edwards, Dr. Roger Hudgins, Dr. Sue Lehr, Dr. J. Gordon McComb, Dr. Marijean Miller, Dr. Marion "Jack" Walker, Dr. Rochelle Wolk, Siobhan Geary, R.N., M.S., Emily S. Fudge, Marcy Sheiner, Cynthia Solomon; Greg Tocco, Debbi Fields, Nancy Bradley, Lynn Power, Kathie Kelley, Chris Riccio, and Jeff Browndyke.

Additional thanks to Nancy Keene, author of *Childhood Leukemia, Your Child in the Hospital,* and *Working with Your Doctor,* for her part in the review of our book and for her editing suggestions. Sections in this book on sources of support, support groups, taking a tour of the hospital, absences from school, who's who in the hospital, and befriending the staff are excerpted or adapted from sections in her book, *Childhood Leukemia.*

We would like to express our appreciation to the members of the hydrocephalus listserv, HYCEPH-L, for opening your lives for all of us, and for bearing with our questions and requests for input for the book. We strongly believe that the stories you've shared with the readers of this book will help countless others to cope with this very unforgiving condition. HYCEPH-L subscribers who contributed their experiences include: Nancy Bradley, Shirley Bricker, Cynthia Burkhead, Ruth Butler, Gina Coats, Don Cook, Geraldine Diehl, Jason M. Dunn, Lynda, Chuck, and Dakoda Eads, Donna M. Ellis, Debbi Fields, Stacy Gaches, Denise Group, Jo Ann Haglund, Mike and Lisa Healy, Joan R. Hendricks, Dara Herman, Paula Jongenburger, Heidi Kanitz, Kathie and Mike Kelley, Gretchen M. Kohl, Karen Langston, Christy R. Little, Chuck Liu, Judy McGhee, Sandra Mallon, Randy Markey, Linda Meehan, Janet Price-Ferrell, Chris Riccio, Carl and Adina Sherer, Brenda Standefer, Christian Stuhr, Greg Tocco, Deanna H. Traxler, Jeannie Washburn, Jim Weaver, Yasushi Yamashita and Shibata Yasuko, Mike and Lisa Zeman, and those who wish to remain anonymous. Also thanks to Kellie's sister Sheri and our good friend Katie Johnson for their support and for contributing stories to our book as well.

Another group of people we would like to thank are the shunt manufacturers who supplied us with photos of their shunts, technical information, instructional videos of surgical procedures, and anything we needed or asked for. The folks who helped us out include:

- Tom Tokos, from Codman/Johnson & Johnson.

- Marie Hatheway, from Medtronic PS Medical.

- Judy Roth and Terry Layton, from NeuroCare Group.

- Courtney Smith, from Phoenix Biomedical Corporation.

- Katrina Halbig, Stephen Farris, and Jim Bazzinotti, from Elekta/NMT Neurosciences (U.S.).

Next, we would like to extend our gratitude to the people at O'Reilly who helped make this book possible. We cannot say enough about the encouragement and support we received from our editor, Linda Lamb. This book started out with a simple one-paragraph email to Linda, explaining, in a nutshell, what hydrocephalus was and why a book about it was so desperately needed. That simple email lead to numerous conversations and meetings to develop an outline for the book. When we first embarked on this project, Linda asked if we thought we could do this together without killing one another. We're happy to report that we've not only survived writing it, but can gladly say we haven't had a single skirmish.

We would also like to thank Carol Wenmoth, editorial assistant, for readying our book for production and her careful attention to detail, from illustrations to permissions to resource listings.

Thank you to both Linda and Carol for believing in us, mentoring us, and for giving us the support (and schedule deviations) we needed when Kellie's health threw us a curve while writing the book. All that positive energy really paid off.

Also thanks to the many people at O'Reilly whom we haven't met who've played a part in the production, copy editing, and design of our book.

Our deepest appreciation to our parents: Greg and Carol Toporek, and Robert and Carole Robinson, for all their love, support, and encouragement over the years and while we wrote this book.

Thanks to our friends, who were there for us when Kellie had her revisions in 1991, and who've faithfully been there through the good and bad times since: Wes Bethel and Jane Lybecker, Shirley Brooks, Anne and Steve Cole, Cathy Goodman, Joe and Katie Johnson, Mary Kay Hasemann, Bob McNamee, Mike "Morty" Morton, Michelle van der Oord, Bob Schmitt, Max and Tonka (the fuzzy buddies), and Troy Colston (wherever you are).

Introduction

EVERY PERSON WITH HYDROCEPHALUS HAS A STORY TO TELL. Many of the particulars—the underlying condition, age at diagnosis, treatment, need for revisions, and side effects—will differ from story to story. But others who have lived with hydrocephalus will recognize in every person's story the impact on patient and family.

So that you can better understand how hydrocephalus has impacted us and our background before coming to write this book, we'd like to let you know where we've been. This is Kellie's story, and my story after I met Kellie.

Early in 1971, a month prior to Kellie's fourth birthday, her parents started to notice a change in the way she was acting. Her sleeping patterns shifted, and she complained of frequent headaches. The symptoms that most worried her parents were that her motor skills were significantly reduced and her gait had become unsteady, causing her to stumble when she walked.

Kellie was given an electroencephalogram (EEG) to see if her physical problems were being caused by something wrong with her brain. The EEG revealed the possibility of a brain tumor, so she subsequently underwent a series of head X-rays to pinpoint the problem (CT scans and MRIs were not yet available back then).

Exploratory surgery revealed a benign cyst in the third ventricle of her brain, which caused aqueductal stenosis and hydrocephalus. Kellie received her first shunt—a ventriculoatrial (VA) shunt—on February 12, 1971, and seven days later had a craniotomy in the right frontal region to drain the cyst. She was released from the hospital after nearly a month's stay, and her recovery was closely monitored by both her parents and neurosurgeon.

At age five-and-a-half, Kellie began to experience the same symptoms as before and was taken to see her neurosurgeon. This time, X-rays of the head revealed an intraventricular tumor, which projected from the third ventricle into the left lateral ventricle of the brain.

The pathology report from a cross-section of the tumor indicated that it was a low-grade astrocytoma, a potentially lethal brain tumor which is derived from cells that support the neurons. Three days later, Kellie received a Torkildson shunt on her left side, and her VA shunt on the right was revised. Kellie's health improved and remained virtually problem-free for nearly 18 years without the need of a shunt revision.

Kellie and I met in 1986, and after four years of dating, we were married in the fall of 1990. Not long after returning from our honeymoon, Kellie began having severe headaches that occurred mostly at night, when she would lie down after standing or sitting all day. She described the pain as extreme pressure, and it seemed like the only way to make the headaches subside was for me to massage her head until she fell asleep.

The headaches continued for a couple of weeks, until one night when massaging near her "shunt bump," I discovered what appeared to be a bubble of fluid beneath her scalp. Not knowing whether this had anything to do with her shunt or not, Kellie called her neurosurgeon the next morning to schedule an appointment.

After performing a neurological examination, Kellie's neurosurgeon ordered a CT scan of her head. Although her ventricles looked normal on the scan, the neurosurgeon suspected the shunt tubing was either cracked or obstructed, causing a subcutaneous buildup of cerebrospinal fluid (CSF).

The neurosurgeon said he would schedule a shunt revision as soon as possible, and that it was "a simple, routine procedure. There's really nothing to worry about." And because neither of us knew any better, we believed him. He explained that if the entire shunt system needed to be replaced, he would reroute the shunt from a ventriculoatrial (VA) path to a ventriculoperitoneal (VP) placement.

Since we were living in Canada at the time, Kellie's case fell subject to one of the hazards of the socialized medical system—waiting lists. Kellie's name was placed on a waiting list for surgery, and we were told it could be anywhere from two weeks to two months before the surgery could be performed. As it turned out, it was nearly four months before she received her shunt revision.

Over the next few months, Kellie's condition continued to worsen: the headaches became unbearable, and her emotions would range from happy one moment to severe depression the next. We called the neurosurgeon's office frequently, asking when Kellie would have her shunt revised. The only reply that Kellie received was, "Your name is on the list and we'll call you when it's your turn."

On Valentine's Day 1991, Kellie finally received a call from her neurosurgeon's office to inform her that her shunt revision was scheduled for the next morning. At the hospital, the neurosurgeon again reassured us that Kellie's operation would be simple, taking anywhere from two to four hours to perform. He asked us if we had any questions; neither of us did, and soon thereafter, Kellie was wheeled down to surgery.

Several hours later, I saw the neurosurgeon walking down the hall toward the waiting room where Kellie's parents and I sat. This was the first time I had ever seen a doctor look scared. He walked into the room, and since we were the only people in there, he closed the door behind him and said:

> There's been a problem. Kellie's shunt practically crumbled in my hands when we went to remove it, and when we started to insert her new shunt, her brain began hemorrhaging. The bleeding was pretty bad, but we think we've managed to stop it. We're going to do another CT series of her head in 30 minutes to see if the bleeding has stopped. If it hasn't, we'll have to open her cranium to try and stop the bleeding, and at that point, I have no guarantees.

"No guarantees" were his exact words. I was devastated. After only recently marrying Kellie, I now faced the possibility of losing the person I loved dearly. Fortunately, the bleeding did stop and additional surgery wasn't required. Kellie was brought up from recovery about an hour later and was placed in the Critical Care Unit (CCU), where she stayed until she was discharged ten days later. She spent most of her time in CCU sleeping and trying to recover from her surgery.

Due to the hemorrhaging in the right hemisphere of her brain, Kellie experienced partial paralysis to the left side of her body. The neurosurgeon hinted that the loss of sensation to her left side might come back over time, but we just had to wait and see.

Kellie took the "baby step" approach to her recovery—pushing herself a little further each day. At first, she needed the assistance of a walker to move about our apartment, but it was only a couple of weeks before she cast it aside for her first solo steps. Once she was able to walk unassisted, she moved on to the pool, where she used the water's resistance to help strengthen the weakened muscles of her left side.

By the end of June, Kellie's parents and I suspected there was something wrong with Kellie again. She was experiencing some of the classic symptoms of a shunt malfunction: neck and back pain, decreased attention span, reduced motor skills, light-sensitivity, headaches, mood swings, and fatigue. Afraid that something could again be wrong with her shunt, we made an appointment with the neurosurgeon for a checkup. We were told that he was out of town at a conference, so she was referred to his partner.

After examining Kellie, the neurosurgeon suspected that her shunt could be obstructed because the fluid reservoir of her shunt didn't fill promptly when he depressed it. He scheduled a CT scan for the next day and asked us to return to his office with the films as soon as they were ready.

By now I was a nervous wreck. In sharp contrast, Kellie remained calm about going to see the neurosurgeon again. After we picked up the films, I took a peek at them while we waited outside and resorted to humor to lighten up the situation. I opened the packet of CT films and started looking at them. Little did we know what we were looking at. I made the comment to Kellie, "You know what? You've got a cute brain," and she started cracking up. It was nice to see her smile and hear her laugh—something neither of us had done much of that morning.

We went upstairs and met with the neurosurgeon, who immediately turned to the CT scans. With his back turned to us, he said, "Young lady, you should be in a coma." We were in shock. He turned toward us and continued talking as he pointed at the CT films on the wall. "There's a problem with your shunt," he said. "You have a buildup of cerebrospinal fluid (CSF) here at the left frontal lobe; that's putting pressure on your brain. Your shunt is malfunctioning, so it will need to be revised again. I'll call emergency and let them know you're on your way. Walk over and check yourself in, I'll be operating on you within an hour."

It's amazing how much detail you can remember when you want to—and sometimes when you don't want to. This happened seven years ago, and yet I remember the details as if it were yesterday. The words. The sounds. The smells of the hospital. And especially the emotions.

CHAPTER 1

What Is Hydrocephalus?

Hope arouses, as nothing else can arouse,
a passion for the possible.

—William Sloane Coffin, Jr.
Once to Every Man

THE WORD HYDROCEPHALUS IS DERIVED from the Greek—*hydro* means water, and *cephalus* means head. It is a neurological condition that occurs when there is an abnormal accumulation of cerebrospinal fluid (CSF) within the ventricles and/or subarachnoid space of the brain. The increase of intracranial pressure (ICP) can be the result of an overproduction of CSF (a condition known as choroid plexus papilloma), an obstruction of the flow of CSF, or a failure of the structures of the brain to reabsorb the fluid. Although there is little public awareness about hydrocephalus, according to recent statistics from the U.S. Centers for Disease Control and Prevention, hydrocephalus affects approximately 1 out of every 1,000 children born each year. Hydrocephalus can also be acquired after birth from a variety of causes.

The goal of this chapter is to provide you with an explanation of the different types of hydrocephalus and how it is caused. Since the focus of treating hydrocephalus is based on CSF dynamics, we begin the chapter with an overview of what CSF is, how it is produced, and the structures of the brain it surrounds, protects, and nourishes. We hope to give enough background so you can communicate better with your neurosurgeon, read medical sources about hydrocephalus with some comprehension, and understand the basic physical structures and fluid dynamics that impact your health.

What is cerebrospinal fluid?

Cerebrospinal fluid (CSF) is a clear, colorless fluid that surrounds the brain and spinal cord, protecting them from injury. CSF is mostly made up of water with a few trace proteins, electrolytes, and nutrients that are needed for the nourishment and normal function of your brain. CSF also serves the brain by carrying away waste products from surrounding tissue.

Cerebrospinal fluid production and absorption

Under normal conditions, the brain produces an amount of CSF equal to what is absorbed by the body each day. Approximately 80 to 90 percent of CSF is produced by the choroid plexus. The choroid plexus—found in the lateral, third, and fourth ventricles—is a network of blood vessels covered by a tissue membrane that secretes newly formed CSF. The average person, including older infants, produces approximately 20 milliliters (ml) of CSF per hour (about 500 ml, or a pint, per day).

The average volume of intracranial CSF (the fluid that is within the brain at any one time) is 125 to 150 ml, of which approximately 90 to 100 ml can be found in the subarachnoid space which surrounds the brain and spinal cord.

CSF is constantly being produced, flowing through, bathing, protecting, and cleansing the structures of your brain before it is reabsorbed into the bloodstream. There is a threefold turnover of CSF within a 24-hour period.

Flow of cerebrospinal fluid

The flow of CSF follows a somewhat predictable pattern throughout the brain and spinal column (see Figure 1-1). Cerebrospinal fluid is produced mainly by the choroid plexus of the lateral ventricles. CSF flows from the lateral ventricles of the brain through the foramen of Monro (a short passageway that extends down from the lateral ventricles) on its way to the third ventricle. From there, the CSF passes through the narrow passageway of the cerebral aqueduct on its way to the fourth ventricle. The cerebral aqueduct is also known as the aqueduct of Sylvius. It is here that the most common cause of hydrocephalus can be found—aqueductal stenosis.

CSF exits the fourth ventricle by way of the foramina of Luschke and Magendie, where it enters the subarachnoid spaces. The fluid continues to flow over the brain to the arachnoid granulations (or villi) in the superior sagittal sinus where it is reabsorbed. The superior sagittal sinus is a venous channel that runs between the left and right hemispheres of the brain. It extends down to the back of the head where it splits in two, creating the transverse sinuses, which then turn into the internal jugular veins that return blood to the right atrium of the heart. Arachnoid villi, located in the

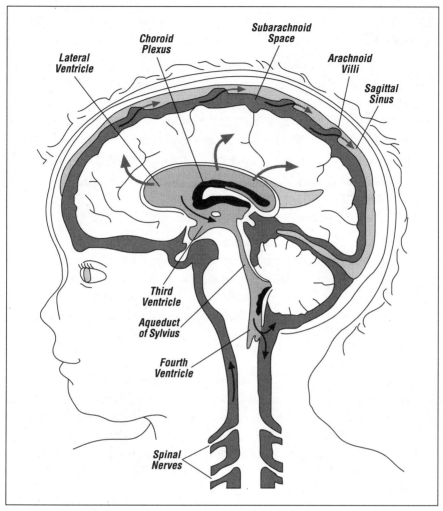

Figure 1-1. CSF circulatory pathway

subarachnoid space, permit the flow of CSF from that space to the superior sagittal sinus, as well as other large channels.

The brain in a nutshell

The brain is the nerve center and is by far the most complex organ in the human body. The primary function of the brain is to control the body. It regulates breathing and circulation, and controls the functions of the body's vital organs. The brain is also responsible for analyzing and remembering everything that you see, touch, hear, taste, and smell. For instance, when you reach down to touch a flower, the nerves in your fingertips send an impulse to the parietal lobe of your brain, which identifies the sensation.

To communicate effectively with neurosurgeons, patients who have hydrocephalus need to become familiar with the basic structures of the brain. Your neurosurgeon will talk about the various structures of the brain, and by being familiar with their location and functions, you will better understand what she is talking about. Learning about some of the terms and functions of the brain will allow you to more actively participate in your care. After some experience with the condition, you will find yourself talking about ventricles, hemispheres, lobes, the cerebellum, cranial nerves, and possibly other parts of the brain you didn't know existed.

The brain is divided into sections that control different bodily functions. The effect that hydrocephalus has on an area of the body greatly depends on where the blockage or abnormal accumulation of CSF is located. If there is a buildup of fluid near the frontal lobes of the brain, you could experience difficulty with motor skills, since the frontal lobe houses the motor cortex. Likewise, if there is a arachnoidal cyst that is placing pressure on the occipital lobe, your vision might be affected.

Responses on one side of the brain control actions on the opposite side of the body. For example, if you want to move your right arm, a signal is sent to the motor cortex of your left frontal lobe. This signal is then sent to the muscles of your arm to perform and control the movement. If there is a cyst or tumor placing pressure on the right side of the brain, it will affect the functions of the left side of the body controlled by the area where the cyst or tumor is located.

This section gives you an overview of the structures of the brain and discusses some of their functions. It first looks at the outermost structures of the brain, the meninges, then at the middle of the brain where the ventricles are located, and finally moves inside to the core of the brain, the brain stem.

Meninges

The meningeal layer surrounds the brain and spinal cord and protects them from injury. CSF acts as a cushioning device between the meninges, gray matter, and the inside of the skull. The meninges consist of three separate layers: the dura, arachnoid, and pia mater (see Figure 1-2).

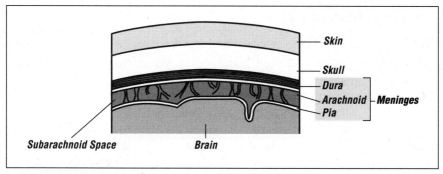

Figure 1-2. Protective coverings of the brain

The outermost meningeal layer is the dura mater. The dura mater is a tough, inelastic membrane that consists of two layers fused together. The outer layer of the dura mater is similar to the periostium (the protective layer that surrounds all bones), and the inner layer is called the dura.

The area between the dura and arachnoid layers is known as the subdural space. When a shunt overdrains, it reduces the volume of CSF within the ventricles, causing the brain to move inward away from the meninges. As the brain moves inward, blood vessels in the arachnoid layer of the meninges are torn, forming a subdural hematoma (a pocket of blood) between the arachnoid and dura layers. Overdraining of the ventricles and subdural hematomas are just one of many possible complications of having a shunt.

The next meningeal layer is the arachnoid. This fine, cobweb-like layer covers the brain and spinal cord, and contains many large blood vessels. Unlike the dura, the arachnoid mater has an elastic quality. The area between the arachnoid layer and the next, the pia mater, is known as the subarachnoid space. CSF flows through the subarachnoid space, over the surface of the brain and spinal cord.

The innermost meningeal layer is known as the pia mater. The pia mater hugs the surface of the brain and spinal cord, and is filled with blood vessels that supply the nerve tissue below.

The meninges extend downward between the cerebral hemispheres (the cerebrum) to create the falx cerebri, and between the occipital lobes of the cerebrum and cerebellum to form the tentorium. The falx cerebri is what divides the left and right hemispheres of the brain, while the tentorium is what separates the upper and lower sections of the brain.

Cerebral hemispheres

The brain is divided into two cerebral hemispheres, which are commonly referred to as the left and right hemispheres. When combined, the cerebral hemispheres make up the cerebrum, which is the largest and most highly developed part of the brain.

The left and right hemispheres are separated by the longitudinal fissure, where the falx cerebri of the dura is located. The left and right cerebral hemispheres are joined together at the center of the brain by the corpus callosum. The corpus callosum is a broad band of fibers which allows one side of the brain to communicate with the other. The cerebral hemispheres are each made up of four pairs of lobes: frontal, temporal, parietal and occipital.

The frontal lobes are located at the front part of each cerebral hemisphere and extend back to about the middle of the brain. The frontal lobes make up approximately one-third of each hemisphere of the brain. The lower region of the left frontal lobe, known as Broca's area, is responsible for initiating speech. The prefrontal cortex, which is located at the front of each frontal lobe, plays a role in memory, social behavior, learning, judgment and personality.

Just forward of the central sulcus, located at the posterior margin of the frontal lobe, is the motor cortex. The motor cortex is responsible for controlling voluntary movements of the muscles and limbs of the body. The central sulcus, which separates the frontal and parietal lobes, begins at the top of the hemisphere and extends downward until it reaches the lateral sulcus.

The temporal lobes are located at the side of the brain, within the temple of the cranium. They are separated from the frontal lobes by a cleft called the lateral fissure. The lateral fissure is an in-folding of the frontal lobe that runs laterally between the frontal and temporal lobes. The upper region of the temporal lobe is associated with the sense of hearing. The inner region of the temporal lobe is responsible for memory.

The parietal lobes are situated above the temporal lobes and between the frontal and occipital lobes. Located within the parietal lobe is the primary sensory area, which is responsible for receiving sensations from the body.

Abnormalities in this area of the brain can be associated with reading and learning disabilities.

The occipital lobe is located in the back of the brain, behind the parietal and temporal lobes and above the cerebellum. The occipital lobe is responsible for interpreting what is seen with the eyes.

Ventricular system

The ventricular system of the brain is made up of four chambers, or ventricles, which are connected to each other by way of narrow passages, called foramen. As mentioned earlier, CSF is produced in the ventricular system by the choroid plexus. The CSF flows from the ventricles into the subarachnoid space and over the surface of the brain and spinal column. Hydrocephalus occurs when there is an obstruction of one of the ventricles or ventricular foramina (CSF passageways) that restricts the flow of CSF within the ventricular system, the subarachnoid space, or the cisterns (reservoirs for CSF). The ventricular foramina consist of the intraventricular foramina (or the foramen of Monro), which connect the lateral ventricles with the third ventricle, and the foramina of Luschke and Magendie (located in the fourth ventricle), which provide a means for CSF to exit the ventricular system. (*Foramina* is the plural of *foramen*.)

The third and fourth ventricles are connected to each other by the cerebral aqueduct, also known as the aqueduct of Sylvius. This is the most common place for non-communicating hydrocephalus to occur, as it is the smallest passageway in the ventricular system. The foramina of Luschke and Magendie are also found in the fourth ventricle. The foramen of Magendie protrudes from the back, and the foramina of Luschke extend from each side of the fourth ventricle. The foramina of Luschke and Magendie are passages where CSF exits the ventricular system over the cerebellum into the subarachnoid space and down to the spinal cord.

The two largest ventricles are known as the lateral ventricles. They are commonly referred to by their left-right position (i.e., left lateral ventricle or right lateral ventricle). The lateral ventricles can also be referred to as the first (left lateral) and second (right lateral) ventricles. Each lateral ventricle lies within its respective cerebral hemisphere (i.e., the left lateral ventricle lies within the left hemisphere of the brain, and the right lateral ventricle lies within the right hemisphere).

The lateral ventricles, although one structure, have three different horns which extend into different lobes of the brain. The anterior horns extend forward into the frontal lobes. The posterior horns extend backward into the occipital lobes, and the inferior horns project downward into the temporal lobes. The area between the posterior and inferior horns of the lateral ventricles is known as the atrium, or trigone, located within the parietal lobes. The structure of the lobes and how they fit together create the chambers of the ventricular system (see Figure 1-3).

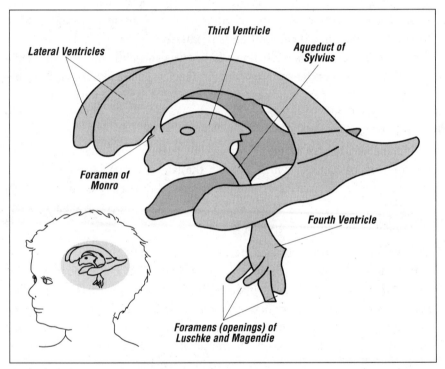

Figure 1-3. The ventricular system

The lateral ventricles are connected to the third ventricle by the interventricular foramen (more commonly known as the foramen of Monro). The third ventricle is located at the center of the brain, which is also home to the hypothalamus and the thalamus. The hypothalamus regulates body temperature, thirst, emotions, sleep, hunger, water balance, and sexual behavior. The thalamus is the relay station of the brain. All incoming messages to the brain, with the exception of the sense of smell, enter the thalamus before being transmitted to the primary sensory cortex in the parietal lobe.

The fourth ventricle is bordered by the medulla and the pons in the front, and the cerebellum behind, with the aqueduct of Sylvius extending upward into the third ventricle.

Cerebellum

Located below the occipital lobes and behind the brain stem, the cerebellum is made up of two distinct-looking hemispheres. The cerebellum is primarily responsible for coordinating movements and muscle tone, and controlling the body's sense of balance.

Hydrocephalus can be caused near the cerebellum when there is an increase of intracranial pressure (ICP) that forces the tonsil of the cerebellum down onto the foramen magnum. The tonsil of the cerebellum is located near the base of the cerebellum. Raised ICP forces the tonsil against the brain stem and can cause an obstruction of CSF flow from the fourth ventricle. This form of non-communicating hydrocephalus can result in severe respiratory and cardiac distress, due to its pressure on the lower region of the medulla.

Brain stem

The structure that connects the brain with the spinal cord is called the brain stem. The brain stem is made up of three sections: the pons, the medulla, and the midbrain. The pons is responsible for control of facial movement, as well as some eye movements, while the medulla controls heart rate and breathing.

Types of hydrocephalus

Hydrocephalus is a condition where the normal drainage of CSF in the brain is blocked in some way. Neurosurgeons classify hydrocephalus according to when the condition was developed (congenital or acquired), and whether it was caused by a reabsorption problem or a blockage somewhere within the ventricles (communicating or non-communicating). Another type of hydrocephalus—normal pressure hydrocephalus—is when the ventricles are enlarged, but there is little or no increase in intracranial pressure. These terms are often combined when referring to a particular type of hydrocephalus. For example, if you have a condition known as aqueductal stenosis (a blockage of the aqueduct of Sylvius) caused by an intraventricular cyst, then your diagnosis would be "acquired, non-communicating hydrocephalus."

Congenital hydrocephalus

Hydrocephalus is considered *congenital* when its origin can be traced to a birth defect or brain malformation that causes an increased resistance to the drainage of CSF. A variety of factors can cause congenital hydrocephalus. Among the possible causes:

- Toxoplasmosis, or *T gondii,* is a type of organism that can be transmitted by eating undercooked meat, contact with contaminated soil, or by direct contact with an animal or bird that already has the infection.

- Cytomegalovirus (CMV) belongs to the herpes family of viruses, and normally produces symptoms that resemble that of the common cold.

- Rubella, or German measles, is known to cause fetal malformations during pregnancy, one of which is hydrocephalus.

- X-linked hydrocephalus is almost exclusively a genetic disorder passed from mother to son on the X chromosome. It is inherited only through the mother, and is predominantly seen in males (approximately one in 20). There is also a small chance that first cousins of children with uncomplicated congenital hydrocephalus can also inherit the disorder.

Congenital hydrocephalus can be linked to other complications. A 17-year study that concluded in 1987 tracked four major congenital neurological malformations: anencephaly, spina bifida, encephaloceles, and hydrocephalus. Of 370 births with these defects, 10.5 percent (39) resulted in stillbirths. Although a majority of live-born infants with hydrocephalus were free of other complications, 37 percent had congenital malformations which were unrelated to the hydrocephalus. Of those, the most common malformations were tracheoesophageal fistula (an abnormal communication between the trachea, or windpipe, and the esophagus), and anomalies with the reproductive, urinary, and cardiac systems (Thomas E. Wiswell et al., "Major congenital neurologic malformations: a 17-year study," *American Journal of Diseases in Children* 144, no. 1, January 1990: 61-7).

Acquired hydrocephalus

Hydrocephalus can be *acquired* later in life if something causes an increase in the resistance to the drainage of CSF, such as an obstruction. Acquired hydrocephalus can also be caused by brain tumor, arachnoid cyst, intracranial or intraventricular hemorrhaging (IVH), trauma to the head, or by infections such as meningitis.

*At the age of six weeks, my mom noticed that my head was unusu-
ally large, and she could lay a finger between the bones in my skull. She
called the neurosurgeon, and met him in the emergency room. He saw me
from across the examination room, proceeded to the phone, and reserved
time in the operating room. To him, it was very apparent that I was in
dire need of a shunt. My head was about the size of the rest of my body.*

· · · · ·

*In 1983, at the age of thirteen, I acquired hydrocephalus when I was
hit in the head by a baseball. It was a freak accident. I was a good player,
and could hit and field well. Unfortunately, that one time the ball was
thrown to me, I looked up and lost it in the sun. My nose bled and immediately swelled; my family and I just assumed that I broke my nose again.
Only later did we realize the true complications that occurred.*

*I went to the doctor and he confirmed that my nose was broken.
However, there was nothing he could do at that time. It would have to just
heal on its own. Approximately a month later, I missed school because I
was very lethargic and had excruciating headaches. At first, they thought
that it might be migraine headaches, however, as I grew more lethargic
and bright lights started to bother me, my family grew very concerned.*

*Since it was at the end of my freshman year in high school, I did not
want to miss much school, so I tried to "work" through the illness. However, when the nausea increased and my vision doubled, I went to my
pediatrician, who sent me to the hospital for tests and a CT scan. As the
result of my scans, I was sent to the Children's Hospital in Boston. It was
there that I was diagnosed with hydrocephalus.*

Bacterial meningitis

Bacterial meningitis is an inflammation of the meninges, the protective layering that surrounds the brain and spinal cord. Hydrocephalus develops when
scarring of the meninges restricts the flow of CSF in the subarachnoid space,
when it passes through the aqueduct of the ventricular system, or affects the
absorption of CSF at the arachnoid villi.

If left untreated, bacterial meningitis can cause death within days. Signs and
symptoms of meningitis include: severe headaches, high fever, loss of appetite, light and sound sensitivity, and tension in the muscles of the neck and
shoulders. In extreme cases, symptoms of meningitis can include vomiting,

convulsions or seizures, and delirium. Once detected, bacterial meningitis can be treated with high doses of antibiotics.

Brain tumors and cysts

Hydrocephalus may also be acquired as a result of brain tumors or cysts. Most brain tumors are detected in children between the ages of five and ten years old. Seventy-five percent of these tumors occur in an area at the back of the brain known as the posterior fossa. Other types of brain tumors that can cause hydrocephalus include intraventricular tumors and, in extremely rare cases, tumors of the choroid plexus (including papilloma and carcinoma).

As the tumor grows in mass, it creates a form of non-communicating hydrocephalus by reducing the flow of CSF within the ventricles. Tumors that are located in the back of the brain most commonly obstruct the flow of CSF through and out of the fourth ventricle. In most cases, the best way to treat hydrocephalus related to a tumor is to remove (excise) the tumor causing the obstruction. However, hydrocephalus does persist in approximately 20 to 40 percent of patients after the tumor is removed.

Cysts are benign sacs or closed cavities that are filled with fluid. Cysts can occur anywhere in the body. With arachnoid cysts, the sacs are filled with CSF and are lined with tissue from the arachnoid membrane. Cysts are commonly found in children, and are located both within the ventricles and on the surface of the brain, or in the subarachnoid spaces. Arachnoid cysts can cause a form of non-communicating hydrocephalus by restricting the flow of CSF within the ventricular system—particularly in the third ventricle. Cysts can also be found in the subarachnoid space.

Depending on the location of the cyst, the neurosurgeon may be able to excise the cyst wall and drain the cyst's fluid. If the cyst is located in an inoperable location (e.g., near the brain stem), the neurosurgeon might decide to place a shunt catheter in the cyst. This catheter is then connected to a shunt system to allow the fluid to be drained. This stops the growth of the cyst and protects the brain stem.

Intraventricular hemorrhages (IVH)

A common complication with premature births is the risk of an intracranial or intraventricular hemorrhage (IVH), bleeding within the ventricles of the brain. IVHs can be found in approximately 40 percent of premature infants. If the IVH is severe enough, it could compromise the ventricles, allowing blood to flow into surrounding brain tissues and lead to neurological changes. The possibility of hydrocephalus developing as a result of an IVH depends largely on the severity of the bleed, and whether or not blood and debris have caused an obstruction in the CSF pathways or reduced the brain's ability to reabsorb the CSF. In many cases, however, hydrocephalus is mild and tends to stabilize. Thus, not all infants who have an IVH will need a shunt system.

Head trauma

Severe head trauma can also cause hydrocephalus, although it is uncommon. The hydrocephalic condition occurs as a result of bleeding into the subarachnoid spaces. Scarring of the drainage pathways from the resulting intracranial bleeding can cause a partial obstruction of the flow of CSF.

Communicating hydrocephalus

The term "communicating hydrocephalus" means that the site of increased resistance to CSF drainage resides outside of the ventricular system in the subarachnoid space. Communicating hydrocephalus is caused in one of three ways:

- An overproduction of CSF (a rare condition associated with a choroid plexus papilloma).
- A venous obstruction (a rare condition known as Otitic hydrocephalus).
- An increased resistance to the drainage of CSF from the subarachnoid space.

"Communicating" means the ventricles of the brain *communicate,* or pass along, the CSF to the surface of the brain. The obstruction of CSF flow occurs not within the ventricles, but within the subarachnoid spaces of the brain. Communicating hydrocephalus can also be the result of a meningeal inflammation, such as an infection, or caused by blood or tumor cells in the subarachnoid spaces.

Non-communicating hydrocephalus

Non-communicating, or *obstructive,* hydrocephalus is caused when there is an obstruction in the flow of CSF within the ventricular system of the brain, including the outlets of the fourth ventricle (the foramina of Luschke and Magendie). The most common place for the non-communicating CSF obstruction is in the aqueduct of Sylvius (also known as aqueductal stenosis). However, the obstruction can also occur in the outlets of the fourth ventricle and from the lateral ventricles into the third ventricle at the foramina of Monro.

An example of non-communicating hydrocephalus is stenosis (or blockage) of the aqueduct of Sylvius. This blockage causes non-communicating hydrocephalus by not permitting CSF to flow from the third to the fourth ventricle. When the obstruction is located in the ventricular system, it causes the ventricles to expand as a result of the accumulation of CSF. Non-communicating hydrocephalus is the most common form of hydrocephalus in fetuses.

Normal-pressure hydrocephalus (NPH)

A person can be diagnosed as having normal-pressure hydrocephalus (NPH) when the ventricles of the brain are enlarged, but there is little or no increase in the pressure within the ventricles. NPH is normally seen in elderly patients, and is most likely caused by an obstruction of the CSF pathways and abnormal brain compliance.

NPH can be divided into two classifications: those where the cause of the hydrocephalus is known, such as a previous history of meningitis or a subarachnoid hemorrhage, and *idiopathic,* where the cause of NPH is not known.

Management of NPH can often be tricky, as the neurosurgeon must try to find the right shunt to treat the condition. If the shunt overdrains, it could result in a subdural accumulation, or pocket, of CSF and/or blood between the dura and arachnoid mater of the meninges. If the shunt doesn't drain enough CSF (known as undershunting), the ventricles may not be allowed to reduce in size. Also, shunting may not improve the situation.

Primary causes of hydrocephalus

Although hydrocephalus can develop for a variety of reasons, congenital hydrocephalus is often a part of other neurological conditions and congenital malformations. Other conditions that hydrocephalus is often associated with include, from most to least common:

- Dandy-Walker syndrome.

- Neural tube defects (NTDs).

- Spina bifida.

- Chiari malformations.

- Vein of Galen malformations.

- Hydranencephaly.

- Craniosynostosis.

- Schizencephaly.

This section briefly describes these disorders and explains how they can cause hydrocephalus, as well as discussing symptoms, treatments, and prognosis. For more detailed information that pertains specifically to your child, talk with your doctor or neurosurgeon.

Dandy-Walker syndrome

Dandy-Walker syndrome is a congenital brain malformation that involves the fourth ventricle and the cerebellum. It is defined as an enlargement of the fourth ventricle and is accompanied by an absence (partial or complete) of the cerebellar vermis (the narrow middle area between the hemispheres of the brain). The combination of these malformations is what causes hydrocephalus in patients with Dandy-Walker syndrome.

Symptoms that often occur in early infancy include slow motor development and progressive macrocephaly (an abnormally enlarged skull). In older children, symptoms of increased intracranial pressure such as irritability, vomiting, and/or signs of cerebellar dysfunction such as ataxia (unsteady gait) and nystagmus (jerky eyes) may occur.

Symptoms of Dandy-Walker syndrome include increased head circumference, bulging occiput (the back of the head), cranial nerve dysfunction, and abnormal breathing patterns. Dandy-Walker syndrome can be associated with other central nervous system structural abnormalities, including malformations of the heart and an absence of the corpus callosum.

In cases where increased intracranial pressure is present, a shunt will most likely be placed to control the hydrocephalus. Even when hydrocephalus is treated early, patients with Dandy-Walker syndrome often face other problems. Prognosis for normal intellectual development is variable depending on the severity of the syndrome and its associated malformations.

Neural tube defects and spina bifida

Spina bifida (SB) is a general term that denotes failure of normal formation of midline structures—in this case, the spinal cord and the spinal column. Those conditions that are of clinical importance include only the neural tube and are collectively referred to as neural tube defects (NTDs). NTDs are best divided into two groups: open and closed.

- **Open NTDs.** These are found in infants with myelomeningoceles. The spinal cord is open and is continuously or intermittently leaking CSF. The entire CNS is malformed, and the myelomeningoceles is likened to the tip of the iceberg above the waterline.

  These infants have a partial or complete paralysis of the lower extremities, which may also be deformed. Bladder and bowel function are almost always severely affected with the infant never becoming continent for urine or stool. The vast majority of infants develop progressive hydrocephalus and will need to be shunted. Because of cortical disorganization, the majority of children will have learning disorders that vary from mild to severe. The medical care required is complex and lifelong.

- **Closed NTDs.** The spinal cord is not exposed, but is covered by skin. CSF leakage is not present. The abnormality is confined to the lower end of the spinal cord, and there is no malformation of the brain. Thus, the Chiari malformation, hydrocephalus, and learning disorders are not a consideration. These infants can develop bladder and/or bowel dysfunction and a mild motor/sensory loss that normally involves only one lower extremity.

At present, there is no cure for myelomeningoceles because the nerve tissue cannot be replaced or repaired. Surgery to close the newborn's spinal opening is generally performed within two days of birth to minimize the risk of infection and to preserve existing function in the spinal cord. Ongoing therapy, medical care, and surgical treatments may be necessary to prevent and manage complications throughout the person's life. Many individuals with myelomeningoceles will need assisting devices such as braces, crutches, or wheelchairs.

The prognosis for children with myelomeningoceles depends on the number and severity of other abnormalities. Prognosis is poorer for those with complete paralysis, hydrocephalus, and other congenital defects. With proper medical care, most children with myelomeningoceles live well into adulthood.

Chiari malformation (CM)

A Chiari malformation (CM; formerly referred to as Arnold-Chiari malformation, or ACM) is a rare congenital anomaly in which two parts of the brain—the brain stem and the cerebellum—are longer than normal and protrude down into the spinal canal. Chiari malformations are divided into two groups:

- Type I. A mild form with the cerebellar tonsils protruding into the spinal cord. This may be asymptomatic or be associated with cranial nerve dysfunction or fluid buildup in the spinal cord (hydrosyringomyelia).

- Type II. A more severe form with an extensive malformation of the cerebellum and brain stem that is seen almost exclusively with an open NTD (i.e., myelomeningoceles). Hydrocephalus is usually present. Some infants may develop difficulty with breathing, swallowing, feeding, etc., as a result of this malformation.

Most patients who have surgery experience an improvement of symptoms almost immediately, and may experience prolonged periods of relative stability, while others may continue to have neurological deterioration. Infants with severe malformations may have life-threatening complications.

Vein of Galen malformation (VGM)

The vein of Galen malformation (VGM) is a rare vascular disorder that is present at birth but normally isn't detected until the child is a few months old. VGMs occur when the vein of Galen, which runs above the aqueduct of Sylvius, balloons to create an aneurysimal sac. This aneurysm often compresses the aqueduct of Sylvius, causing hydrocephalus.

Vein of Galen malformations are commonly diagnosed in infants by a cardiologist, as the infant often suffers heart failure (a heart attack) because of the rapid heart rate. Another symptom that aids in the detection and diagnosis of a VGM is macrocrania (an enlarged skull). Macrocrania is caused when the ventricles enlarge due to the obstruction of CSF flow, causing increased intracranial pressure.

Symptoms often include headache (due to increased intracranial pressure), lethargy (due to an enlarged heart), and vomiting. One of the primary concerns in the diagnosis of a VGM is the enlarged heart, which may lead to heart failure. VGMs are easily diagnosed with contrast-enhanced CT or MRI. X-rays of the chest will confirm whether the heart is enlarged or not.

Shunting is often required to treat the hydrocephalus, but may not be necessary if ICP is reduced when the VGM is treated.

Hydranencephaly

Hydranencephaly is a rare condition in which the brain's cerebral hemispheres are absent and are replaced by sacs filled with cerebrospinal fluid. An infant with hydranencephaly may appear normal at birth. The infant's head size and spontaneous reflexes, such as sucking, swallowing, crying, and moving the arms and legs may all be normal.

Due to the lack of cerebral hemispheres, there is no significant neurological development, with the infant's function remaining at the newborn level forever. Hydrocephalus frequently develops, and a shunt is inserted to keep the child's head from becoming abnormally large.

Diagnosis may be delayed for several months because early behavior appears to be relatively normal. Some infants may have additional abnormalities at birth, including seizures, myoclonus (spasm or twitching of a muscle or group of muscles), and respiratory problems. There is no definitive treatment for hydranencephaly other than to place a shunt to prevent the head from becoming large, and surgery to treat other malformations.

Craniosynostosis

Craniosynostosis is a congenital anomaly which is characterized by the premature closure of one or more cranial sutures before the brain has fully grown. The disorder results in an abnormal head shape, and may be a feature of a chromosomal or genetic syndrome or abnormality. Treatment for craniosynostosis generally consists of surgery, usually performed early in life. This allows the skull to accommodate brain growth and improves the appearance of the child's head.

Prognosis for craniosynostosis varies depending on whether single or multiple sutures are involved and the presence of associated abnormalities. The prognosis is generally better for patients with single suture involvement and no associated abnormalities. Hydrocephalus is rarely present with single-suture involvement and is occasionally seen with some other forms of craniosynostosis.

Schizencephaly

Schizencephaly is an extremely rare developmental disorder characterized by abnormal slits, or clefts, in the brain's cerebral hemispheres. Individuals with clefts in both hemispheres (bilateral clefts) are commonly developmentally delayed, and have delayed speech and language skills. Individuals with smaller, unilateral clefts (clefts in only one hemisphere) are often paralyzed on one side of the body and may have normal intelligence. Patients with schizencephaly may also have varying degrees of microcephaly, mental retardation, hemiparesis or quadriparesis, reduced muscle tone, and hydrocephalus. Most patients with schizencephaly experience seizures.

Individuals with schizencephaly are generally treated with physical therapy, anticonvulsants to control seizures, and placement of a shunt for hydrocephalus.

CHAPTER 2

Getting the Diagnosis

Omne ignotum pro magnifico.
(Everything that is unknown
is taken to be grand.)

—Pliny the Elder

BY THE TIME YOU RECEIVE THE DIAGNOSIS for the condition of hydrocephalus, it is very likely that you or your child have been through a gamut of tests. You know something is wrong. Your doctor knows something is wrong. But until the results come back, you're in limbo.

Even after a diagnosis, neurosurgeons still can't answer all your questions about the condition. There is no cure for hydrocephalus, and the options for treating the condition are limited.

This chapter examines the hardest aspect of this potentially life-threatening condition: facing the unknown. We start by describing the symptoms of hydrocephalus and medical tests that are used to diagnose the condition. We look at several conditions that share some symptoms with hydrocephalus. We briefly discuss getting a second opinion. Then we turn from the medical aspects of diagnosis to the personal, looking at the diagnosis experiences of three different people. The chapter ends with descriptions of the range of responses by patients and families to receiving the diagnosis.

Symptoms

With newborns, hydrocephalus is detected almost immediately, as the child's head may be larger than normal or misshapen. However, with older children or adults, hydrocephalus usually starts to reveal itself with a variety of signs and symptoms weeks or months before it is detected.

Common symptoms of an increase of intracranial CSF pressure include:

- Abnormally large head or increased head growth in infants or children (macrocephaly).

- Frequent headaches, particularly late at night or early in the morning.

- Awkwardness or stumbling when walking (gait disturbance).

- Vision problems, including double vision (diplopia).

- Concentration or mental difficulties.

- Nausea or vomiting.

- Incontinence.

- Lethargy.

- Neck pain.

Persons with hydrocephalus might not have all of these symptoms. With infants and small children, the most visible symptom will be macrocephaly. In teenagers and adults, headaches, gait disturbance, and concentration and mental difficulties are likely to be more prominent.

In order to help your doctor or neurosurgeon diagnose the condition quickly, keep track of symptoms that you observe on a daily basis. Keep a notepad handy and write down the symptoms that occur, noting the date and time they happen. This information helps your doctor or neurosurgeon see if there is a pattern to when certain symptoms occur, and can prove to be quite valuable in evaluating the situation.

Abnormal head growth

With infants and small children, the primary indicator that hydrocephalus could be present is an abnormally large head (macrocephaly). Unlike adults, the sutures of a child's skull aren't fused together. It is important for your pediatrician to track the growth rate of your child's head to ensure that the slow progression of macrocephaly can be detected early. If left undetected and untreated, your child's skull could continue to expand because of abnormally large ventricles (also known as ventriculomegaly). Macrocephaly can cause the following signs and symptoms:

- Irritability.

- High-pitched crying or screaming.

- Split sutures of the skull.

- Distended veins in the scalp.

- Bulging or widening of the fontanels that would cause the head to be misshapen.

- Absence of upward gaze, which is known as sunsetting; most frequently present in the instance of acute non-communicating hydrocephalus.

- Impaired lateral gaze (sunsetting of one or both eyes).

- Loss of vision.

- Weakness or spasticity of the limbs.

Head sizes for male and female infants grow at different rates. Your child's pediatrician should have current head growth charts for each sex, not one chart that offers a median value for both. With infants who were born prematurely, head size should be charted by age according to conception, not by birth age. Your child's pediatrician should continue to chart and monitor the growth of your child's head until he reaches six or seven years old.

> My son was five months old when they started thinking it was time to shunt him; his head circumference had been borderline since birth but it was at that age it really took off in size.

If you notice the head of your child is abnormally large, it is advisable to seek medical attention as soon as possible. Keep in mind that head size is something that is attributable to many causes; if both parents have large heads, it could be possible that your child's head size is genetically determined and normal. When in doubt, check it out.

> Since my daughter was two weeks old, I had been going to her pediatrician complaining that something was wrong with her. They told me it was colic. We lived with that explanation for some time, then they told me it was probably a reaction to her formula. Again, we bought that for a while. The only symptom our daughter had was piercing screams in the night and never sleeping . . . and I mean never! The doctor said this was very common, so we tried to go on with our lives coping with a sleepless child.

> When she was around six months of age I asked the pediatrician to check her head—it looked a little odd—but the doctor said nothing was wrong and that I was being over-protective and too critical of her.

At 13 months old, she was finally diagnosed with hydrocephalus and then needed three operations in 18 days.

Headaches

Headaches are a common symptom of the onset of hydrocephalus, particularly with adults. Headaches can be caused as a result of increased cranial pressure (ICP), either within the ventricles or on the surface of the brain. The actual headache occurs when pressure of surrounding fluid and brain matter places pressure on blood vessels and the meninges.

The severity of headaches can range from mild, dull headaches that come and go intermittently, to ones that are debilitating. It may be difficult to tell the difference between a regular headache and a headache caused by increased ICP.

Gait disturbance

Gait disturbance—a reduction or loss of walking motor skills—is usually the first symptom in adults. As intracranial pressure increases, nerve fibers (axons) of the brain become stretched as the ventricles enlarge. Axons take a long course around the ventricles to reach the motor cortex in the frontal lobe. Thus, when the ventricles expand, the axons are stretched, causing ataxia (a lack of control of voluntary muscles).

If hydrocephalus remains undetected and untreated, a person's gait will worsen. Gait disturbance can reveal itself as poor coordination, imbalance, stumbling, falling down for no apparent reason, and even loss of the ability to walk or stand.

> *My mom had shunt surgery in March. After about five months, she started to show NPH [normal pressure hydrocephalus] symptoms again. She cannot walk or eat, and is semi-conscious, exactly like before the first shunt surgery. The doctor said she will be fine again after she has her shunt revision tomorrow. I hope he is right.*

Vision problems

Vision problems often occur in patients who have or are developing hydrocephalus. Increased intracranial pressure can cause the following vision-related symptoms:

- Non- or slow-reacting pupils.

- Sunsetting of the eyes (also known as Parinaud's syndrome).

- Light sensitivity.

- Impaired lateral gaze.

- Rapid, involuntary eye movements (nystagmus).

- Double vision.

Papilledema, swelling of the optic nerve, indicates ICP. If absent, it does not exclude elevated ICP, as it occurs in the minority of patients. Papilledema is diagnosed by looking in the eye with an ophthalmoscope. Symptoms for papilledema include decreased visual acuity, blurring vision, and light sensitivity. Decreased visual acuity first presents itself with intermittent light sensitivity that progresses. If hydrocephalus is not treated promptly, papilledema can lead to blindness. For additional information about vision problems as a side effect of hydrocephalus, see Chapter 7, *Side Effects*.

Concentration or mental difficulties

Concentration and/or mental difficulties often develop in patients with hydrocephalus. Unfortunately, these effects can also last well after shunts have been placed.

Family members will need to help monitor symptoms. Look for any deviation from normal behavior, such as problems with visual and spatial relations, short-term memory loss, or difficulty with verbal and nonverbal problem-solving. Also be alert for signs of lethargy. For example, you might have a difficult time waking your child. Or you might notice a change in social activities; she might become withdrawn and easily lose interest in whatever she's doing.

How hydrocephalus is diagnosed

Initially, hydrocephalus is detected when one or more of the symptoms of the condition become evident. For example, in an infant, you might notice that your child's head is bulging or is larger than normal (macrocrania or macrocephaly). In a small child, you might notice that your child has painful headaches, gait disorder, or vision problems.

When hydrocephalus is first suspected, your primary care physician should then refer you to a neurosurgeon for further evaluation and testing. A neurosurgeon is a doctor trained to operate on the brain, spinal cord, and other nervous structures of the body. If other problems are present, such as seizures or vision problems, the physician should also refer you to a neurologist or a neuro-ophthalmologist.

Neurological examination

Before the neurosurgeon orders any tests, such as a CT or MRI scan, she will likely perform a neurological examination. This exam includes a history of neurological milestones and a physical examination to check for possible neurological deficits. Below are some of the signs the neurosurgeon will look for as an indicator that hydrocephalus could be present.

Premature infants

Premature infants are more likely to develop hydrocephalus as a result of an intraventricular hemorrhage (IVH), which can cause posthemorrhagic hydrocephalus. The neurosurgeon will feel the fontanel, or soft spot on the cranium where the sutures of the skull are still open, to see if it is fuller than normal. She will also check the infant's head circumference to see if it is within the normal range. Fullness of the fontanels and a large head are indicators that hydrocephalus is present.

Additionally, she will check to see if muscle tone is normal. If an IVH or hydrocephalus is suspected, the neurosurgeon may first order an ultrasound of your child's head rather than order a CT or MRI scan.

Full-term infants (from birth through 1 year old)

As with premature infants, your child's neurosurgeon will check the size of the cranium and the fontanel for fullness. Since your child is older and more developed, the neurosurgeon will also check his eyes and reflexes. One of the things the neurosurgeon will look for is whether or not your child has a startle response. If he lacks a startle response, it may indicate loss of sensation to that part of the body.

As your child grows, some indicators of a possible neurological deficit are that he is not meeting some of his developmental goals. These include smiling, crawling, walking, and being able to roll over.

Children (ages 1 through 12)

After your child is one year old or older, the neurosurgeon will examine him to see if he is reaching mental and physical developmental milestones.

Mental milestones:

- Is your child communicating verbally?
- Is your child doing well in school? Has he fallen behind his peers in recent months?
- Does your child have a hard time remembering things?
- Has there been a noticeable change in your child's personality in the past few weeks or months?

Physical milestones:

- Did your child begin to show signs of walking by the time he was one year old?
- Is your child's gait steady or unbalanced? Does he tend to drift to one side when he walks? The neurosurgeon will be looking closely to see if your child moves symmetrically.
- Can your child balance on one foot?
- With his eyes closed, can your child place both feet together, side by side, and maintain his balance?

The neurosurgeon will check your child to see if his arms and legs are strong, or if there is a deficit in one side or the other. She will test tendon and muscle reflexes, and will also check for any loss of sensation in the extremities.

By looking into your child's eyes, she will be able to check for papilledema. The neurosurgeon will place an index finger in front of your child's face and ask him to follow its movement from side to side, and up and down. This is to check for possible paresis (paralysis) of the abducens (or sixth cranial) nerve. The sixth cranial nerve controls lateral (side to side) eye movements.

The neurosurgeon will also ask your child to walk heel-to-toe with head up and arms extended, forward and backward, to evaluate his gait and balance. If he has difficulty performing this test, it could be an indication that there is pressure on the cerebellum.

The neurosurgeon will check the plantar, or Babinski, reflex. This reflex test is done by drawing a blunt object, such as the handle of an instrument, along the outer edge of the foot from the heel to the little toe. The normal, or flexor, response is to have the toes bunch together and move in a downward motion. However, if the big toe moves upward, the result is an extensor response, or Babinski reflex. A Babinski reflex is a clear indication of some form of brain or spinal cord disease. It should be noted that infants will normally have a positive, or upward, Babinski reflex, whether hydrocephalus is present or not. As a result, the neurosurgeon will probably skip this test until your child has reached his first birthday.

The neurosurgeon will test finger-to-nose reaction by holding up an index finger and asking your child to touch his index finger to the doctor's finger and then his own nose, as quickly as possible. This test is primarily performed to see if there is any type of cerebellar impairment on either side of the brain. If he cannot perform this test and misses either the doctor's finger or his own nose, it could indicate the presence of some form of visual impairment (e.g., papilledema).

The neurosurgeon will also test for pronator drift. In a standing position, the doctor will ask your child to close his eyes, then extend both arms in front, palms up. The neurosurgeon will be looking to see if one arm wavers or drifts down and to the side, which can be an indication of injury to the motor areas of the brain.

Adults

For teens and adults being tested for hydrocephalus, many of the same tests will be done as are done for older children.

Radioisotope cisternography

Radioisotope cisternography, or nuclear cisternogram, is a test often performed when normal pressure hydrocephalus (NPH) is suspected. Radioisotopes are used to help the radiologist and neurosurgeon monitor the flow of CSF within the subarachnoid spaces, ventricles and the basal cisterns.

In a cisternogram, the patient is injected with anywhere from 85 to 500 microliters of either radioiodine serum albumin (RISA) or indium diethylenetriamine pentaacetic acid (DTPA) in the lumbar subarachnoid space following a lumbar puncture. A scintilliscope is used to scan for the isotopes at various timed intervals to track the flow of the radioisotope through the shunt system. In a person without NPH, the radioisotope can be detected flowing into the subarachnoid spaces and basal cisterns, with little accumulation in the ventricles. However, if the radioisotope stays primarily within the ventricles and little or no radioactivity is detected over the hemispheres of the brain, then NPH can be assumed.

You can expect a brief moment of discomfort during the initial lumbar puncture; however, the injection of the radioisotope does not hurt.

Ultrasonography (ultrasound)

Ultrasonography uses high-frequency sound waves to outline the structures within the body. The resulting ultrasound is caused by the reflection of the sound wave bouncing off the part of the body being studied.

Ultrasound is used to diagnose congenital hydrocephalus in utero (when the child is still within the mother's womb). Hydrocephalus can be detected in utero during normal prenatal screening in the 28th week of pregnancy and sometimes earlier. The obvious indication that hydrocephalus is present is that the fetus will have an abnormally large head.

When hydrocephalus is detected in utero, the parents will normally be referred to a pediatric neurosurgeon who will work with the obstetrician to provide proper care for the mother and unborn child.

Ultrasound is used most often on infants, as their cranial sutures have not yet joined together. Ultrasound cannot be used once the soft spot has filled with bone. The primary benefit of using ultrasonography on infants is that they can be imaged while awake from portable equipment that can be brought crib-side, unlike CT and MRI scans which may require infants to be sedated for testing. Although the ultrasound allows the ventricle size to be measured accurately, it cannot image the surface of the brain and some of the posterior fossa.

CT and MRI scans

Until the introduction of computed tomography, or CT, scanners in 1971, the only option for imaging the brain of a child or adult was with traditional X-rays. Diagnosis of hydrocephalus and other brain malformations was difficult because X-rays do not provide enough contrast to see the tissues of the brain.

Within a few short years of introduction, CT imagery became a household word as CT scanners became more common in university and medical research facilities. Since CT scans provided clearer pictures of the body's internal organs, tissues, and bones, they quickly became a standard diagnostic tool for surgeons, significantly reducing the need for exploratory surgery.

Magnetic resonance imaging, or MRI, received FDA approval for clinical use in the United States in 1985. Instead of using X-rays, MRIs use radio waves in combination with a magnetic field to create pictures of the body's internal structures. These images provide a clearer view of gray and white matter of the brain, as well as the vascular system. Though expensive, MRIs are the primary diagnostic test used by most neurosurgeons today.

Preparing yourself or your child for CT or MRI scans

CT and MRI scans are relatively painless procedures, unless your neurosurgeon orders the imagery to be contrast-enhanced—then you'll receive an injection or temporary IV, which allows the contrasting agent to flow into the bloodstream.

On the day of the procedure, arrive at the imaging center 15 to 30 minutes prior to the time of the appointment. This will allow you time to complete the necessary paperwork and to meet with the technician to go over medical history. If the imaging series is to be contrast-enhanced, arriving early will give the technicians extra time to get an IV started.

If your child is being tested and has any apprehension about the procedure, ask the technician to explain the test to her. If asked, most technicians will give children a tour of the imaging console and of the equipment in the scanner room before the test to help allay any fears.

In order to perform the test, the patient will be asked to disrobe and change into a surgical gown, and to remove any type of metallic jewelry. Adults should refrain from wearing makeup or using hair spray, as these may interfere with the imaging device. Next, the patient will be asked to lie on the scanner table, which slides inside the circular drum that houses the imaging equipment, and asked to lie perfectly still while inside the CT or MRI machine so the images don't blur. Infants and small children may be given a mild sedative to help keep them still.

CT and MRI scans take pictures of the complete cranial and intracranial anatomy, including the subarachnoid spaces and the structures of the posterior fossa. These pictures, called slices, are taken in sections laterally (side-to-side) and sagittally (front-to-back) at different intervals.

How long does a CT or MRI scan take?

With modern scanners, a CT scan can be as quick as a simple two-to-five-minute procedure, while an MRI series can take as long as an hour, depending on the type of scan and whether or not enhancement materials are used. To pass the time, some CT and MRI machines come equipped with headphones so patients can listen to favorite music while in the chamber. This can be especially comforting to young children who receive MRI scans, as the "clunking" noise from the magnets can be loud and scary.

Risks of CT and MRI scans

Two possible risks for patients who undergo CT scanning are exposure to radiation and a reaction to the use of iodinated contrast material.

CT scans use low doses of ionizing radiation to do the imaging. The average CT scan exposes the patient to radiation doses of five to ten rads (an absorbed dose of radiation) per slice. Although any damage is a rare occurrence, frequent head CT scans can place the patient at risk of radiation exposure which can damage the eyes and possibly cause cataracts. One way of reducing the risk of radiation exposure to the eyes is a method called angled gantry, in which the CT scanner is angled away from the eyes, reducing the dose of radiation the eyes receive.

The chance of radiation damage is minimal compared to the benefit of an accurate diagnosis.

> After my daughter had undiagnosed symptoms for a year, I was at my breaking point and wanted action taken. I went in to see the doctor and told them to run some tests like a CT scan immediately. Their response was, "Why expose a child to radiation?"
>
> Dumb question when you are talking about a life. The CT scan confirmed that she had hydrocephalus since birth. They shunted her immediately.

Another risk of CT scanning is the use of iodinated contrast material, which is administered intravenously. This type of imaging series is known as "contrast-enhanced." Although the amount of iodine used is relatively low, there is a 1 in 10,000 chance of a patient experiencing anaphylactic shock (an allergic reaction), and a 1 in 40,000 chance of death. Other possible reactions to contrast material include damage to the kidneys (nephrotoxity) and/or damage to nerve cells (neurotoxity).

Since MRIs use powerful magnets to help produce the images, MRIs should not be performed on patients who have pacemakers or metallic implants, such as aneurysm clips (more commonly known as brain clips). Patients with pacemakers should not be subjected to MRI scans as there is a possibility that the magnetic field of the machine could render the pacemaker inoperable.

Neurosurgeons sometimes use brain clips in operations on people with hydrocephalus or who have had tumors or cysts removed. Brain clips might be used to deal with an intracranial bleed, complication in surgery, stroke, or even sometimes to attach a ventricular catheter. However, most brain clips today are made of a nonmagnetic material, so this shouldn't be an issue. If you know you have brain clips, but are unsure what type of material they are made of, ask your neurosurgeon.

CT versus MRI: advantages and disadvantages

CT scanning requires patients to remain motionless for the duration of the test; however, the scan may take only two to five minutes. There is the small risk of exposure to radiation. MRI scans also require patients to stay motionless during the test, which can last anywhere from 30 to 60 minutes, depending on the type of contrast or imaging being done. Since an MRI can take so long to perform, infants and young children often require sedation so they won't move during the procedure.

A concern shared by many families and their doctors is the cost of a CT versus an MRI scan. The average CT scan costs only $300 to $500 to perform, while an MRI could run as high as $2,000. If cost is a limiting factor for you, talk this over with your physician before he orders any diagnostic tests. Also, it is a good idea to check with your medical insurance provider to find out whether they will cover the cost of an MRI. Some insurance companies may cover only a portion of the cost, so it's important to find out what portion you will be required to pay, if any.

For routine, annual examinations, our insurance company will only cover 80 percent of the cost for an MRI. However, if the MRI is being done for an emergency—something they consider a legitimate reason—then they will cover it 100 percent.

Both CT and MRI have their advantages, but what it really boils down to is which image will give the neurosurgeon the best view of the problem he is trying to diagnose. Until there is an accepted and set standard for the treatment and monitoring of hydrocephalus, neurosurgeons will continue to differ on their choice of imaging device. Ask your doctor to explain his thinking on which test to order. If you have serious concerns, consider getting a second opinion before proceeding.

Possible misdiagnoses

Although rarely misdiagnosed with today's modern imaging techniques, the condition of hydrocephalus is occasionally mistaken for benign extra-axial fluid of infancy, and Alzheimer's disease in adults.

Benign extra-axial fluid of infancy

At birth and for the first few months, the child's head circumference will be normal, but will suddenly start to grow rapidly over a short period of time. Since abnormal head growth is an indicator that hydrocephalus may be present, the child should be referred to a pediatric neurosurgeon for further evaluation. A CT series of the head will be ordered to check the size of the ventricles and for the presence of cysts or tumors.

When CT images return, the neurosurgeon will see that the size of the ventricles are normal or slightly enlarged, and there is no indication of an intracranial mass. What they will notice, however, is an abnormal accumulation of cerebrospinal fluid in the subarachnoid space (the area between the skull and the hemispheres of the brain). This is known technically as benign extra-axial fluid of infancy, and can also be called a benign subdural hygroma, or external hydrocephalus.

In cases of benign extra-axial fluid of infancy, the subarachnoid accumulation is normally reabsorbed by the time the child reaches 18 to 24 months of age. Once the benign extra-axial fluid has been detected, your child's neurosurgeon will require follow-up scans to ensure the fluid accumulation is being reabsorbed by the brain.

Alzheimer's disease

Alzheimer's disease is commonly confused with normal pressure hydrocephalus (NPH), as some of the symptoms of both are the same. Indicators of NPH include urinary incontinence, gait disturbance, and dementia—one of the prime symptoms of Alzheimer's disease.

When NPH is suspected in an adult or elderly patient, it is recommended that a CT or MRI of the head be conducted to evaluate ventricular size. If scans of the head are inconclusive (i.e., ventricles seem to be of normal size), it is recommended that a lumbar puncture be performed to determine the CSF pressure within the subarachnoid space. Another test that can be performed to differentiate between the two is a radioisotope cisternogram to monitor the flow of CSF within the brain.

Asking for a second opinion

Once hydrocephalus is detected, and if shunting is recommended, it is important to act upon the neurosurgeon's recommendations as soon as possible. The longer the condition is left uncontrolled, the greater the risk of neurological damage.

It is your right to ask for a second opinion. Neurosurgery, whether performed on a child or an adult, has inherent risks and many possible complications. Ask your neurosurgeon if there is time for you to obtain a second opinion. If there is, your neurosurgeon should assist you in finding another neurosurgeon in your area. Your neurosurgeon should also assist you in arranging the appointment, since the medical records and any CT or MRI films will need to be transferred. If the neurosurgeon indicates there is some urgency in performing the shunt placement or revision, ask him if it is possible to have another neurosurgeon meet with you as soon as possible.

It is in your best interest to make sure that the neurosurgeon explains hydrocephalus to you clearly, in terms you can understand.

> I have gone for third, fourth, and fifth opinions until I found someone who I could connect with and believe that they were treating my son like they would treat their own. You have to follow your gut feelings when it comes to this stuff. We are just parents, many without fancy medical degrees, but we know our kids. We have that "parental radar" that goes off when we are concerned . . . follow that feeling.

Three people, three diagnoses

Although many cases of hydrocephalus are diagnosed either in utero or at birth, it can also affect people at any age. There are three possible times when a person could be diagnosed with hydrocephalus: at or before birth (known as congenital hydrocephalus), as a child (known as childhood onset hydrocephalus), or later in life as an adult (known as adult onset hydrocephalus). Although the basis of the condition is the same—an abnormal accumulation of cerebrospinal fluid—the situations in which a person is diagnosed can differ sharply.

Diagnosis 1: Congenital hydrocephalus

Each year, 1 in 1,000 children are born and diagnosed with hydrocephalus. That seems like a fairly high number, especially when the latest statistics reveal that a child is born in the U.S. every 8.1 seconds. This would mean that a child is born with hydrocephalus every 135 minutes. With statistics like that, it's amazing just how few people know what hydrocephalus is, and how little information there is out there for people to find out more about it.

> Cameron was a total surprise to us. You see, we already had four children, the youngest being 13, so we were sure our baby-raising days were over. In my seventh month, I began to feel that something was wrong. The baby was still moving, but the quality of the kicks had changed. My obstetrician kind of blew me off. He did a few non-stress tests, but they were inconclusive.

> On January 9, 1996, our son Cameron was born at 4:30 a.m. Our tears of joy quickly turned to tears of fear when Cameron went into respiratory distress. He was rushed into the nursery where they could work on him, and later taken to another hospital 20 miles away which had a neonatal intensive care unit (NICU). I was left to recover from the birth and pray for our little boy. The prognosis was not good.

> My husband went to the other hospital with our son, and when he came back, we were both sad and afraid. He brought me a Polaroid picture of Cameron they took in the nursery. I held that picture all night long and cried. The nurses in the hospital didn't know how to handle me, so they just closed the door and left me alone.

Two and a half weeks later, they started to wean him from the ventilator, and he started to breathe on his own. They did an MRI to see why he had a seizure on the day he was born. That is when they found out that he had a stroke before he was born. Because of the damage that was done, they said Cameron would never walk or move his left side. They were pretty sure he had cerebral palsy. Our world stopped at that moment. I felt like someone had punched me in the stomach.

On February 5, the pediatrician called in a neurosurgeon because the ultrasound of Cameron's head was abnormal. They did a spinal tap two days later and informed us that Cameron had hydrocephalus. However, they said the fluid looked fine, so the neurosurgeon discharged him. We finally got to take our baby home! Four days later they did another ultrasound. The neurosurgeon's office phoned and told me to bring him back for emergency surgery. They did the surgery that night at 8 p.m., and by 10 p.m. we were in the recovery room holding our baby. He was supposed to be in the hospital for five days after they placed the shunt, but he was doing so well they sent him home the following day.

Cameron has continued to surprise everyone. Every time he sees any of his doctors, they shake their heads in amazement. There is no sign of cerebral palsy. Our life with him has been a wonder. He really is a miracle and a blessing. There isn't a person who meets him who doesn't tell me he is the most beautiful boy. I am still afraid every minute that our luck will change. Every day seems like a time bomb. I know that the shunt could cause problems at any time. I look at Cameron and believe in miracles. I pray every day that God will continue to watch over our baby.

Cameron experienced an intracranial hemorrhage either prior to or at the time of birth, causing acquired communicating hydrocephalus.

Diagnosis 2: Childhood onset hydrocephalus

Many factors can cause hydrocephalus in children. The most common cause of hydrocephalus is the result of a congenital form of aqueductal stenosis that restricts the flow of cerebrospinal fluid within the ventricles of the brain. With some, hydrocephalus can be caused as a result of other congenital defects, such as myelomeningoceles.

Other fairly common causes of hydrocephalus in children are cysts and brain tumors. Porencephalic cysts are commonly found within the brain, next to the ventricular system. Arachnoid cysts can be found either within the ventricular system or in the subarachnoid space. Brain tumors in children are most frequently found in the posterior fossa. Since cysts and brain tumors can grow over a long period of time, they are difficult to detect until they begin to block the passage of cerebrospinal fluid.

As a parent, it can be difficult to understand why one day your happy, active child has suddenly changed.

> At the end of July 1996, late on a Wednesday afternoon, B.J. complained of a headache and did not feel well or hungry. He had a little soup, I told him to drink some water, and he went to lie down. I thought he just got too much sun—we live in Jerusalem, Israel, and the summer sun here is fierce. He was up all night with a steadily worsening headache and vomited a few times. That night I thought he wasn't feeling well because of his exposure to the heat and sun, but by Thursday morning I was beginning to fear that it could be meningitis.

> I called my pediatrician. She said to bring him in right away. She examined him. About five minutes later she was on the phone with the local hospital asking if they had a CT scan—she used to be a pediatric neurologist. After a few simple neurological tests, she asked him to touch his chin to his chest—he couldn't. When she looked into B.J.'s eyes, she saw massive papilledema (swelling of the optic nerve) from high intracranial pressure (ICP). My pediatrician knew right away there was a blockage, probably based in the third ventricle. This is where his tumor actually was.

> We went to the main medical center in the city where they handle all of the neurosurgery cases. After a few hours the doctors came and told us there was definitely something wrong, but first they needed to deal with the immediate crisis of the extremely high ICP.

> The neurosurgeon said that inserting the shunt would be a simple procedure that would give B.J. immediate relief and solve the pressing issue of his severe headaches. After that, the doctor said, they could take their time and do careful diagnostics to figure out what the underlying cause of his headaches were. His shunt, a PS Medical high-pressure system, was inserted around midnight of the same day. We were extremely fortunate. He started to feel ill and was diagnosed within 24 hours, which is extremely rare.

It wasn't until later that B.J.'s neurosurgeon discovered that he had a benign juvenile pilocytic astrocytoma (JPA). The tumor filled the third ventricle and extended out of all three openings into both lateral ventricles and down into the fourth ventricle.

B.J. is now nine years old. In the weeks and months since B.J. received his first shunt, he has had others placed and removed—being shunt independent for a month or so over the summer. However, when he began showing signs of intracranial pressure again, his neurosurgeon placed another shunt system. Aside from having a slight headache when he wakes up in the morning—which is normally gone by the time he gets to school—he feels absolutely wonderful.

Diagnosis 3: Adult onset hydrocephalus

The two most common forms of hydrocephalus in adults are hydrocephalus ex-vacuo and normal-pressure hydrocephalus (NPH). Hydrocephalus ex-vacuo occurs when there is damage to the brain caused by stroke or injury. In some cases, there may also be shrinkage of brain substance, particularly with the elderly and individuals with Alzheimer's disease. When reduction in brain matter occurs, the amount of intracranial CSF increases to fill up the space. NPH is caused when there is a gradual blockage of the CSF drainage pathways in the brain, such as in the subarachnoid space or within the ventricular system. Although the ventricles may become enlarged, the pressure of the CSF remains within normal range.

The symptoms first started to appear when I was about 40 years old. My feet would tingle and feel totally numb when I was working out in aerobics class. I was certain the numbness was caused by the running shoes I was wearing, so I started buying new ones, trying to find the perfect fit. But that didn't work either. A few months and four pairs of shoes later, the tingling and numbness were still there.

That spring, we went on a holiday to Disney World with our 16-year-old daughter, and we stayed in the same hotel room. At the time, I was experiencing "urine hesitancy," or incontinence, during the night. I didn't think much of it, but it really bothered my daughter and my husband. They suggested I get this problem checked out. I went to a bladder specialist when we got back home and all of the tests came back negative, so I decided it was just the way I urinated. I never dreamt the numbness in my feet and bladder problems were related to one another.

A few months later I was going down some steps in our home, and my legs completely disappeared from beneath me. I dropped everything and collapsed. I just figured I was really clumsy. The same thing happened during the middle of the night when I got up to go to the bathroom a few times. I collapsed, but thought it was caused by my legs being asleep.

This continued on for a few more months, and during this time I also suffered from nagging headaches—not excruciating by any means, but my husband noticed how much Tylenol we were going through, and I was the main person in the family taking it. Still, I didn't put all these symptoms together.

Then one day, I was driving to work, and lost sensation in my hands; they felt like pins and needles. I went to rub my right hand on the steering wheel, and to my surprise, my hand was not on the steering wheel, it was on the seat beside me. This really gave me a scare, so I headed straight to my family doctor's office. She was not too pleased with me, because in one of my previous visits, she arranged for me to see a neurologist—an appointment which I had canceled because I didn't think there was anything wrong with me. She made another appointment with a neurologist, but it took another month for it to be scheduled.

The neurologist did a bunch of tests. I believe she was testing me for multiple sclerosis (MS) as I had all the symptoms of that disease. The final test was a CT scan, which I had to wait three months for. We lived in Edmonton, Alberta, at the time and it was impossible to get tests like that unless you were practically dying.

During those three months, my condition kept getting worse. I would double-book appointments at work (I was a sales representative for a large international corporation). I would phone my friends twice in a row and repeat the same conversation. They were very worried about me, but figured I was just being absent-minded.

My husband and I went on another holiday to San Francisco. This holiday was about two weeks before my scheduled CT scan. My condition during the trip was really bad. I passed out at the airport in Vancouver *while waiting for our connecting flight. I walked like a total invalid (I guess they call that "gait"). We visited an aunt while in San Francisco and she really noticed that something was wrong. My condition was gradually deteriorating—something that my family didn't notice because they saw me every day. The symptoms would come and go. One day my eyesight could be practically gone, and the next it could be perfectly fine.*

I had the CT scan when we returned from San Francisco, and was immediately admitted to the hospital for surgery. According to my neuro-surgeon, the ventricles of my brain were so large they were ready to explode. I had quite a few complications after the surgery as my body tried to reject the foreign object, but after a month everything seemed to settle down.

I was diagnosed with adult onset, normal-pressure, communicating hydrocephalus and received a ventriculoperitoneal (VP) shunt. I was 42 years old at the time and am now 44. I had one revision a year later when I began experiencing the same symptoms again. I had another CT scan just recently and the ventricles are back to normal size, but I still suffer from frequent headaches.

Responses to the diagnosis

When the diagnosis is made, there is a wide array of possible responses: relief, shock, denial, sadness, anger, fear, and hope. All these responses are natural, common responses to a stressful situation. You also may have physi-cal responses such as weight loss/gain, or even illness. The diagnosis trau-matically affects not only the patient, but family and friends—even the fam-ily pets. The important thing to remember is to take care of yourself and your family. This is a stressful time.

Relief

While waiting to be diagnosed, patients are often run through a battery of tests so their physicians and neurosurgeons can make an accurate diagnosis. Tests may be given within a few days or stretch over weeks or even months. The tests themselves can be stressful. Waiting for results and living with the unknown is usually very difficult. You may not know what is happening. Symptoms may continue to progress. When all the tests are done and you finally hear the diagnosis, there is a strong possibility that you will feel a huge sense of relief because now the waiting is over.

> I was very relieved. My symptoms were very much like those experienced if you had a brain tumor or multiple sclerosis. I was diagnosed with normal-pressure hydrocephalus, which usually can be kept under control with the placement of a shunt, which is what I had done. I felt a brain tumor or multiple sclerosis would have been a lot more devastating for me and my family.

Confusion and numbness

At the time of diagnosis, you might hear what the doctor is saying without really comprehending a word. This dreamlike state is an almost universal response to shock. The mind provides protective layers of numbness and confusion to prevent emotional overload. This allows you to examine information in smaller, less threatening pieces. It is sometimes helpful to write down instructions, record consultations on a small tape recorder, or ask a friend to help keep track of all the new and complex information.

> My daughter was diagnosed with hydrocephalus in utero at 19 weeks. It came as a shock to both my husband and me. It was not something we were expecting. My obstetrician didn't really give us a lot of information, or maybe he did, but we were just so shocked that nothing made sense.

· · · · ·

> I was 37 when diagnosed with hydrocephalus. It's thought that I was actually born with the condition and that my body compensated until it could no longer do so. Everything else was ruled out. I was only working on about one or two cylinders. I was shocked that they wanted to open my head up!

Denial

It's easy to ignore something that is obvious—people do it every day. However, when it comes to hydrocephalus, it is important to trust your instincts. Problems within the brain, including hydrocephalus, often make the body react in ways it otherwise wouldn't. If you see the signs of a possible problem, it's best to check it out.

I didn't want to believe that my daughter was having problems with her shunt again. All of the signs were there, but I continued to ignore them. She was walking differently, and her normally bubbly personality had changed. But she wasn't sleeping very much either, so we assumed that was the cause. By the time we took her to see her neurosurgeon, it was almost too late. Two days after her shunt was revised, you'd never know that anything was wrong with her. I will never ignore these signs again.

After an initial diagnosis, you might use denial to shield yourself from the frightening medical situation. Denial may serve as a useful method to survive the first hours or days after diagnosis, but a gradual acceptance must occur so that you and your family can begin to make the necessary adjustments to treatment. As a parent, once you accept the doctor's encouragement about prognosis and treatment, push fears into the background, and begin to believe that your child will survive, you will be better able to provide support for your child.

My parents' reaction to finding out that I had hydrocephalus was denial, at first. An obstetrician noticed my slightly larger head when I was born in 1955, but my parents didn't believe it, so nothing was done. But when my family was told why I blacked out in 1972, my parents accepted the diagnosis and a shunt was implanted.

Sadness

A diagnosis of hydrocephalus often brings a sense of loss, even when the prognosis is very good. You grieve the loss of normalcy, the realization that life will not be the same. Fortunately, as you or your child's prognosis changes for the better and as you meet or read about other people living with hydrocephalus, these feelings of sadness will slowly fade.

When I first found out my son had hydrocephalus, it was during the Gulf War—which is a blur to me—I knew nothing about hydrocephalus at all. Any information I found was so depressing I could not even read it without crying.

· · · · ·

At the time of the diagnosis, I was told that I needed surgery. I felt so awful that it really did not faze me; I was numb to what the doctor was

saying. After he left the room, about a half hour later, I looked at my
father and we both started to sob.

A woman recalls the sadness she felt when her friend underwent emergency surgery:

> *We had only been friends a short time, and yet it felt as if I had*
> *known this person for an eternity. To look at her, you would never know*
> *that anything was wrong with her. When her boyfriend called to tell me*
> *that she had been taken to emergency surgery because of a problem with*
> *her shunt, I was saddened to think that this person who I felt so in tune*
> *with might possibly die. But thankfully, that didn't happen.*

Fear

A natural response to a diagnosis of hydrocephalus is feeling fearful or helpless. Life feels out of your control. There can be fears about the threat to health or life, surgery and hospitalization, and an uncertain future. You may fear that you cannot deal with the problems facing your family or that you cannot cope with a condition that threatens your child.

> *My son Mike acquired a cold and his first shunt placement was*
> *delayed a week because of the congestion. I panicked and thought it was*
> *dangerous to wait, but they said the fluid had been there all that time and*
> *it would be more dangerous to operate with the bad cold. It was the long-*
> *est week of my life. I did jigsaw puzzle after jigsaw puzzle. To this day I*
> *still cannot do them without flashing back to that horrible waiting period.*

Fear usually stems from the unknown. It's vital to become educated and informed about hydrocephalus, for your own peace of mind and so that you can translate what you know to children, friends, and family. Once diagnosed, it is important to understand what is going to happen during and after the surgery. If this means getting your neurosurgeon to explain it step by step to ease your fears, ask him to do so. Showing you or your child what a shunt looks like, how it works and where it is placed will make the surgery seem a little less frightening. When you have a better understanding of what lies ahead, the apprehension and fear will slowly become more tolerable.

> *My baby was diagnosed in utero as having hydrocephalus. I was*
> *scared for my baby—mostly that he wouldn't live. I have worked with*

children who have hydrocephalus, but all of them have some other dis-
abilities, and I was not too aware that hydrocephalus could be a condi-
tion in and of itself. I was most frightened by what I didn't know.

Anger

Anger is a common and natural response to a diagnosis of hydrocephalus. You might get angry because of the uncertainty: waiting for test results or not knowing when another shunt revision might be needed. You might get angry because hydrocephalus makes life difficult: a symptom is causing discomfort, a revision is needed right before a planned vacation or business trip, an activity isn't possible because it could affect the condition. Or you might get angry just because it seems so unfair.

> *During the in-and-out hospitalizations over the summer, our son has developed quite a little attitude. As he has gotten older, the merry-go-round of surgeries has really ticked him off. He is angry that he has hydrocephalus. He is angry that his shunt fails. He feels badly he can't play all of the time with his friends. This is a lot for a six-year-old to cope with.*

Since you cannot direct your anger at the condition of hydrocephalus itself, you might target doctors, nurses, or family. Because anger directed at other people can be very destructive, it is necessary to devise ways to express the anger. Some suggestions for managing anger follow.

When there is anger toward your doctor:

- Look for ways to improve communication between you and the neurosurgeon.
- Talk to other parents of children with hydrocephalus (having someone who understands what you are going through is a great source of comfort).
- Discuss your concerns and feelings with one of the nurses on staff.

When there is anger toward your family:

- Take a deep breath and wait before speaking, or walk away.
- Get outdoors or exercise.
- Join a support group.

- Keep a journal to write your feelings in.

- Reduce your caffeine intake.

- Listen to music.

- Talk with friends.

- Get a massage.

- Improve communication within the family.

- Seek individual or family counseling.

- Find one positive thing out of each day.

- Learn more about the condition.

> *I am angry that I have this disease, but I realize that my condition could have been worse. At first not much information was provided by my neurosurgeon except for a small booklet on shunts. But as time has passed, I have collected two more books and two more pamphlets on hydrocephalus as well as a web site.*

Physical responses

Reaction to the initial diagnosis can be traumatizing. There could be a long, stressful period of symptoms and worry before the diagnosis is made.

The weeks following the diagnosis—testing, hospitalization, and recovery—could make you literally ill, even if you are not the person diagnosed with hydrocephalus. Eating and sleeping patterns may change dramatically. You may stop eating or grab only fast food; normal sleep patterns are a thing of the past; staying in the hospital exposes you to all sorts of illnesses. Waking moments are filled with emotional stress, which makes the physical stress more potent.

> *I am angry. I feel guilty for not being more persistent with my pediatrician. In the year we were trying to find out what was wrong, I have lost at least 15 pounds, and I was only 110 to begin with. I haven't slept well the whole time. My husband is a basket case over all this. Our marriage has been severely strained, but we are slowly picking up the pieces and trying to get back to a somewhat normal life. On the positive side, our daughter is responding well. The neurosurgeons were great as far as educating us about hydrocephalus.*

To attempt to prevent illness, and to give you strength to deal with problems that can arise, it is helpful to try to eat nutritious meals and snacks, get a break and take a walk outdoors, and find time to sleep. Exercise is a great way to relieve stress and clear your mind, making it a little easier to enjoy a good night's sleep. Care needs to be taken not to overuse drugs or alcohol. Physical illnesses usually end after a period of adjustment.

Hope

Never give up hope. Hope is the belief in a better tomorrow. Hope sustains the will to live and gives the strength to endure each trial. Since the 1950s, treatment for hydrocephalus has steadily improved and is still improving. Your family and friends can offer support. Other families who have been in the same place you are can offer much hope.

> We read many medical documents, but our uneasiness couldn't go away. We really wanted to hear anything from people who had a VP [ventriculoperitoneal] shunt operation, and about their life with it. Finally, we found a hydrocephalus listserv on the Internet, and many people responded to our request for information. It has been so helpful to us, and has given us hope for our young daughter.

How hydrocephalus affects the patient

Unless you have hydrocephalus yourself, it can be extremely difficult to understand how another person with the condition feels. There are a range of possible complications from hydrocephalus and shunting. What affects one person only slightly may play a major part in how another person lives from day to day.

> Aside from the occasional headache, I had pretty much been problem-free for nearly 20 years when I had two revisions in 1991; one of which has forever changed my life—not only physically, but psychologically. Due to all of the sudden trauma I experienced, I now contend daily with a form of post-traumatic stress disorder. I am hyper-vigilant; noises seem amplified and any sudden movement or element of surprise makes me want to jump out of my skin. Sometimes I wish I could just run out of my body to escape the constant anxiety. I've tried medications like BuSpar, a tranquilizer, but all they seemed to do was leave me feeling like a space cadet, so I've stopped taking them.

Concentration is difficult for me on a day-to-day basis. I've noticed that with a lot of stress or lack of sleep, my concentration level is practically nonexistent. It seems as though I'm only good for 15 or 20 minutes at a time, and then things just start to get jumbled. I have to walk away and come back when my head's clear.

Though it was very traumatic for me to learn about my condition later in life, I believe it was a blessing in disguise. I've always thought of myself as being the same as everybody else. I am slowly learning to accept that I simply have to function to the best of my abilities—not someone else's. I am a capable young woman. It may take me a little longer than someone else, but I can do it.

How hydrocephalus affects others

Hydrocephalus doesn't just affect the person with the condition, it affects siblings, friends, other family members, relationships, and marriages. As a parent or patient, you will find yourself quickly consumed by many needs—doctor visits, countless tests, imaging exams—all of which usually need to be performed in a relatively compressed time frame. This is a very stressful period for everyone, and time is critical.

Whether hydrocephalus is being diagnosed initially or the decision is made to replace a failing shunt system, friends and family have no choice but to sit back and watch their loved one struggle with symptoms and go through a very serious operation.

The best thing that family and friends can do is communicate with each other about feelings and fears. Rather than trying to hold everything inside and cope with it on your own, share your feelings with others around you. Talk with your friends and family members to help educate them about hydrocephalus and how it affects you or your child. While some may be afraid to talk about the condition, others will be right there by your side. The more people understand about the condition, the more they will be able to provide support.

Siblings

Siblings of children with hydrocephalus may experience an array of emotions during the hospitalization of their ill brother or sister. These feelings can range from worry and fear to resentment and jealousy.

Children also have very active imaginations. Often, their fears about what is happening to their brother or sister are actually far worse than reality. As a parent, talk with your other children to discuss their fears and explain to them in terms they can understand how their brother or sister is doing. By talking through their fears and concerns, you can help prepare them for visits to the hospital, letting them know what to expect.

Siblings may feel completely overwhelmed when a brother or sister is ill. Visiting their sibling in the hospital can also be very stressful. They may see their brother or sister going through the pain and discomfort of surgery and treatment, and may notice their physical changes too. Weight gain or loss, a shaved head, bandages and IVs are also upsetting for children to see. Well siblings may worry that their brother or sister won't get better, or that they might catch hydrocephalus from them.

Siblings all cope differently with illness. If the sibling is a child, chances are his imagination is running wild. Answering his questions will require a detailed and honest approach. The condition of hydrocephalus will need to be explained in simple, age-appropriate terms. The answers should alleviate some of the child's fear.

> When my sister was in the hospital for her last shunt revision, our brother, who also has a chronic illness, was acting very immature and unsupportive. This really angered me. I felt that as a family member, he could put his jealousies aside and be a better brother. Instead of being there by her side in the hospital, he was out partying with his friends. My sister's condition was very serious, and none of us knew if she would ever walk again due to a complication during the revision.

> It wasn't until years later that he apologized for his behavior. He said that he was afraid of what might happen to his older sister, and that he couldn't bear to see her in the hospital, even though he was accustomed to having her visit him there.

Resentment and jealousy are common feelings experienced by siblings. These feelings are amplified when a brother or sister is suddenly hospitalized or undergoes an operation. Though the sibling who is well may truly be concerned about his brother or sister, there could be an element of jealousy involved. These are very confusing emotions for a child to deal with. A child may worry about his ill sibling, yet resent all the attention, gifts, and conversations that revolve around the ill sibling. Jealousy is usually compounded by the additional feeling of guilt for having these emotions.

Siblings of an ill brother or sister need to have the lines of communication open at all times. Let them know that they are deeply loved and valued. Many siblings are very compassionate and display a tremendous amount of strength.

> My sister has had hydrocephalus for many years. At first, I was not aware of the symptoms and complications as we were both very little when she had her first operation. As a child, I knew she had some restrictions, such as not being able to do gymnastics or "head" the ball in soccer, but not much was explained to me.

> I always wished I could find the right words to say to my sister when she would be self-conscious about the scars on her head, or when she would have to explain to a hairdresser where the scars came from.

> I was away at college when she had two shunt revisions as an adult. When I first visited her in the hospital, it was distressing for me to see the hair shaved off half of her head, a large bandage around her head and tubes in her arms and nose. I prayed that this shunt would last at least 20 years (which is how long the previous one was supposed to last). I was scared for her, but wanted to be supportive and strong. I don't know if I achieved this.

> My mom helped tremendously in terms of nursing her and helping her rehabilitate. In hindsight, it struck me as odd that she didn't receive any form of physical therapy. I tried to walk with my sister when I could. I felt bad that this had to happen to her at all. I don't like to sound full of pity, because I admire what my sister can do and how she copes with having hydrocephalus. I am proud of her.

> I am always concerned about my sister; perhaps I feel that I need to protect her, but I know that she can take care of herself. Perhaps my need to protect is a way to feel like I am actively doing something.

It's good to be aware of these varied and normal emotional responses. Siblings of children with hydrocephalus need lots of love, attention, and comfort.

Friends

During times of serious illness or hospitalization, it becomes remarkably clear who your true friends are. American journalist Walter Winchell once said, "A real friend is one who walks in when the rest of the world walks out!"

> *A friend of mine, someone I knew since grade school and have shared many good and bad times with over the years, was my closest confidante. I could share anything and everything in my life with her. I was really hurt when she suddenly disappeared when our daughter, Kaylie, went into the hospital to be treated for a vein of Galen malformation and to be shunted for hydrocephalus. As a family unit, we were all upset about what could happen during the surgery, and when I turned to my friend for support, she wasn't there.*

> *Months later, after Kaylie was back at home, my friend showed up at our doorstep one afternoon in tears. She said she was afraid that Kaylie might die, and she didn't know how to deal with it at that time. It didn't take long before we were both crying and hugging each other. We are true friends, so there were no grudges to hold or reasons to be upset with her. Life is too short for those kinds of things.*

During the enormously stressful times of illness, friends play a key role in lifting your spirits and making you forget—even if for just a little while—what you are contending with on a daily basis. Friends play a major role in recovery. Friends can serve as a link and convey to others what might be too draining for you to talk about at the time. Friends can also lighten the load at home by helping out with household chores such as laundry, feeding family pets, shopping, or preparing meals. Often just lending a listening ear and a shoulder to cry on is the best thing a friend can do.

> *I was unaware that my friend was having problems with her shunt until her husband phoned with the news that she had been hospitalized. He explained to me that her shunt was revised and that her brain hemorrhaged when the surgeon attempted to remove an old shunt. I was shocked and horrified. I had no idea what to say or do to help make the situation any better.*

> *At this point, no one knew whether she was going to stabilize and fully recover, or whether there would be serious and lasting effects from*

the hemorrhage. I was 3,000 miles away and wanted nothing more than
to be there for her. I wanted to do anything to make the situation easier.
Although I could not physically be with them, I wanted my friends to
know that I would always be with them in spirit.

I called practically every night to find out how she was doing. I
prayed and cried often. She had been there for me during many rough
times in my life, and I wanted her to know that I cared about her deeply. I
knew that she had a long haul ahead of her, and I never wanted her to
feel isolated or alone with her condition.

Marriage

Somewhere in your marriage vows the words "in sickness and in health"
were probably mentioned. A diagnosis of hydrocephalus can truly be a test
of your marriage, either bringing you closer together or pushing you apart.
Emotions are high, and coping skills differ. Couples must simply survive the
first few overwhelming weeks, then work together to rearrange the pieces in
a new pattern.

If you or your spouse is the person with hydrocephalus

Hydrocephalus will affect you and your spouse differently; you will have different ways of coping with the stress. How hydrocephalus impacts each of
you, and how you respond, also impacts the two of you as a couple.

If you have hydrocephalus, it is important that you talk openly with your
spouse about your condition. If you haven't already done so, share information about your medical history. If you have copies of your medical records,
let your spouse read through them to understand better what you've been
through. By knowing more about your condition, your spouse can help you
cope with the condition and help keep an eye out for the signs and symptoms of possible problems with your shunt.

If your spouse has hydrocephalus and is hospitalized, you may find being
separated from your loved one for an extended period of time to be physically and emotionally draining. Even though you may have the support of
family and friends, chances are you are still going home to an empty house
or to children with many questions about the absent parent.

Utilize your individual strengths to make it through this rough time. Remember that your spouse is your best friend, and you should be able to talk together about how you are feeling, good or bad.

> *I have been married for one year, and my husband has to have neurosurgery. I am frightened by people having surgery in general. The surgery he probably has to have involves taking his whole shunt out, being in the hospital for 10 days on antibiotics and then putting a new sterilized shunt back in. He has been in the hospital four times since January, and has been on intravenous antibiotics at home since March. We have been married since July 1996. So, as you can see, it has not been an easy first year. However, we plan on sticking it out.*

> *We believe that this will make our marriage stronger; it probably already has. But I definitely need support. I feel like I can't deal with my husband being sick anymore. Why can't we just have a break? We are only newlyweds! He is 33 years old and has never had a shunt infection until all this trouble started. We are both tired of hospitals and doctors.*

> *Even though he has been sick, we still have plenty of good times. He has a great sense of humor, which also brings my humor out. I know that humor has been getting us through these rough times.*

If your child has hydrocephalus

It is easy for worry and the extra strain of frequent doctor visits and hospitalization to take their toll on your marriage. Your child will be seeing his doctors and will also need to be taken to imaging centers and to the hospital. Once your child is out of the hospital, he will probably need some form of therapy, whether it is physical or psychological, to help him recover from surgery.

Those medical appointments, tests, hospitalizations, and advocating for and soothing your child take a lot of time and are stressful. More often than not, one parent is left to take the child to examinations or to visit the child in the hospital during the day while the other parent is at work. If at all possible, don't let this happen. Try to share responsibilities. While your child is in the hospital, take turns or alternate the days that you visit your child during the day so one parent doesn't feel responsible for spending all day there.

If the strain of seeing your child go through a shunt placement or revision is becoming too much for you, let your spouse know. Perhaps let your spouse take care of everything for a day to let you wind down or attempt to relax. When visiting the hospital, remember that your child will need rest to recover. Take time when your child is resting to go for a walk together or with friends.

In some ways, having an ill spouse or child is often harder on the people who are well than on the person who has the condition. It's very easy to let the condition get the best of you. Be open about your feelings. Ask for support.

Informing your child

Mark Twain once said, "When in doubt, tell the truth."

If your child is an infant or very young when first diagnosed with hydrocephalus, and she is fortunate not to have any shunt complications until later in her life, the question arises, "When do I tell my child about her condition?" The obvious answer is to explain the condition to her when she is old enough to begin understanding. If you are unsure about when or how to explain this, consult with your child's pediatrician or neurosurgeon and ask for advice. Do not wait to tell your child about her condition until there is a need for another shunt revision. This could traumatize your child.

> I knew I'd been in the hospital for something when I was little, but was unaware of what actually happened to me. I had strange memories as a young child. I was in a big crib. My arms were tied to the side rails. The air was filled with the smell of rubbing alcohol. I was wearing a knit cap. I had the vivid memory of my mother crying as I hugged her, telling her, "I'm okay, Mommy." It wasn't until I was eight or nine years old that I found what I thought looked like a mosquito bite just above my hair line. As I took a closer look, the mark on my head wasn't so small after all. The scar went all the way across the front of my head. I then found more all over my scalp. I remember being very confused and upset by what I had discovered. What had happened to me? My parents then told me everything they knew in terms they thought I'd understand.

If you explain hydrocephalus to your child in terms she can understand, she will have a healthier attitude toward the condition and be able to better cope with it later in life.

> *I started when Carolyn was two to three. It happened that one of her shunt sites on her head got bumped and hurt. I called it her "shunt bump," and went on to have a long conversation with her about how she got the bump. I explained that the doctor put it there. As she got older, we went on to talk about the shunt line that is visible on her chest and that it was to drain fluid from her brain. That went along with the fact that the doctor looked at CT scans to see how well the shunt was working and what her brain looked like. We certainly surprised the neurosurgeon on a routine visit when Carolyn told him she knew he was the one who put the bumps on her head.*

Since most children have vivid imaginations and cope differently from adults, it is important to talk to them truthfully about hydrocephalus in terms that they will understand. Medical terminology can be very complex, and it is important that the condition of hydrocephalus be explained to your child in a simple manner, using terms that are easy for the child to comprehend.

As a parent, you may be sorting through your own emotions, and having to provide an explanation to your child may prove to be overwhelming. If this is the case, it might be wise to ask your child's neurosurgeon to help explain the condition to your child with both parents present. One suggestion would be to create a forum, where the neurosurgeon explains the condition to the child and allows her to ask questions along the way. With the parents present, the child will be more relaxed and secure in the knowledge that everything will be okay. If your child's neurosurgeon is not able to talk with your child about hydrocephalus, ask the neurosurgeon if there is a counselor or neurological psychologist on staff who could.

Another suggestion is to find age-appropriate literature to help explain the condition to your child. *Just Like Any Other Beagle* is a coloring book which is published by Cordis Corporation, a shunt manufacturer. This coloring book explains what hydrocephalus is and how it is treated. *The Human Brain Coloring Book*, published by HarperPerennial, provides detailed illustrations of the structure of the brain, including the ventricular system and an explanation about cerebrospinal fluid. Ask your child's neurosurgeon or neurological psychologist for recommended age-appropriate books.

Reading and talking about hydrocephalus with your child will allow her to be more knowledgeable about her condition and helps her to dispel any fears or misconceptions she may have.

CHAPTER 3

Selecting a Neurosurgeon

If you listen carefully to the patient, he or she
will tell you the diagnosis.

> —Dr. Richard Smith,
> Editor, *British Medical Journal*
> *London Times,* August 10, 1993

NEUROSURGEONS ARE DOCTORS WHO ARE TRAINED to operate on the brain, spinal cord, and other nervous structures of the body, making neurosurgery one of the most complex and challenging of medical specialties. As such, neurosurgeons are often considered the best of the best—the "top guns" of surgical specialists.

One of your most difficult decisions will be to choose the right neurosurgeon. You will want the neurosurgeon to have top-notch training, to be knowledgeable about hydrocephalus, and most importantly, to be an excellent communicator.

In this chapter, we discuss how to go about finding the right neurosurgeon for you. We provide you with tips on how to locate a neurosurgeon through referrals, and some questions you could ask him to help you make your final decision. We also discuss ways for you to find out more information about your neurosurgeon's medical background and training.

Having a good doctor-patient relationship can make all the difference. How you communicate with your neurosurgeon, and how he communicates with you, is very important. We'll show you ways you can build a solid and lasting relationship with your neurosurgeon to ensure you are informed, educated, and a partner in the decision-making process.

We close with some suggestions on how to find a new neurosurgeon when relocating to a new area.

When you need a neurosurgeon

Upon first identifying the presence of hydrocephalus, your family physician or neurologist will refer you to a local neurosurgeon to examine and evaluate your condition, and then talk with you about surgical solutions.

The best time to look for a neurosurgeon is when you can do so at your leisure. If you have the time, you can check credentials and, most importantly, meet and talk with candidates. However, you sometimes won't have the luxury of getting to know a neurosurgeon before he needs to perform a shunt placement or revision. You will need to trust the referring doctor, the neurosurgeon who was recommended, your own judgment, and your instincts.

The following scenarios illustrate circumstances under which you might find yourself in need of a neurosurgeon for treatment of hydrocephalus.

Scenario 1: Newly diagnosed patient

You visit your family physician because in recent weeks your child has been walking oddly, her personality has changed, and she's started to fall down for no apparent reason. Recognizing these symptoms as possible signs of a neurological problem, your doctor asks you to take your daughter to a neurologist for an electroencephalogram (EEG). Your doctor also schedules your daughter for a head computed tomography (CT) series, just in case it's necessary.

The EEG comes back inconclusive, but the CT series indicates that your daughter's ventricles are enlarged—a symptom of hydrocephalus. The neurologist explains the condition to you briefly and says he is going to refer your daughter to see a pediatric neurosurgeon to talk about surgical options.

When you visit the neurosurgeon, she informs you that your daughter will need to have a ventriculoperitoneal shunt placed as soon as possible. After talking with the neurosurgeon at length about hydrocephalus, shunts and possible complications, you need to make a decision on whether to go ahead with the surgery. The neurosurgeon offers you the option of getting a second opinion for your daughter, and even offers to call another neurosurgeon in the area for you to take her to that day or the next.

Realizing that there is some time to work with, you opt to take your daughter for a second opinion. After looking at the CT scans and performing a brief exam, the second neurosurgeon confirms the initial diagnosis. This neurosurgeon recommends that your daughter be shunted as soon as possible to treat her hydrocephalus. He says he would happy to perform the operation, but also reassures you of the first neurosurgeon's reputation as a skilled surgeon.

Since it is apparent that your daughter needs to be treated fairly soon, you choose which neurosurgeon you want her to have, and then call to schedule the operation.

Scenario 2: Receiving emergency treatment

You are on a three-week vacation with your wife traveling across the United States and Canada. Near the end of your first week, you start to experience headaches and feel nauseated, especially in the mornings. Since you are away from your home, you brush the symptoms aside and consider them due to being on the road, not eating properly, and not being used to the time difference. However, these symptoms begin to worsen over the next 48 hours, and you find yourself bedridden.

Concerned, your wife convinces you to go to the local hospital to be examined for food poisoning. During the initial screening in emergency, you reveal to the attending physician that you have a ventriculoatrial (VA) shunt and hydrocephalus. Soon after, you find yourself in the chamber of a CT scanner. Thirty minutes later, the attending physician approaches with another doctor. He introduces the second doctor as a neurosurgeon, who explains to you that the symptoms are probably associated with either an obstructed or infected shunt.

At this point, you are more than a thousand miles away from home, have a shunt problem, and know absolutely nothing about the neurosurgeon who is attending you. You inform the neurosurgeon that you're on vacation and ask what the options are: can you return home for surgery, or is it of immediate concern? The neurosurgeon says that although you could make it home in time to have a shunt revision performed without any problems, there is also a chance that your condition could worsen. Your wife wants you to have the revision done, but you have your doubts.

Scenario 3: Finding a new neurosurgeon

Your son has had hydrocephalus since the age of five, and you've recently relocated to a new town. Once you have found a family doctor, you ask him if he could recommend a local neurosurgeon to manage your son's case. Your family doctor schedules you and your son for a consultation visit with a neurosurgeon the following week.

After waiting an extra thirty minutes in the waiting room, you and your son are finally taken back to an examination room where you spend another twenty minutes waiting for the neurosurgeon. When he does arrive, he seems short with you and isn't particularly nice with your son either.

You ask him if there is a problem, but he offers no explanation and continues to flip through your son's medical records. When he does speak to you, you feel as if you are being talked down to.

Lessons learned

The first scenario illustrates an example of a great working relationship between a doctor and a patient's family. Here, your family physician realizes there is a problem and takes the necessary steps to ensure that your child is diagnosed and treated properly. When hydrocephalus is detected with the CT scan, your daughter is referred to a pediatric neurosurgeon who then reviews the condition, discusses surgical options, and offers you an opportunity to have a second opinion. All of the doctors involved worked together with you to ensure prompt and proper treatment.

In the second scenario, you are diagnosed as having a probable shunt obstruction or infection while many miles from home. You are faced with making the difficult decision of whether to have the surgery in a foreign environment or fly home for the operation where you are familiar with the neurosurgeon and medical staff. In this instance, you should have the attending neurosurgeon consult with your neurosurgeon back home. Medical records can be faxed and, if necessary, previous CT or MRI films can be sent via Federal Express overnight. If immediate surgery is required, you could still request a second opinion or, knowing that this surgeon has consulted with your neurosurgeon at home, could forego the second opinion and have the operation. One thing that would have benefited you would have been if you could have obtained a copy of a baseline CT scan from your neurosurgeon prior to going on vacation, or you could obtain a wallet-sized card of your most recent scan. (For more information about how to obtain a wallet-sized card of your CT or MRI scans, see Chapter 11, *The Well-Informed Patient*.)

With the final scenario, you meet a neurosurgeon to handle your son's care, but find that he is a poor communicator. In this case, you should call the family physician back and explain to her what happened when you went to see the neurosurgeon. Don't worry, it isn't like you are tattling on the neurosurgeon. You are simply relaying the situation to the family physician. At this point, your doctor can do one of two things. She can act as a mediator and help in identifying any problems, or she can simply refer you to a different neurosurgeon. If you are a member of a hydrocephalus support group, you could contact a few of the members, find out who their children's neurosurgeons are, and relay those names to your doctor for a possible referral. Also, the Hydrocephalus Association maintains an active directory of pediatric neurosurgeons in North America. Since time is on your side, you could contact the association and request they send the directory to your doctor on your behalf. Remember, in this scenario there is no immediate cause for medical attention, just a need to locate a new neurosurgeon for follow-up care.

Referrals

The amount of investigation you will have time to do will vary. In the most rushed scenarios, you will be referred to a neurosurgeon who will perform emergency surgery. With slightly more time, you can check the technical credentials of the neurosurgeon through an interview with him and/or through physician directories. There are particular considerations for a pediatric neurosurgery. Ideally, if you have time, try to end up with two or three recommended neurosurgeons to investigate further.

Physician referrals

If hydrocephalus is suspected, your family physician or neurologist will provide you with a referral to a neurosurgeon. Your family physician probably knows the best neurosurgeons in your area, but may or may not be aware of their familiarity with treating hydrocephalus.

> The neurosurgeon our family doctor referred us to was a real problem. This guy had no personality, and wasn't interested in fielding questions from us about how many patients he's treated with hydrocephalus. We knew after a few short minutes we were in the wrong doctor's office, so we thanked him for his time and left—and never returned.

Your doctor will probably know which doctors have good reputations in the medical community, which hospitals they have admitting privileges to, and most importantly, who has the knowledge and ability to manage your case. If your doctor cannot immediately recommend a neurosurgeon, chances are he can find out this information by making one or two phone calls.

When we got home, we called our family doctor and relayed our experience with the first neurosurgeon to her. She apologized (though we weren't blaming her for anything), and said that she'd do a more thorough check before giving us the name of another.

After a few days, she called us and gave us the name of another neurosurgeon. But instead of just giving us the name and number, our doctor told us that she had interviewed three neurosurgeons in our area, looked into their background, and found out which hospitals they worked out of. In her opinion, this neurosurgeon was the best of the three. Needless to say, we were impressed. We trusted her opinion, even more this time since she'd taken the time to find the right doctor for Amy.

Insurance provider/HMO referrals

If your family doctor isn't familiar with the neurosurgeons in your area, try calling your insurance provider or HMO. Your insurance company will have a list of neurosurgeons who participate with their plan. The best way to do this is simply to call your provider's customer service number and ask them if they could recommend a neurosurgeon in your area. Explain to them that you are interested in finding a neurosurgeon who specializes in the treatment and care of patients who have hydrocephalus.

Your insurance provider has a business relationship with the neurosurgeons it covers. All physicians covered by a medical insurance company or an HMO have been screened to ensure their quality and credentials meet the guidelines of the plan. By contacting your insurance provider's customer service center, you can also ask some preliminary questions about the neurosurgeon, such as:

- Do you know if this neurosurgeon treats patients with hydrocephalus? If so, do you know how many patients are under her care?
- Does the neurosurgeon have more than one location for her practice?
- Which hospitals does she have admitting privileges for?

- How long has this neurosurgeon been covered by your insurance?

- Have you had any patient complaints against this doctor?

This information can be helpful, especially if the neurosurgeon has multiple practices.

It is also a good idea to ask your insurance provider or HMO if it provides coverage for neurosurgeons who are located out of your plan area, and what its terms are for seeing a physician outside the plan. This is particularly important if you want to see a neurosurgeon at a university medical center.

Word-of-mouth referrals

You might also receive a word-of-mouth referral from others who are patients. For example, if a parent has taken her child to see a particular neurosurgeon before, she will be able to tell you honestly how she feels about the way the neurosurgeon handled the surgery and how he treated her child.

> While sitting in the waiting room at the neurosurgeon's office, I noticed another mom sitting across from me with her son. His head was partially shaved, and he had a fairly large scar at the top of his head. This was only our second time to see this neurosurgeon, and we still weren't sure whether we liked him or not. I asked the mother if her son had hydrocephalus, and she said yes. When I asked her what she thought about the neurosurgeon, her face lit up, and she went on and on about how wonderful he was with her son. That pretty much sealed the deal for us.

However, it is important to keep in mind that one person's experience with a neurosurgeon will not necessarily predict what your experience with him will be. Before taking another patient's advice on a physician referral, you should ask questions such as:

- How long have you been seeing this neurosurgeon?

- Did he diagnose your condition (or shunt malfunction/infection) promptly and accurately?

- Do you feel comfortable talking with this neurosurgeon about problems you are experiencing?

- Does this neurosurgeon communicate well with you and with other members of your family?

- Do you feel the neurosurgeon shares information with you openly and honestly?

- How does this neurosurgeon relate to children? (If applicable.)

- How does your child like this neurosurgeon? (If applicable.)

- Does he believe your concerns and answer your questions in a manner that you find acceptable?

- Has this neurosurgeon ever operated on you? If not, what is your relationship as a patient with this neurosurgeon? If so, when was the last operation performed, and what was it?

- How many times has this neurosurgeon operated on you? Did you feel the operation was necessary? Did the neurosurgeon attempt to treat the problem by another means prior to opting for surgery?

- Do you know other patients who see this neurosurgeon? If so, what are their opinions of him?

By asking these simple questions, you can ascertain whether or not the person who is giving you the referral has a strong relationship with this particular neurosurgeon. You are looking to find out what they are basing their recommendation on—skills, knowledge, ability to communicate with the patient, etc.—which will help you make your own decision when the time comes.

I advise a person to contact Best Doctors, the American Medical Association (AMA), or simply do some calling around. If the office secretary is unable to provide you with some simple facts, etc., then see if you can get an appointment for an interview of sorts. Some doctors have no problem with doing this. An excellent way of getting a referral is to go to the neurosurgical ward/floor of a hospital or medical center and speak with the head nurses (or neurosurgical nurses) to see who they would recommend. (This is an excellent way to find a neurosurgeon as the nurses really know who is the best surgeon, if he cares, if he deals only with children, etc.)

Neurosurgery for infants and children

Infants and children with hydrocephalus have a different set of primary care needs, are more prone to having learning disabilities, and can lag behind in social activities. Because neurosurgeons who concentrate on pediatric care attend to more infants and children than other neurosurgeons, they are more capable of meeting the patient's and the family's needs for physical, emotional, and psychological care.

Over the past few years, neurosurgeons who treat predominantly pediatric patients (children and infants) organized the American Board of Pediatric Neurological Surgery (ABPNS). Although not yet recognized as a separate specialty by the American Board of Medical Specialists (ABMS), ABPNS began certifying pediatric neurosurgeons in 1996. A list of board certified pediatric neurosurgeons can be found in Appendix A, *Pediatric Neurosurgeons*. This information is updated on the Internet at: *http://www.abpns.org/*.

Under the proposed petition, candidates who apply for certification as a pediatric neurosurgeon will have to meet one of the following criteria to become board certified:

- Complete an accredited postgraduate fellowship in pediatric neurosurgery as outlined by the Accreditation Council for Pediatric Neurosurgical Fellowships, Inc.
- Successfully complete the written examination of the ABPNS.
- Acquire certification by the American Board of Neurological Surgery (ABNS) or the Royal College of Physicians and Surgeons of Canada (RCPSC).
- Submit surgical logs indicating a practice of pediatric neurosurgery for the year prior to submitting their application. These logs must demonstrate that 75 percent of their cases were age 21 or under, or they must have treated 125 patients who were below the age of 12.

Under the proposed petition, certification will also be considered for senior neurological surgeons who have established themselves as practitioners of pediatric neurosurgery and have:

- Had the requirement for accredited fellowship training waived by a special review of the ABPNS.
- Successfully completed the examination in pediatric neurosurgery which is given by the ABPNS.
- Acquired certification by the ABNS or the RCPSC.

- Submitted surgical logs indicating a practice of pediatric neurosurgery for the year prior to submitting their application. These logs must demonstrate that 75 percent of their cases were age 21 or under; or they must have treated 125 patients who were below the age of 12.

Since pediatric neurosurgery is a specialty, you may want to consider having this kind of specialist operate on your infant or child. If your child's neurosurgeon is not certified by the ABPNS, ask the neurosurgeon how much of his practice is with infants and children, and how many shunt operations for hydrocephalus he does in a year.

Finding out more

As patients, we often entrust our health to people we hardly know. One reason we don't know more about our doctors is because we don't take the time to find out more about them. This can be done by interviewing them or by doing some basic research about their medical background at your local library or online. Unless you ask questions or do some research on your own, your doctor probably isn't likely to share that information with you.

Commercial resources

An easy way to check on your doctor's credentials is to call Medi-Net, a consumer information service that provides healthcare consumers with a background check on any doctor who is licensed to practice in the U.S., including credentials, degrees, training, board certification(s), as well as any disciplinary actions or sanctions taken against the doctor. Each complete Medi-Net physician profile costs $15.00 per doctor. Preliminary information is provided on the telephone, with detailed reports mailed or faxed to callers, usually on the same day. To order a report, call toll-free 1-888-ASK-MEDI (275-6334) or 1-800-972-MEDI (972-6334). Medi-Net is also available on the Web at *http://www.askmedi.com*.

Print resources

Most public libraries in the U.S. receive physician directories that are kept in the reference section. Here you can find detailed information about your neurosurgeon's background, experience, and where he has worked previously.

- *AMA Directory of Physicians in the United States* (35th Edition). This four-volume set lists all physicians practicing in the United States, Puerto Rico, the Virgin Islands, and certain islands in the Pacific, or who are temporarily located in foreign countries. The books include listings for both members and nonmembers of the AMA.

Volume one is an alphabetical listing of physicians by last name. Each listing includes the city and state, and the name of the foreign country where the doctor is located (if applicable).

Volumes two through four are broken down by geographical area. Volume two contains listings for physicians who are providing care under federal services—either working for the Veterans Administration (VA) or as a military doctor—and those located in the states of Alabama through Illinois. Volume three lists physicians in Indiana through New York, while volume four contains listings for North Carolina through Wyoming and those who are in temporary foreign locations.

The listings in volumes two through four provide more detailed information than can be found in volume one. Physicians are listed alphabetically by last name according to the city and state in which they are located. Each listing also includes the following information:

— Primary mailing address for the doctor's practice.

— Medical school code and year of graduation.

— The year the doctor obtained his license to perform medicine in that state.

— Designation of his primary and secondary medical specialty.

— Type of practice.

— American Specialty Board Certification code.

— Listing of any physicians' recognition awards.

For example, a listing for a neurosurgeon in the *AMA Directory of Physicians* might be as follows:

DOE, Jane M. 321 ANYPLACE DR. 98227 #026-08-78 L85 NS *20 †25

All of the information to decipher the codes that make up the physicians' listing in the *AMA Directory* can be found in the front of each volume. In the above example, the code #026-08-78 indicates that this particular physician graduated from Mayo Medical School in Rochester,

Minnesota, in 1978 (026 is the state identifier; 08 is the code for the medical school; 78 is the year of graduation). L85 means that Dr. Doe received her license in Washington state in 1985. The designator NS means that she is a licensed neurosurgeon. *20 indicates that her type of practice is direct patient care, while the †25 indicates that she is certified with the American Board of Neurological Surgeons.

- *The Official ABMS Directory of Board Certified Medical Specialists.* Published annually by the American Board of Medical Specialists, the *ABMS Directory* is a four-volume set that lists all board certified medical specialists in the United States. The section on neurological surgeons can be found in volume two (beginning on page 3,673 in the 1998, 30th edition). The *ABMS Directory* lists the qualifications of each doctor and describes the process that a neurosurgeon must go through to become board certified.

All practicing neurosurgeons who are certified by the ABMS are listed in this book alphabetically by city and state. Information in each listing includes:

— Year of board certification (or recertification).

— The doctor's birth date or year, and where he was born.

— Medical school.

— Place of internship, residency, and fellowships.

— Current and past hospital appointments.

— Academic appointments.

— Professional organizations the neurosurgeon is a member of.

— Type of practice.

— Contact information, including mailing address, and phone and fax numbers if available.

A sample listing for a neurosurgeon in the *ABMS Directory* could be:

DOE, Jane M.
Cert NS 85. b 08-30-45 Dearborn MI. MD NYU Sch Med 70.
Int 70-71 (U Minn Minneapolis MN) Res NeurS 75-79 (Mass Gen Hosp) Fell NeurS 80-81 (Stanford U).
Cur Hosp Appt (U Hosp-U Calif, San Francisco, CA). AANS - AMA - CNS - ASA - ACS. U Calif Med Ctr Dept NS 94143 (415) 555-0000.

In this example, Dr. Doe received her board certification as a neurosurgeon (Cert NS) in 1985; she was born in Dearborn, Michigan, August 30, 1945. She received her M.D. from the New York University School of Medicine in 1970; interned from 1970-1971 at the University of Minnesota in Minneapolis; was a neurosurgical resident at Massachusetts General Hospital from 1975-1979. She also had a neurosurgery fellowship at Stanford University from 1980-1981. Dr. Doe is currently associated with the University Hospital at the University of California, San Francisco, and is a member of five different professional organizations. Her mailing address and telephone number are listed last.

Some of the more common professional organizations that you will find in a neurosurgeon's listing are:

— American Association of Neurological Surgeons (AANS).

— American College of Surgeons (ACS).

— American Medical Association (AMA).

— American Surgical Association (ASA).

— Canadian Medical Association (CMA).

— Congress of Neurological Surgeons (CNS).

• *16,638 Questionable Doctors* (and state editions). Public Citizen: Health Research Group, founded by Ralph Nader in 1971, publishes a three-volume set of books which lists doctors who have been disciplined by state or federal agencies for incompetence, negligence, substance abuse, patient abuse, or the misprescription of prescription drugs. The title of the 1998 edition is *16,638 Questionable Doctors*. They also publish state editions of *Questionable Doctors*. Check the reference section of your library for the latest edition or call (202) 588-1000 to order. PCHRG can also be contacted by email at *public_citizen@citizen.org*, or through their web site at *http://www.citizen.org/*.

Online resources

The Internet opens a new way of researching and relaying information that can otherwise be difficult to locate. If you cannot find a copy of the *AMA Directory of Physicians* or the *ABMS Directory*, you can go on the World Wide Web (WWW) and find the information online. Two sites you can use to look up information on neurosurgeons follow. As with all online sites, the address of the page or the particulars of the interface are subject to change.

- American Association of Neurological Surgeons (AANS). The AANS web site has a searchable directory of neurosurgeons available at *http://server400.aans.org/FindaNeurosurgeon/*.

  Here you can search by area code, last name of the neurosurgeon, city and state, or by country (for locating neurosurgeons outside the United States). When you click on the "Search" button, you will be taken to another page that lists the name, phone number, and address for the neurosurgeons that match your search criteria.

- American Medical Association (AMA). The AMA's Web site offers a greater amount of detail than the AANS site. If you go to the AMA homepage (*http://www.ama-assn.org/*), click on the "Doctor Finder" link to the physician search page.

  Once at the search page, you can either enter the name of the physician you are trying to find more information about, or enter your city and state for a list of physicians in your area. For example, if you enter your city and state and click "Neurological Surgery" for the medical specialty, the search results page will list all of the neurosurgeons in your city. If you click on the link for the name of the neurosurgeon, you will be taken to another page that lists the following information:

  — Address and phone number for the neurosurgeon's office, including a link to a location map.

  — Neurosurgeon's gender.

  — Year and name of the medical school the doctor graduated from.

  — Listing of where the doctor performed his medical residency training.

  — Primary and secondary practice specialties.

  — Major professional activity, i.e., type of practice.

  — Board certification confirmed (this should say "Yes" next to it; if it says "No," you should look for a different neurosurgeon).

National Practitioner Data Bank

Since 1990, the U.S. Department of Health and Human Services (DHHS) has been collecting information on all physicians in the U.S. Any disciplinary actions by state licensing boards or medical societies, malpractice payments, and revocation or limitation of a doctor's license by a hospital or clinic must be reported. One of the purposes of the data bank is to provide health care providers with a method of identifying possibly incompetent practitioners. In the past, doctors could simply cross a state line and continue to practice, with state authorities ignorant about their past problems. Unfortunately, consumers do not have access to this information. If citizens pressured their elected representatives to eliminate the restrictions on access to the data bank, it would be possible to make a more informed choice of medical care providers.

Interviewing the neurosurgeon

It might sound strange, but interviewing your neurosurgeon makes a lot of sense. It gives you an opportunity to find out more about the neurosurgeon—her background and interests—as well as to see how open she is with her patients.

Whether you have an existing relationship with a neurosurgeon or are a new patient, it is always good to know who you are dealing with. Often, your neurosurgeon will know far more about you than you know about her. If you are going to see the neurosurgeon for the first time, there are some very simple questions you could ask to help you get to know her better.

Before you start asking questions, ask your neurosurgeon if she has time to answer them, or if she would prefer you schedule another appointment when you could come back to talk with her. Neurosurgeons are often short on time and book appointments close together on days they are seeing patients in their office. If the sole purpose of your visit is to ask questions, let your neurosurgeon's receptionist know that your visit is for a consultation and that you have some questions you would like to ask. The receptionist might try to get you to ask her the questions, but be persistent on scheduling an appointment with the neurosurgeon. After all, if you need surgery, the receptionist won't be the person performing the operation.

Once you have an appointment with your neurosurgeon, it is a good idea to make a list of questions that you want to ask. Possible questions are:

* Where did you go to medical school?
* Where did you perform your internship and residency?
* What are your research interests?
* Do you specialize in any other form of surgery (i.e., vascular surgery)?

- Are you board certified?

- Which professional medical organizations are you a member of?

- How many years have you been a practicing, licensed neurosurgeon in this state/province?

- How many patients under your direct care have hydrocephalus?

- How many shunt placements/revisions have you: Assisted on? Performed?

- How many shunt operations have you performed: In the last year? In your career?

- When was the last time you placed or revised a shunt?

- Which hospital or hospitals in this area do you have admitting privileges for?

- Are you familiar with the third ventriculostomy procedure? If so, have you ever performed one? Was it successful?

By asking these and other questions, you will be able to find out information about your neurosurgeon's background. You will also be able to find out how familiar she is with treating patients with hydrocephalus.

If a neurosurgeon performs very few shunt operations in a year (less than ten or twenty), you might want to look for another neurosurgeon. You need to have a neurosurgeon whose shunt placement and revision skills are up to date. For some neurosurgeons, particularly pediatric neurosurgeons, it's not uncommon for them to perform fifty or more shunt operations per year.

Knowing how many patients with hydrocephalus your neurosurgeon has under her care is also important. Some neurosurgeons would rather focus on treating conditions of the brain other than hydrocephalus. If the neurosurgeon indicates that she doesn't treat many hydrocephalus cases in a year, ask her if she could recommend another neurosurgeon in the area who does.

You can also find out many facts about a neurosurgeon before you go in for an interview—including education, certification, and pending legal actions.

Developing a relationship

Having confidence in your neurosurgeon's background and expertise is just one element in forming a solid and lasting relationship. The psychological environment in which you or your loved one is treated also plays a vital role in mental health and recovery. A successful doctor-patient relationship is attainable when the parent and neurosurgeon respect each other.

As well as having a skilled surgeon, look for a neurosurgeon who believes in including you as a partner in decision-making—discussing surgeries and follow-up—and one who closely monitors your care. You need to feel comfortable in discussing your questions and concerns. You want any quality-of-life issues you have to be listened to and taken into account. If your child is the patient, the neurosurgeon needs to recognize that you are the expert on your child.

> *The bottom line is obviously technical and medical expertise. The best bedside manner in the world is meaningless if the surgeon's lack of skill places a child in the hospital in the first place!*

> *But given any sort of choice or range of options, then of course the neurosurgeon should have a pleasant personality. He should also have the ability to relate to children and be able to reassure them that everything will be all right. He should be someone who can listen and respond to the parents.*

Communication skills

Finding the right balance of medical and communication skills is key to a successful relationship. Here are some communication skills to look for:

- Uses language that is easy to understand.
- Communicates effectively and compassionately.
- Answers all of your questions openly and honestly.
- Respects your values and beliefs.
- Establishes good rapport with you or your child.

Range of personalities

Most people want a neurosurgeon who believes in patient education, provides excellent care and follow-up, offers support, and most importantly, communicates truthfully and respectfully with patient and family. A good neurosurgeon not only possesses good technical skills, but takes an interest in his patients' lives, carefully follows up on the progress of their recovery, offers advice and counseling if needed, and communicates well.

Our neurosurgeon considers himself partners and equals with the medical staff and the parents of his patients in his fight for a child's health. He is on a first-name basis with most people on the nursing staff and with practically all of the parents with whom he has any sort of extended contact. You can call him whatever you wish, and at any hour. He gives all patients his office, home, beeper and cellular phone numbers, as well as his email address.

Sometimes your neurosurgeon might be rushed when seeing patients in the office if his appointments are scheduled close together. When he has little time to spend with his patients, he will often have the nurses on his staff answer questions from the patient. These nurses are highly trained as neuro-surgical nurses and can often answer a majority of your questions regarding hydrocephalus. Everyone in the neurosurgical practice is looking out for your best interest. If the nurse cannot answer your question, she will bring the neurosurgeon back in, if possible, or have him contact you at a later time.

However, problems do happen. These parents felt their concerns were not respected or acted on.

We had one really bad experience with our son's neurosurgeon—it forced us to leave our hospital to look for a new one. The neurosurgeon we had went on vacation right after a revision, leaving Shaun supposedly in the care of another neurosurgeon. This doctor never came in to see him. The residents were very rude and were not concerned with him. My husband and I were getting very frustrated as his recovery was not the norm, and he was having a lot of problems—overdraining, vision distur-bances, vomiting, fever, etc. The residents were worthless, and the attend-ing physician was nowhere to be found. The residents did not know what to do, they did not or could not get the attending physician to come in, and we were left in the middle.

Adult patients can also have difficulties getting listened to. Finding a neuro-surgeon who listens to you and not just to the "normal" person who accom-panies you to the appointment can be a challenge. You know your body bet-ter than anyone else. Your concerns should be trusted, especially when you are complaining of symptoms associated with hydrocephalus.

Just once I would like to reverse the roles between me and my neuro-surgeon. When I see him with a reasonable complaint, he tries to brush it over as something else. I trust him to know what he's doing. Why can't he trust me to know how I'm feeling without having to have my wife present at the doctor's visit to corroborate my story?

Neurosurgeons, like other surgeons, need to have a lot of confidence to do their job well. Their self-selection and training emphasize this confidence. However, too much confidence can sometimes get in the way of including you in the decision-making process.

Keep in mind that you are a part of your health care. You deserve to be treated well. If the analogy helps, think of yourself as the customer; you have to be satisfied with your care. Neurosurgeons need to understand their patients' needs, and should take the time to get to know their patients well. The relationship that you have with your neurosurgeon is one that will hopefully last a very long time.

Although any type of surgery has its possible complications, neurosurgery brings with it a greater risk of complications and problems. If you are having reservations about the neurosurgeon you or your child is seeing, don't ignore that instinct. However, don't be too quick to cast aside your neurosurgeon solely because you don't like his personality.

Working on the relationship

If you feel your neurosurgeon is not treating you with respect, you could try to work it out or find another neurosurgeon. Switching neurosurgeons, however, is not trivial. It takes time. Your current doctor has some familiarity with your case. He might have real technical skills that you'd hate to give up. You might end up with a new neurosurgeon who doesn't have significantly better communication skills.

Before blaming communication problems on the neurosurgeon, step back and take a look at the way you are communicating with him. If you are feeling anxious and stressed prior to your visit with the neurosurgeon, your feelings are likely to come through in the way you react to the situation at hand, especially if you are hearing bad news for the first time. If you find yourself in a heated or tense conversation with your neurosurgeon, it is probably be a good idea to call a time-out, head to neutral corners, and wait until you both have calmed down enough to continue the conversation.

If you are having problems relating with your neurosurgeon but you think his technical skills are good, try to resolve the personal issues. Request a meeting and be open about what is causing a problem for you. Phrase your issues as "I" statements so they are easier for him to listen to without taking them personally. ("I feel confused," rather than, "You never explain anything.") For example, if you are feeling rushed and talked down to, you might say:

• I feel rushed and intimidated during our meetings.

• I would like to feel that I can predict the amount of time I will have and to get through a list of my questions and concerns.

• I hear your explanations, but they are too technical for me to understand. Could you explain things to me in terms I can comprehend?

• How much time do you usually allow for a follow-up meeting? Can I schedule extra time?

• I realize you have a very busy schedule, so would it help if I faxed my questions to your office ahead of time?

If you are unable to come to a resolution with your neurosurgeon, you will have to ask yourself if the personality conflict seriously impacts your medical care. There could be instances where you decide to stay with the neurosurgeon even though the relationship is not satisfying. For example, if you live in a rural area and the neurosurgeon you have is the only one within a hundred-mile radius, or if the neurosurgeon is so skilled that you don't want to see anyone else, you would probably think twice before going with another neurosurgeon. If you cannot resolve the conflict, if you have the luxury of living in an area where there are many skilled neurosurgeons to choose from, and if your insurance company allows you to schedule consultations with physicians, then it is a good idea to shop around for another neurosurgeon.

Not everyone has the same idea of what makes a good relationship with a neurosurgeon. Some people might want and expect an authoritative doctor and be perfectly comfortable in a situation that you don't like. Neurosurgeons have different personalities and styles, just as other people do. If you are not comfortable with the neurosurgeon you or your child is seeing, it is in your best interest to find another one. You can stay with your current neurosurgeon temporarily while seeking out another.

Relocating and finding a new neurosurgeon

When relocating to a new area, it is a good idea to establish a relationship with a neurosurgeon as soon as possible in case there is an emergency. By doing so, you will already have a neurosurgeon you can turn to. He will be up to date on your medical history and should have all of your medical records, including CT and MRI films. How do you go about finding a neuro-surgeon in a town where you barely know anyone?

The first person you could ask would be your present neurosurgeon. The neurosurgery community is fairly tight-knit, and it's possible that either he or another neurosurgeon he knows may know of someone in the area where you are relocating.

> In preparing for a move from Washington state down to California, we asked my wife's neurosurgeon at the University of Washington if he could recommend a neurosurgeon in northern California. As it turned out, one of his colleagues had just accepted a position in the neurosurgery department at the University of California, San Francisco, so he gave us his phone number and email address. He also helped transfer her records down to the new neurosurgeon as soon as we had made an appointment.

If your neurosurgeon is unable to suggest someone in your new area, the next person you could ask would be your family physician or pediatrician. Let him know everything you or your child has been through, and ask him if he could recommend one or two neurosurgeons in the new area. It would also be wise to ask him if there is anyone he could refer you to at a university medical center or children's hospital, if that's what you desire.

Next, you will need to call each of the neurosurgeon candidates to schedule appointments. When you call to make the appointment, be clear with the receptionist that you are new to the area and that the purpose of your visit is for consultation purposes only. If possible, try to see all candidates on consecutive days. That way, your medical records and films can be transferred from one to the next, allowing the new neurosurgeon to have enough time to review them. Scheduling the appointments a day apart also helps you keep your impression of them fresh in your mind, and makes it easier for you to make your final decision of who will be your neurosurgeon.

When we relocated to a new city, I had a terrible time trying to find a new neurosurgeon. I was told by my previous neurosurgeon to locate a new one as soon as possible. He said the main reason for doing this would be so he could transfer my records and MRIs so the new neurosurgeon would be up to date on my case history. I tried to schedule a consultation visit with a new neurosurgeon, but it took over a month to get the appointment. On the morning of the appointment, the new neurosurgeon's office called to tell me that they had not received my medical records or MRIs yet and asked me to track them down. When I phoned my previous neurosurgeon's office, they informed me that the doctor I was about to see had never requested any records or films! Luckily, I had copies of my records with me, so I just brought those to the appointment.

When I got to my appointment, the neurosurgeon's receptionist was rude with me, and so was the neurosurgeon. Talk about making a bad first impression. And to make matters worse, the neurosurgeon actually had the gall to ask me what I was doing there. When I told him that I had just moved to the area from out of state and that I wanted to establish a rapport with a new neurosurgeon in the area, he went off on a tangent about only being available to his family "twenty-four hours a day, seven days a week, and not to patients." All I was looking for was to have a neurosurgeon who would know my case history in case of an emergency, not someone I could call every time I had a headache! He must have thought I was a hypochondriac or something, but I can tell you, I'm never seeing him again or recommending him to anyone else.

When you meet with a new neurosurgeon for the first time, you should inform him that you are new to the area and that you are trying to decide whom you would like to manage your case. For instance, you could say, "I'm new to town and am looking for a neurosurgeon to provide follow-up care for my hydrocephalus. I had a wonderful relationship with my previous neurosurgeon, and was hoping to have a similar one with you. I tend to ask quite a few questions. How do you feel about that?"

Then gently explain the other issues. This way, you are stating in a positive manner what you hope for and need. Most doctors (and other people as well) are uncomfortable if they are grilled but are perfectly willing to talk about how they feel or operate if asked politely.

CHAPTER 4

Treating Hydrocephalus

There is one singular ingredient of the art of healing that should not be allowed to vanish...the transmission of a few encouraging words.

—Sherwin B. Nuland, M.D.
Doctors: The Biography of Medicine

THE METHODS OF TREATING HYDROCEPHALUS have evolved greatly through history, with the most progress being made since 1955 when John Holter invented a ball-and-spring valve system to be implanted in his son. Since that time, great strides have been made in improving shunt technology and learning more about the causes and effects of hydrocephalus.

This chapter begins with an overview of the parts of a shunt system, how they work, and where they can be placed in the body. We include a discussion about the different types of shunt systems—how they are manufactured and tested—and provide you with an overview of the types of shunts available from five manufacturers.

We next take a look at the operations, including pre- and postop, and an introduction to anesthesia. The procedures described include those for implanting a ventriculoperitoneal (VP) and ventriculoatrial (VA) shunt, and the third ventriculostomy procedure.

The intent of this chapter is to give you the background needed to discuss treatments and procedures with your neurosurgeon, to help envision how a shunt will help relieve fluid buildup, and to understand what will happen during a surgical procedure.

The shunt system

A shunt is a micromechanical device that is used to divert the buildup of cerebrospinal fluid to another area of the body where it can be reabsorbed. A shunt system consists of three parts: two catheters made of silicone (approximately 1/8" in diameter), with a one-way valve placed between the two catheters to allow cerebrospinal fluid (CSF) to flow out of the brain.

The three parts of the shunt are:

- **Proximal catheter.** The section of shunt catheter tubing that is placed within the ventricles or lumbar region of the spine is called the proximal catheter. The term *proximal,* which means nearest, is used because it refers the end of the shunt system that is closest to the affected area. The proximal catheter, which may also be referred to as the ventricular catheter, is used to drain CSF from the ventricles of the brain.

- **Shunt valve.** The shunt valve is what regulates the flow of CSF between the proximal and distal catheters.

- **Distal catheter.** The section of shunt catheter located furthest away from the affected area is called the distal catheter. The distal catheter can be placed in the peritoneal cavity of the abdomen (ventriculoperitoneal, or VP), into the right atrium of the heart via the internal or external jugular vein (ventriculoatrial, or VA), or in the pleural space that surrounds the lungs (ventriculopleural, or VPl). The most common placement of the distal end of the shunt is in the peritoneal cavity because of the ease of insertion and reliable long-term function.

How shunts work

When the flow of CSF is normal and unobstructed, new CSF is constantly produced, flowing into the ventricles and out of the brain again. Hydrocephalus can occur for one of two basic reasons: there is an obstruction in one of the CSF pathways, or CSF is not permitted to be reabsorbed. Figure 4-1 shows a CT image of a brain with CSF buildup in the ventricles (dark area in the middle).

When a shunt is implanted in a person with hydrocephalus, the goal is for the shunt system to mimic what would occur in the body naturally. CSF will be drained by the shunt, and the flow will be regulated so that a constant intracranial pressure (ICP) is maintained within the brain. Figure 4-2 shows

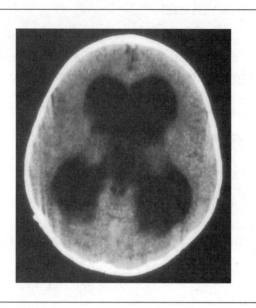

Figure 4-1. Before shunt placement

a postoperation CT image of the same patient's brain. The ventricles have drained and have resumed their normal size. The white area in the middle of the image is the shunt valve.

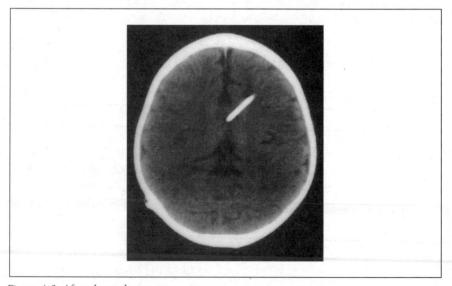

Figure 4-2. After shunt placement

CSF enters the shunt system through small holes or slits near the tip of the proximal catheter. As CSF is produced by the choroid plexus, the shunt valve will regulate the amount of ICP by draining fluid from the ventricles. From the proximal catheter, CSF flows through the valve system and into the distal catheter, which drains CSF into another area of the body where it can be reabsorbed (directly or indirectly) by the bloodstream. For instance, in a person with a VP shunt, CSF would flow out of the distal catheter into the peritoneal cavity. This causes the body no harm, because CSF is normally reabsorbed by the superior sagittal sinus, a large venous structure that carries the blood flow away from the brain.

Valve pressure ratings

Most shunt valves are known as *differential pressure* valves. This means the valve is self-regulating. It is capable of gauging the amount of ICP and can adjust to differential pressures (DPs) between the ventricles and the distal cavity the shunt drains into. This allows the right amount of CSF to be drained based on ICP.

The most common pressure ratings for differential pressure valves are:

- Extra-low-pressure: 0-10 mm H_2O.

- Low-pressure: 10-50 mm H_2O.

- Medium-pressure: 51-100 mm H_2O.

- High-pressure: 101-200 mm H_2O.

The values listed above are a median range and are based on information supplied from various shunt manufacturers. The amount of fluid that is allowed to flow through the shunt valve depends on the specific design characteristics of the valve, as well as levels that are rated by the manufacturer of the shunt valve. Check with your neurosurgeon to find out the type of shunt you have and its pressure setting. The flow of CSF through the valve can be changed by the pressure of tissue or debris in the shunt system.

Changes in body position

Intracranial pressure is measured according to atmospheric pressure. The atmospheric pressure relates to the location of the ventricular system and the distal end of the shunt catheter. When you are lying down, your ventricles are considered to be level with the distal end of the shunt. In this position, the normal range of ICP can range from anywhere between 50 mm H_2O and 200 mm H_2O. For infants, the normal ICP is generally less than 60 mm H_2O, and less than 40 mm H_2O for premature infants (P. H. Chapman et al., "The relationship between ventricular fluid pressure and body position in normal subjects and subjects with shunts: a telemetric study," *Neurosurgery* 26, no. 2, February 1990: 181-89).

When you sit or stand after lying on your back, the distal end of the shunt system is below the ventricles. This sudden change in body position can cause your ICP to drop momentarily to a level between -50 mm H_2O and +50 mm H_2O. In order to compensate for this drop in pressure, shunt valves not only need to be able to accommodate a wide range of atmospheric pressures as the patient changes position, but they also need to adapt to the differential pressures of CSF production. Fortunately, most shunt valves today are differential pressure valves. This means the valve has the ability to adjust automatically to a range of pressures to maintain ICP at the correct level for your body.

Without a differential pressure valve (as with some older shunt systems), changes in body position can sometimes cause a siphoning effect in the distal catheter. The siphoning effect occurs when CSF from the distal catheter flows into its drainage cavity (e.g., right atrium of the heart or the peritoneal cavity), causing fluid from the ventricles to drain suddenly. When this happens, you will probably feel a sense of light-headedness. This is normal, and should only last for a few seconds. Your shunt just needs a chance to respond to changes in elevation brought about by a change of body position.

Placement of shunts

As stated earlier, a shunt has three parts: the proximal catheter, which drains excess fluid, the valve that regulates the flow of CSF from the ventricles, and the distal catheter, which deposits the fluid elsewhere in the body. In some types of shunts, like the Codman Uni-Shunt from Johnson & Johnson, slits near the tip of the distal catheter control pressure.

The proximal catheter is placed in the ventricles of the brain or in the lumbar region of the spine. The shunt valve is placed in a pocket under the scalp. The distal catheter can be placed in a variety of locations, depending on the specifics of that person's case.

This section describes the three most common types of shunt placements: ventriculoperitoneal (VP), ventriculoatrial (VA), and ventriculopleural (VPl).

Ventriculoperitoneal (VP) shunt

VP shunts divert CSF away from the ventricular system of the brain and drain into the peritoneal cavity. The peritoneum lines the abdominal cavity, which is where the digestive organs (i.e., stomach and intestines) are located. The CSF is then absorbed into the bloodstream by blood vessels in the wall of the abdomen.

When the distal end of the shunt system is placed in infants and small children, it is a common practice for the neurosurgeon to leave an extra 120 centimeters (almost 4 feet) of tubing into the peritoneal cavity. This extra tubing allows the system to lengthen as the child grows, eliminating the need for lengthening procedures.

A variety of complications can occur when the distal end of the catheter is in the peritoneal cavity. These include:

- Formation of abdominal pseudocysts (cysts filled with CSF).
- Penetration of an organ in the peritoneal cavity, such as the bowel, bladder, vagina, uterus, or umbilicus.
- Obstruction of the catheter, caused when the tip of the distal catheter is occluded by scar tissue, fatty tissues that surround organs and the bowel, or by a reaction of the abdominal contents (i.e., intestines, stomach, etc.) to a foreign body. The obstruction occurs when CSF isn't permitted to flow out of the holes or slits at the tip of the distal catheter.
- Peritoneal shunt infections.

In cases where the distal catheter has penetrated the bowel, it is necessary to replace (revise) the shunt system.

Figure 4-3 shows examples of VP and VA shunt placements.

Ventriculoatrial (VA) shunt

VA shunts are often used when the peritoneum no longer absorbs the CSF. Like VP shunts, VA shunts drain the cerebrospinal fluid away from the ventricular system. However, the distal end of the VA shunt enters the bloodstream via the internal jugular vein. The catheter is then inserted so that the

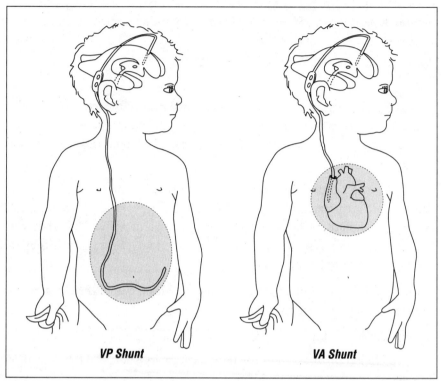

VP Shunt   VA Shunt

Figure 4-3. VP and VA shunt placement

tip of the distal catheter lies in the right atrium of the heart. This enables the CSF to enter the bloodstream directly.

One of the disadvantages of VA shunts in infants and young children is that they usually require more revisions than VP shunts because the neurosurgeon cannot place additional tubing to allow for growth in children.

Problems that are associated with VA shunts tend to be more severe because they involve the cardiovascular system. Some problems that can occur include:

- Separation of the catheter with migration into the pulmonary artery.

- Abnormal heart rhythm (cardiac arrhythmia).

- Shunt infections leading to an inflammation of the heart (endocarditis).

- An increase in the pressure of the blood supply to the lungs (pulmonary hypertension).

Prior to receiving a VA shunt, all patients should have an echocardiogram (an ultrasound of the heart) to rule out the possibility of a hole in the right atrium or ventricle of the heart. This could allow foreign material, known as *emboli,* to travel through the blood to the brain.

Ventriculopleural (VPl) shunt

The distal catheter of the VPl shunt is placed in the pleural space surrounding the lungs. The VPl placement is not recommended for infants and small children, because the pleural space may not be able to reabsorb the CSF fast enough. In this case, the fluid could build up around the lungs, causing hydrothorax (excessive fluid in the pleural space).

Other placements

There are times when placing the distal catheter of the shunt system in one of the traditional locations (i.e., the peritoneal cavity or the right atrium of the heart) cannot be used by the neurosurgeon. However, these aren't the only places where your neurosurgeon can place the distal catheter. The distal catheter can actually be placed in any vein, artery, or open cavity in the body as long as it provides a way for CSF to be reabsorbed or excreted.

Other possible placements include:

- **Lumboperitoneal (LP).** LP shunts are usually placed when the ventricles of the brain are too small for shunt placement, or when a VP or VA shunting has failed. The only difference between the LP and VP shunt is that the proximal catheter is placed in the lumbar region of the spine; the distal catheter is placed in the peritoneal cavity. LP shunts are useful only for treating communicating hydrocephalus.

- **Ventriculofemoral (VF).** The VF shunt is similar to the VA shunt system, except that the distal catheter is run down the length of the patient's body and is inserted into the femoral vein near the groin. Once the distal catheter is inserted into the femoral vein, it is passed up into the right atrium of the heart, similar to a VA shunt placement. Another reason the neurosurgeon might choose to place a VF shunt is that one of the other areas of the body, such as the pleura, peritoneum, and/or venous system in the neck, has been compromised or is diseased. A possible complication of VF shunts is immobilization of the legs.

- Ventriculo-gallbladder (VGB). The VGB shunt procedure involves placing the distal catheter of the shunt within the patient's gallbladder. This procedure can also be referred to as ventriculocholecystic shunting. VGB shunts are commonly used in patients if the hydrocephalus is difficult to manage using one of the more common distal catheter placements.

- Ventriculoureter (VU). The distal catheter of the VU shunt is placed in the ureter. Ureters are a pair of long tubes which carry urine from the kidneys to the bladder. This type of shunt placement allows CSF to be stored in the bladder until the patient urinates. The main problem associated with VU shunts is salt loss in children and infants. VU shunts are a good alternative for a VP shunt when the abdominal cavity is scarred and cannot absorb CSF.

- Ventriculogastric (VG). The distal catheter of the VG shunt is placed in the patient's stomach. The VG shunt placement is sometimes used as an alternative to having the shunt drain into the peritoneal cavity. One risk of VG shunt placement is an infection that migrates from the stomach into the distal catheter.

- Ventriculofallopian. An alternate path for women is to have the distal catheter placed in one of the fallopian tubes.

Differences among shunts

Not all shunts are created equal. How are you, as the patient, to know which shunt valve has tested better, is more reliable, and is best for you? Choose a good neurosurgeon and trust his recommendations. However, this does not mean that you have to be in the dark about which shunt is recommended for you or how it works. Being informed—able to visualize how the shunt works, and able to ask questions about it—helps many people relax, trust, and get on with treatment. Your neurosurgeon may have samples of the shunts he recommends. You can ask to see models in order to understand how the shunt will operate.

Check with your neurosurgeon to see what type of shunt will be used (e.g., flow-control, anti-siphoning, programmable, etc.) and who manufactures it. Although your neurosurgeon will keep records of the type of shunt valve you have, knowing this information can be useful later in case of an emergency.

Shunts can vary by the materials they are made of and standards they are manufactured under, as well as by their features.

Materials and components

Nearly all shunts used for treating hydrocephalus today are made out of or contain silicone and plastic. Some shunts are made entirely of silicone and plastic to reduce the risk of metal components interfering with CT and MRI equipment, while other shunts contain some nonmagnetic metal components in addition to the silicone and plastic. Most shunt valves and catheters contain dots or stripes of barium sulfate, a radiopaque material.

Manufacturing and testing standards

Shunts are manufactured and tested in various ways. Some shunt manufacturers build their shunts in clean rooms similar to those used by most computer chip manufacturers. These clean rooms meet strict international standards for a sterile, dust-free environment. Unfortunately, not all shunts are made this way.

Some shunt manufacturers test each and every valve they make by putting them through a series of rigorous tests. These tests include not only pressure testing to verify the valves' pressure, but subjecting shunts to extreme heat and cold, shock tests, and numerous CT and MRI scans to ensure they work properly. In these cases, if a shunt valve passes all of the tests, it is then sterilized and packed for distribution. If it fails, the shunt valve gets tossed (as it should). However, some shunt manufacturers test only a few shunt valves from a specific batch or may only pressure test them prior to sterilization. Again, trust your neurosurgeon to use shunts that are produced by a manufacturer who adheres to strict production and testing practices.

Common features

Shunt valves share many common features. For instance, most shunt valves and catheters are equipped with a radiopaque material, usually barium sulfate, which allows them to be viewed in the body by X-rays and CT scans.

Most shunt valves include a bulb reservoir so that surgery doesn't need to be performed to test the shunt system. The reservoir gives your neurosurgeon access to CSF in the shunt, enabling him to perform a shunt tap. A shunt tap is done by inserting a small-gauged needle through the scalp, penetrating the bulb of the reservoir. By performing a shunt tap, your neurosurgeon can:

- Measure ICP.

- Remove CSF from the shunt system for analysis.

- Inject a radioisotope into the shunt valve to follow and quantitate the flow of CSF with an isotope camera (gamma camera).

The bulb reservoir is designed to enable small-gauged needles to be inserted, and this in no way compromises the function of the shunt valve. However, shunt taps need to be performed under sterile conditions to reduce the risk of introducing bacteria directly into the shunt valve.

Warning: Do not depress the bulb reservoir of your shunt. This should be done only by your neurosurgeon. Improper or unnecessary depression of the bulb reservoir can overdrain the ventricles or cause an obstruction in the shunt.

Manufacturers

There are a number of companies around the world who manufacture shunts and catheters for treating hydrocephalus. Five major manufacturers of hydrocephalic shunt systems are:

- Johnson & Johnson, manufacturers of Codman systems.

- Medtronic, manufacturers of PS Medical shunts.

- NeuroCare Group, manufacturers of Heyer-Schulte® shunts.

- NMT Neurosciences (U.S.), Inc. (formerly Elekta Instruments, Inc.), manufacturers of the Cordis® line of shunt products, including the Orbis-Sigma Valve.

- Phoenix Biomedical, manufacturers of the Diamond Valve and shunt systems.

This section gives information on only these five commonly used shunt manufacturers, because of space limitations. We are not endorsing these manufacturers or their products; we are making no claim that one valve or system is better than another. The systems are listed as samples only. We have included this information so you can be aware that there is a range of different shunt systems available, with various features. The information is listed alphabetically by manufacturer.

Descriptions of particular models of shunts are current at the time of writing. Features, materials, and manufacturing will continue to change; shunt design is a dynamic area for research, testing, and improvements. It is hoped that features, materials, and manufacturing methods of shunts will continue to improve with time.

Johnson & Johnson

Johnson & Johnson makes the Codman line of shunt products, including the Hakim™ Precision Valve System, the Uni-Shunt®, and the programmable Medos shunt valve.

In the Codman Hakim™ Precision Valve System, a small ruby ball-and-spring mechanism regulates the flow of CSF through the valve. The ruby ball rotates freely, with a self-cleaning action to minimize protein buildup as CSF flows through the valve. When the pressure exerted by CSF exceeds that of the spring mechanism, the ruby ball rises from its seat, permitting CSF to flow through the valve. The spring mechanism is precisely calibrated to one of five pressure levels ranging from very-low-pressure (10 mm H_2O) to high-pressure (130 mm H_2O). See Figure 4-4, shown approximately actual size.

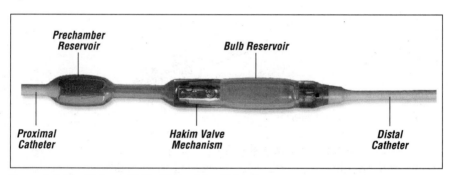

Figure 4-4. The Codman Hakim™ Precision Valve System

The Uni-Shunt (see Figure 4-5) is a one-piece shunt system in which the ventricular catheter, shunt valve, and distal catheter are all one unit. This design eliminates the risk of catheter disconnection. The Uni-Shunt has dual-distal slit valves that are spaced one inch apart. The slit valves closest to the distal end of the catheter do most of the work, while the set of proximal slit valves act more as a backup in case the lower valves fail to work. The Uni-Shunt also uses an elliptical reservoir that conforms to the skull and permits the neurosurgeon to flush the shunt system to test if it is working properly. This system is available in three infant lengths and two adult lengths, as well as three different pressure settings (low, medium, and high).

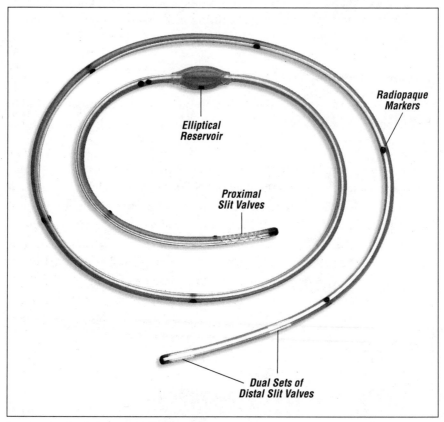

Figure 4-5. The Codman Uni-Shunt®

The Codman Medos shunt (not shown) is available in two models: programmable and nonprogrammable. Both are based on a Hakim ball-and-spring valve system similar to the one used in the Hakim Precision Valve System. The only difference between the two is that the Medos valve is programmable, and the Hakim Precision Valve System is not. The Medos programmable shunt has 18 different pressure settings, ranging from 30 mm H_2O to 200 mm H_2O in increments of 10 mm. This means the neurosurgeon has the ability to adjust the pressure setting after the shunt has been implanted. In adults, the Medos programmable shunt would be set to 200 mm H_2O, and shunts for infants and children are set to age-appropriate settings.

The programmable mechanism is based on a noninvasively adjustable pressure setting of a flat spring in the inlet valve of the unit. A stepper motor within the valve housing changes the pressure setting of the spring if activated by an external programmer. The external programmer emits a magnetic signal to the motor which changes the setting up or down in incremental steps. After implantation, the pressure can be adjusted by positioning the external programmer above the inlet valve. The pressure setting is indicated on a white ring located near the inlet valve, which can be viewed by X-ray to ensure the required pressure has been set. Since the programmable shunt is adjusted with the aid of magnets, the valve will need to be readjusted after an MRI scan.

Johnson & Johnson is also developing a new type of shunt catheter that is impregnated with an antimicrobial agent (a combination of the antibiotics rifamycin and clindamycin) to prevent catheter-related shunt infections. Johnson & Johnson is presently seeking FDA approval to use this new catheter in patients. If approved, neurosurgeons and patients could expect to see them being used sometime in 1999.

Medtronic

Medtronic makes the PS Medical line of hydrocephalus shunts, which includes the Delta™ Valve. (The "PS" in PS Medical stands for "Pudenz-Schulte.")

The Delta™ Valve (see Figure 4-6) automatically adjusts for increasing negative pressures in the distal catheter by proportionally increasing its resistance to the flow of CSF. When the patient is lying down, the Delta™ Valve performs as a differential pressure (DP) valve by providing a set resistance to flow depending on the valve chosen. However, when the patient stands and negative hydrostatic pressure is created in the distal catheter, the resistance to flow increases proportionally, thus creating a near-constant level at any flow rate. The Delta™ Valve is made of a combination of plastic and silicone components, so it doesn't interfere with CT or MR imaging devices. The valve is available in pediatric and adult sizes, including a burr hole valve and an LP configuration.

NeuroCare Group

NeuroCare produces the Heyer-Schulte® line of shunts, including the Novus™ shunt valve system.

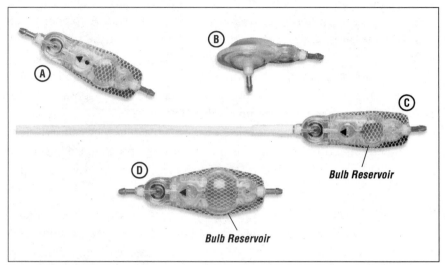

Figure 4-6. Delta™ Valve shunt systems: (A) Contoured Delta™ Valve, small (for infants and children); (B) Delta™ Burr Hole Valve; (C) Delta™ shunt assembly with a peritoneal distal catheter connected; and (D) Contoured Delta™ Valve, regular size (for adults and young adults).

The Novus shunt valve regulates the physiological flow of CSF within normal ranges of ICP, whether the patient is lying down, sitting, or standing. The Novus shunt features a patented physiological flow device that adds variable resistance to the flow of CSF to prevent overdrainage when the patient sits or stands from a supine position. The Novus shunt has a reservoir dome for flushing, and is made from a combination of silicone and plastic components. Available in two pressure settings, low and medium pressure, the Novus valve is also available in adult and pediatric sizes (see Figure 4-7, shown slightly larger than actual size). All NeuroCare Heyer-Schulte ventricular and peritoneal catheters contain a stripe of barium to allow the entire system to be viewed when the patient undergoes X-ray or CT scan.

NeuroCare is also testing a new shunt valve system called the Beverly Referential Valve (not shown). This new valve, currently pending FDA approval for use in the U.S., consists of a calibrated spring-like mechanical reference coupled to a lever-and-piston valve element. Because resistance to gravitational flow is provided primarily by the internal reference, the effect of subcutaneous pressures on the valve mechanism is lower than in other valves. In experiments, the Beverly valve produced inlet pressures within normal ICP ranges in both supine (50 mm to 150 mm H_2O) and standing (-100 mm

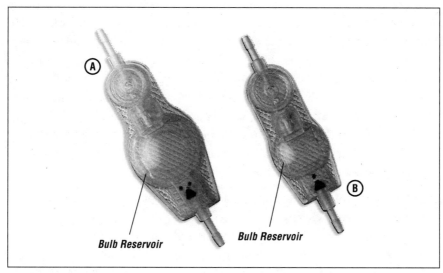

Figure 4-7. The Novus™ (A), and Novus™ Mini (B) shunt valves

to 50 mm H$_2$O) positions through a range of flow rates (K. M. Jaeger and T. N. Layton, *New shunt system for treatment of hydrocephalus: in vitro testing*, Consensus Conference on Complex Hydrocephalus and Hydrocephalus Complications, Assisi, Italy, April 1997).

NMT Neurosciences (U.S.), Inc. (formerly Elekta Instruments, Inc.)

NMT Neurosciences manufactures the Cordis line of shunt valve systems, including the Orbis-Sigma® and Omnishunt® systems. (Photos of these shunt systems were not available.)

The Orbis-Sigma Valve is designed to regulate automatically the flow of CSF through the valve. It provides CSF drainage control over a range of conditions and differential pressures (DPs). The DP control helps to maintain a constant IVP, which reduces the risk of over- or underdrainage by the system. The Orbis-Sigma Valve regulates the CSF pressure using a valve diaphragm and seat that moves along a graduated pin. When IVP increases, the diaphragm moves downward and allows CSF to flow out of the valve around the graduated pin. When IVP starts to go down, the diaphragm will move upward to help maintain a constant IVP. This type of shunt system is known as a flow-control valve system.

The Cordis Omnishunt™ is a one-piece system, which means that the proximal and distal catheters are already connected to the shunt valve. The Omnishunt uses a ball-in-cone design and is available in three different pressure ranges (low, medium, and high). In a ball-in-cone–designed shunt—also known as the Hakim valve—the opening pressure of the valve is adjusted by a precisely calibrated spring which maintains a constant pressure for different CSF flow rates. One benefit of the Omnishunt is that it is all in one piece and doesn't require the neurosurgeon to connect the ventricular and distal catheters to the valve, lessening the chance of the catheter becoming disconnected from the valve.

Another feature of the Omnishunt is a right-angle guide which is placed over the burr hole site where the proximal catheter passes through the skull. When the proximal catheter exits the burr hole site with other systems, it is bent at a 90-degree angle to allow the catheter to run along the outside of the skull beneath the scalp. The right-angle guide keeps the ventricular catheter from pinching or kinking when the catheter is bent, and also helps to keep the ventricular catheter from moving within the ventricle when it is bent.

Phoenix Biomedical

Phoenix Biomedical makes the Diamond™ valve and shunt systems, which are designed to provide one-way flow control for treating hydrocephalus. (See Figure 4-8, shown approximately one and one-half times actual size.)

The Diamond™ valve is made of two silicone domes with two crossed slits and a differential pressure valve mechanism. The shunt valve and differential pressure valve mechanism are connected by an elastic tube with an aperture in the side wall which acts as a flow-control mechanism. The valve mechanism is contained within a silicone chamber that is secured to a plastic base. The valve base and catheters contain small amounts of radiopaque material to assist in their detection by imaging devices. The valve is also marked with a radiopaque flow direction arrow on top of the bulb reservoir.

The Diamond™ valve incorporates the Newton SaFR™ (Self-adjusting Flow-Regulating) flow-control mechanism that regulates ICP and the flow of CSF within physiological limits, regardless of whether the patient is lying down or standing.

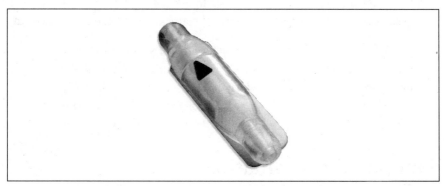

Figure 4-8. The Diamond™ valve

Questions to ask before surgery

Before surgery, it is best to consult with your neurosurgeon to ask any questions and hopefully to allay any fears you may have about the procedure. Some questions you could ask your neurosurgeon include:

- Are there any reasons why I should not have this operation? Is this operation absolutely necessary?

- How long will the shunt procedure take?

- How long will I be in recovery?

- How long can I expect to be in the hospital?

- What are the possible complications of this surgery? Are there any that I should be more worried about than others?

- Will you be using sutures or staples to close the wounds on my head and abdomen (or neck or chest, as appropriate)?

- How much of my hair will be clipped away to prepare me for surgery? Should I have my hair cut prior to being admitted into the hospital?

- How soon after surgery can I have visitors?

- Will I need any physical therapy after the operation?

- How long will it be before I can resume my normal activities following the operation?

Knowing these answers should better prepare you for surgery and recovery. For instance, finding out whether your neurosurgeon uses sutures or staples can help alleviate any shock you or your family might have if you are expecting to see sutures and instead see a row of staples in the head and abdomen.

When I went up to see my wife following her shunt revision, I was floored when I saw the row of staples in her head! Her scalp was an orangy-red color from the Betadine, and the staples were in plain view— all 18 of them! My first reaction was to look away, and I nearly cried when I saw her like that. I had no idea this was how she would look.

Preoperative evaluation

Prior to surgery, a clerk or member of the hospital's medical staff will review your paperwork to ensure all preoperative instructions have been followed and the surgical consent form has been signed. One or both parents are required to sign the surgical consent form if the patient is under the age of 18.

A member of the nursing staff will review your medical history and ask if you have any allergies or are taking any medications. It is very important to inform the nursing staff and surgical team if you are allergic to latex. Exposure to latex can cause the patient to go into anaphylactic shock. Many children with myelomeningoceles (which is associated with hydrocephalus) develop latex allergies as a secondary condition.

You will then be examined by a nurse on the floor. The nurse will check your vital signs (i.e., blood pressure, pulse, temperature, and respiration). If you haven't already done so, you will be asked to remove any jewelry and makeup, and change into a hospital gown.

Once you have been prepared for surgery, the next person you talk to will be the anesthetist, who is either a physician (an anesthesiologist) or a member of the nursing staff who is trained in anesthesiology (a Certified Registered Nurse Anesthetist, or CRNA).

Anesthesia

Shunt placement procedures are normally performed under general anesthesia. Prior to being taken to the operating room, the patient and designated members of the family (particularly if the patient is an infant or small child) will meet with an anesthetist.

Your anesthetist needs to know your height, weight, and age. She will also need to know about your prior operations, whether you've had any problems in the past with anesthesia, if you are taking prescription medications, and if you are allergic to any medications.

The following list of questions is from the "Pre-Anesthesia Questionnaire," posted on the web site of the American Association of Nurse Anesthetists (*http://www.aana.com*). Answering these questions prior to your surgery will prepare you for the meeting with your anesthetist:

- Have you recently had a cold or the flu?
- Are you allergic to latex (rubber) products?
- Have you experienced chest pain?
- Do you have a heart condition?
- Do you have hypertension (high blood pressure)?
- Do you experience shortness of breath?
- Do you have asthma, bronchitis, or any other breathing problems?
- Do you (or did you) smoke? If so, how long have you (or did you) smoke, and how many packs per day?
- Do you consume alcohol? If so, how many drinks per week?
- Do you or have you taken recreational drugs?
- Have you taken cortisone (steroids) in the last six months?
- Do you have diabetes?
- Have you had hepatitis, liver disease, or jaundice?
- Do you have a thyroid condition?
- Do you have or have you had kidney disease?
- Do you have ulcers or any other stomach disorders?
- Do you have a hiatal hernia?
- Do you have back or neck pain?
- Do you have numbness, weakness, or paralysis of your extremities?
- Do you have any muscle or nerve disease?
- Do you or any of your family have sickle-cell anemia?
- Have you or any blood relatives had difficulties with anesthesia in the past?

- Do you have bleeding problems, such as hemophilia?

- Do you have loose, chipped, or false teeth? Do you have bridgework?

- Do you wear contact lenses?

- Have you ever received a blood transfusion?

- For women: Are you pregnant, or do you suspect that you may be pregnant? If so, when are you due?

It certainly is a long list, but knowing this information helps the anesthetist determine which type of anesthesia is best for you.

Questions you should ask your neurosurgeon and anesthetist regarding anesthesia include:

- How will the anesthesia be induced? Intravenously or by mask?

- What are the risks or side effects of anesthesia?

- What type of drugs are being used? What are the alternatives if my child is allergic to them?

- How will I be monitored during the surgery?

Once you are wheeled down to the operating room and placed on the operating table, you will be hooked up to an IV. Additionally, you will be hooked up to the following devices either before or after being given anesthesia:

- An electrocardiogram (EKG), used to monitor your heart rate. This is done by placing electrodes that connect to the EKG machine on your chest and back.

- An automatic blood-pressure (BP) cuff, used to monitor your blood pressure at timed intervals throughout the procedure. The BP cuff will be placed on your left arm so it doesn't interfere with the surgeon's approach during the operation.

- A pulse oximeter, used to measure the amount of oxygen in the bloodstream. The pulse oximeter will be clipped onto the tip of your index finger and is held in place with a piece of surgical tape.

There are many different drugs used for anesthesia. Your doctor will make the best choice for your situation and will administer the drugs either with gas or through your IV. Under general anesthesia, you will experience a total loss of consciousness. You will not feel any physical pain during the procedure.

Recovery and postoperation

After surgery, you will be moved from the operating room into the recovery room. Depending on your condition, you can be transferred to a regular hospital ward and, in most instances, you will be discharged within a day or two.

> *A shunt surgery was performed, and a few days later I was sent home. I was sore from the incisions, but my vision was restored to normal. I was fortunate that school only had a few weeks remaining, as I was able to miss the rest of the academic year and spend my summer recovering. After the scars healed and my hair grew back, you would never know that I had hydrocephalus. At that time, I thought very little of hydrocephalus and its possible effects. At the age of 13 I felt almost invincible and this "water on the brain" was nothing. I resumed life as normal after that summer.*

If there have been any complications that require close monitoring of your neurological status, you may be transferred to an intensive care unit (ICU), where you will remain until your condition improves.

> *ICU is tough on any child. I regretted not being able to spend the night with my son, and I insisted that I be called as soon he woke up, no exceptions. Shaun found ICU to be very frightening. I tried to be on the regular floor as much as possible.*

The nursing staff will check your vital signs and monitor your neurological condition. The neurosurgeon will decide when you can be moved out of ICU and into a regular ward prior to being discharged.

Shunt placement operations

The following brief descriptions of typical shunt placements can provide you with a general overview of the procedures for placing a VP or VA shunt.

There are two general approaches your neurosurgeon can take when it comes to placing the proximal catheter. The first, referred to as a *posterior approach,* is where the proximal catheter is inserted into the lateral ventricle from an opening the neurosurgeon makes at the back of your head. The other, referred to as a *frontal approach,* is where the neurosurgeon places the proximal catheter into the lateral ventricle from an opening made at the top of your head, just forward from one of the cranial sutures. The terms used for the different surgical approaches are in reference to the area of the brain the proximal catheter must pass to reach the ventricles.

Before beginning the procedure, your hair will be clipped or shaved to allow the neurosurgeon an unobstructed area for the operation. The amount of hair that is clipped away depends greatly on the type of operation being performed, and upon the personal preference of your neurosurgeon.

> When my son had his revisions they shaved half of his head; one time they shaved the entire thing except a stripe in the middle (when he had subdural hematomas drained and a revision at the same time). I commented to the doctor about the hair and was told that they only remove what they must and it is not done for cosmetic reasons. As soon as he got out of the hospital we shaved the rest and let it all grow in at once. In his last three revisions, only a tiny area was shaved. It looked like it would if, for example, a kid fell and needed stitches. No big deal.

The opening your neurosurgeon makes in your skull to allow access to your brain and ventricles is called a burr hole. This is a very small opening that is made using a surgical drill. Your neurosurgeon may also need to make a burr hole if you have a subdural hematoma (SDH). He would drill a burr hole over the SDH, which would allow him to relieve intracranial pressure.

The techniques described below may vary from the way your neurosurgeon performs the shunt placement operation. Consult with your neurosurgeon on the specifics of how your particular operation will be performed.

Ventriculoperitoneal (VP) shunt placement

Once your neurosurgeon has created the burr hole, his next step is to make an opening in your abdomen where the distal catheter will be placed. A small incision will be made in your abdomen, just below the rib cage, to allow your neurosurgeon access to your peritoneal cavity. The peritoneum is a membrane that covers vital organs in your abdomen, including the intestines, stomach, and liver.

His next task will be to place the shunt system. Using a device called a stylet, your neurosurgeon will insert the proximal catheter through the burr hole and into the lateral ventricle of your brain. Next, he will remove the stylet and attach the proximal and distal catheters to the shunt valve. Your neurosurgeon will secure the catheters to the shunt valve using nonabsorbable sutures. Once the catheters are connected, he will test the shunt system to ensure that CSF is flowing through the valve. If fluid flows through the shunt system without getting obstructed, his next task will be to place the distal catheter in your peritoneal cavity.

Your neurosurgeon will use a tunneling device to pass the distal catheter under your skin from the incision in your head to the incision in your abdomen. He will then make a very small incision into your peritoneum and insert the distal catheter.

> Shaun's neck and abdomen were extremely sore after the initial placement of the shunt. He was a toddler—just 16 months old—and it bothered him greatly. I think my greatest heartache at the post-surgery time was this soreness. His head did not hurt at all, just his neck where the catheter had been passed.

With both catheters in place, your neurosurgeon will clean the areas around the incisions he has made, and will use surgical staples or sutures to close the wounds. The final step is to cover the staples or sutures with a sterile gauze bandage to help protect them from becoming infected.

Ventriculoatrial (VA) shunt placement

The only difference between a VP and a VA shunt placement procedure is the operation performed for placing the distal catheter.

To begin the procedure, your neurosurgeon will place the proximal catheter in the same fashion as described above. The proximal and distal catheters will be connected to opposite ends of the shunt valve and secured in place with nonabsorbable sutures.

Next, he will need to make a small incision on your neck to allow him access to either the internal jugular vein or the common facial vein. Using a needle, your neurosurgeon will insert a guide wire and vessel dilator into the chosen vein. The guide wire and vessel dilator allow your neurosurgeon to carefully guide the distal catheter through the wall of the vein and into the right atrium of your heart. In an infant, it will be necessary to briefly expose the facial vein or internal jugular vein in order to insert the shunt.

As with the VP shunt placement, your neurosurgeon will use a tunneling device to pass the distal catheter beneath your skin between the incisions in your head and neck. The tunneling device will be removed, and the distal catheter will be slipped over the guide wire and into the vein in your neck. Your neurosurgeon will then use a fluoroscope (an imaging device that takes X-rays without using films) to ensure that the tip of the distal catheter lies within the right atrium of your heart.

Once the distal catheter is in its proper place, he will remove the guide wire and vessel dilator, and close the incision in your neck, as well as the one on your head. Your neurosurgeon may use either surgical staples or sutures to close the incisions.

Endoscopic third ventriculostomy

An alternative to shunt placement for some patients is the third ventriculostomy, which is often referred to as either 3V or third-vent. Although this procedure has been done since 1922, in early years it was usually not successful because medical instruments and imagery of the brain at the time were inadequate. However, the third-vent has been used more often since the mid-1980s after the introduction of neuroendoscopic surgery.

In performing a third ventriculostomy, your neurosurgeon will make a small hole in the floor of the third ventricle of your brain. This hole, which is several millimeters in size, allows CSF to flow from the blocked ventricles into the open spaces surrounding the brain.

Neuroendoscopic third ventriculostomies are performed by using an endoscope to navigate through the ventricular system and puncturing a small hole through the floor of the third ventricle.

If successful, the third ventriculostomy procedure will eliminate your need for a shunt. However, not everyone with hydrocephalus can receive this procedure. The patient must have non-communicating hydrocephalus (the obstruction of CSF flow is within the ventricular system).

It is mainly recommended for children older than six months of age who have been diagnosed with aqueductal stenosis. Many neurosurgeons, however, prefer to hold off on performing a third ventriculostomy on a child until he is two or three years old because the holes in the floor of the ventricle tend to close up as tissues in the brain grow.

In the short run, a third ventriculostomy is more risky than a shunt, but just the reverse in the long run. Complications of a third ventriculostomy include:

- Hemorrhage.
- Aneurysm formation.
- Cranial nerve palsy, particularly causing double vision.
- Diabetes insipidus (water, not sugar disorder).
- Memory deficits.

Although a third ventriculostomy eliminates the need for a shunt, it is still not a cure. Even patients who receive a successful third ventriculostomy must be monitored closely following the procedure to ensure that the holes in the floor of the third ventricle don't become obstructed or close from scarring. The overall success rate is about 50 percent. Previous history of meningitis or subarachnoid hemorrhage will reduce the success rate.

Nonsurgical treatments

In an attempt to reduce the risk of surgery and shunt complications, neurosurgeons have tried a variety of nonsurgical treatments to control hydrocephalus. These treatments include a combination of different pharmacological products, including acetazolamide (Diamox) and furosemide (Lasix) to reduce production of CSF by the choroid plexus, and serial lumbar punctures of the spine to drain CSF.

Acetazolamide and furosemide, both of which are diuretics used for treating other conditions, are given to hydrocephalus patients to control intracranial pressure and fluid retention. These drugs may be used to provide temporary relief of increased ICP, but usually they are not helpful.

Serial lumbar punctures are predominantly used on premature infants who had an intraventricular hemorrhage. Repetitive lumbar punctures are performed to drain excess CSF within the ventricles. Often, an intraventricular hemorrhage will block CSF flow within the ventricles or in the basal cistern, causing non-communicating hydrocephalus, making serial lumbar punctures ineffective.

Nonoperative treatments of hydrocephalus have seen only moderate success rates, often postponing surgery to implant a shunt system.

CHAPTER 5

Hospitalization and Recovery

Everyone who is born holds dual citizenship,
in the kingdom of the well and in the kingdom
of the sick. Although we all prefer to use only
the good passport, sooner or later each of us
is obliged, at least for a spell, to identify
ourselves as citizens of that other place.

—Susan Sontag
Illness as Metaphor

WHEN YOUR DOCTOR GIVES YOU THE NEWS that neurosurgery is required, you may feel shocked, alarmed, or relieved to know that your suspicions have finally been confirmed. You may be anxious about the surgery itself, and feel pressure to arrange work, school, or family life in the face of uncertainty. If you or your child have not been to the hospital before or haven't had neuro-surgery, you will probably have many questions regarding the hospital stay.

In this chapter we take a look at hospitalization and recovery after surgery. We first answer common questions about hospitalization, including how long you can expect to be in the hospital, who decides when you get dis-charged, how to make your hospital room more homey, and what personal items and clothing to bring to the hospital. We next discuss ways to prepare your family for the experience.

We provide you with some insight on hospital admissions, who the different doctors and nurses in the hospital are, and talk about hospital food, park-ing, and some of the general rules for visiting. The chapter ends with a dis-cussion of follow-up care: monitoring following surgery, recovery in the hos-pital and at home, and follow-up visits with your neurosurgeon.

When neurosurgery is required

Many patients and their families have learned that it's hard to anticipate everything that will happen when you are admitted to the hospital for a shunt placement or revision procedure. You will have to restructure your life temporarily and, in some cases, permanently. In many instances, you may not have time to prepare much before surgery. Correcting a problematic shunt or decreasing intracranial pressure (ICP) may have to be done under emergency surgery, which adds to the stress on your family.

> *My wife's last revision was a complete surprise to all of us. She had been experiencing headaches and nausea in the morning for about a week, but since we were trying to have a child, we thought we had been successful in achieving our goal. However, when she went to the doctors for a blood test to see if she was pregnant, the test came back negative, so her doctor sent her to the lab for a quick CT scan. Her ventricles were compressed. That sure took us by surprise.*

Some of the stress can be relieved by getting as much information about the surgical procedure as possible. Your neurosurgeon can provide you with literature or videos on the procedure, so you can know what to expect before being admitted to the hospital. Make a list of questions or concerns you have about the operation. Having a list prepared will enable you to remember everything you wish to discuss with your doctor. You can write down the surgeon's responses as well.

It can be helpful to take a friend or relative with you to the neurosurgeon's office or to the hospital for any checkups or tests. A relative or friend can offer moral support, take notes, or simply act as another set of ears to recall important points you might have missed.

> *My husband and I were not really in a mental state to understand everything. We were not advised of the high possibility of shunt revisions. We were led to believe the initial shunt would be all that was needed to make our son better. Then, ten months later, the neurosurgeon had to revise the entire system. I wish we'd been prepared.*

Some sources of information for educating yourself and your family about the condition and operation include your primary care physician, your neurosurgeon, books or web sites, and hydrocephalus support groups. See

Appendix B, Associations and Organizations, and *Appendix E, Internet Resources,* for helpful resources.

When surgery is required, the following suggestions will help make life less stressful:

- **Arrange for child care.** Children may not be allowed to visit the hospital. However, some hospitals—particularly children's hospitals—offer a day care center where you can sign your children in for the day while you are visiting. Here, your children will be able to play with other children who are in a similar situation. The people providing the child care are trained to handle children whose parents or siblings are in the hospital, and can talk with them about their anxieties or fears.

- **Establish a phone tree.** Call one or two family members or close friends to let them know about the upcoming operation. Give them the hospital's name and general information number. Ask them to phone other family members and friends to spread the word. After you have established the initial phone contacts, let them know that you will provide them with updates when you can, and that when you do, you'd like them to pass along the information. You can also leave updates on your telephone answering machine.

    The hardest thing I had to do when my husband needed to have his shunt revised was to call family and friends to let them know he was in the hospital. It didn't help that his operation was a complete surprise to both of us. I thought I could make all the calls, but by the third one, I was a wreck.

- **Communicate with your child's school.** Shunt replacements and revisions can often require your child to be away from school for a while. Your child may miss more school to go to doctor appointments or for follow-up tests. Contact the school as soon as possible to tell them of your child's condition and pending absence. Staying connected with his teacher, classmates, and friends will help make things easier when your child returns to school. Find someone to act on your behalf as a liaison between the family, school, and hospital, such as a parent of one of your child's friends, a hospital social worker, or the school nurse. Communicating with the school and reentering school after surgery is covered in Chapter 9, *School.*

- **Communicate with your workplace.** Many people with hydrocephalus who work don't tell their bosses or coworkers about the condition. They fear their condition might be used against them, or that they may get some form of preferential treatment or retribution in the workplace.

Depending on your work circumstances, you can contact your direct supervisor or the company's human resources manager to tell her about the situation. She can make arrangements for sick leave or a medical leave of absence as covered by the Family and Medical Leave Act. Your employer cannot legally terminate your employment because of an illness or because you need to take care of a sick family member. The human resources manager can notify the appropriate people in the workplace. She can also answer any questions you have about your health plan, and make arrangements for help through the Employee Assistance Program (EAP), if your employer has one.

Before returning to work, contact your human resources manager to let her know of any special needs you may have. Under the Americans with Disabilities Act (ADA), your employer may be required by federal law to accommodate any short- or long-term needs you may have for the workplace. If you need to work part-time, your human resources manager may be able to arrange this for you.

Common questions

When being admitted to the hospital for a shunt placement or revision, you may not have enough time to plan ahead. You will probably have a lot of questions to ask, for yourself or on behalf of your child. The following are some commonly asked questions regarding hospitalization.

How long will I be in the hospital?

Expect to be in the hospital for at least two days—and possibly longer—after a placement or revision. If there are complications during the operation, such as an intracranial hemorrhage, you may be in the hospital for weeks.

Who decides when I can be discharged?

Your neurosurgeon will make the final decision on when you can be discharged after the operation. During your stay in the hospital, your neurosurgeon will continue to monitor your recovery by checking in with you when she makes daily rounds. The neurosurgeon will check your chart to see how you've progressed, and will check your cognitive and motor skills to make sure that your neurological condition either has improved or hasn't worsened since surgery.

Can I decorate the hospital room?

Hospital rooms usually appear bland or institutional. Since you or your child will probably be in the hospital several days, you may want to decorate the room. You might:

- Put up large, bright posters.
- Tape cards on the walls, hang them from strings like a mobile, or arrange them around the windowsills.
- Put up pictures of your family, friends, and/or pets. Hospitals can be lonely places, and being able to see pictures of family and friends can be very comforting, especially for children.

> We brought in lots of pictures and stuff to brighten up the room. This allowed the staff to see our son with family and friends in the context of his life, and not just as another shunt patient in bed 3C.

- Bring bouquets of balloons or flowers. Keep in mind that most hospitals don't allow flowers or plants in an intensive care unit.
- Bring a favorite pillow, blanket, or quilt to place on the hospital bed. You may have to make sure your linens aren't accidentally carted away with the hospital linens.

> We put Shaun's football blanket on his bed and it makes him feel very comfortable. The doctors will always have something to talk to Shaun about with the blanket there. They ask what his favorite team is, and tell him about theirs. It's a great thing!

> We also make a point of never letting him get an injection while he's in his bed, as this is his "safe place." All shots are done in the treatment room.

Not all hospitals, or roommates for that matter, are warm to the idea of decorating.

*We were never allowed to do anything special to our room. In fact,
our son shared a room with the child of another family who didn't want
the television turned on. When we would turn the television on so our son
could watch a program he liked, they would complain to the nurse or talk
so loudly that we couldn't hear the sound. After a couple days of this, the
TV was "conveniently" broken.*

It is best to check with the nurses on the floor, or with other patients who
are sharing the same hospital room, before bringing in lots of decorations.
Most, however, will welcome the warmth and change from the drab hospital
color scheme.

What should I bring to the hospital with me?

When preparing to enter the hospital, bring whatever you use every day.
Bring enough supplies to last at least two to three days. Friends and other
family members can always bring more later if your hospital stay is
extended.

- Eyeglasses, or contact lenses and cleansing solutions.
- Toothbrush and toothpaste.
- Dental floss.
- Soap, shampoo/conditioner.
- Hand lotion or skin cream.
- Brush or comb.
- Nail clippers.
- Powder.

Here are some suggestions for additional items to bring along, for yourself or
visiting family:

- Books, magazines, newspapers, crossword or puzzle books.
- Walkman with headphones, and tapes or CDs to listen to.
- Drawing paper or coloring books, pencils, pens, or crayons.
- A journal or diary to keep notes about your stay in the hospital. Even if
  you don't feel like writing your thoughts down, a friend, spouse, or par-
  ent could enter them for you.
- Puppets, stuffed animals, or other small toys.

What clothes should I bring to the hospital?

You will be asked to change out of your clothes and into a hospital gown shortly after being admitted to the hospital. Even after your surgery has been completed, you will probably be required to wear the hospital gown so that the nurses can check your vital signs and change any bandages when necessary.

Many hospitals provide brightly colored smocks for young patients, but many children and teens prefer to wear their own clothing. This can pose a laundry problem, so check to see if the floor has washers available for families—otherwise, you could find yourself hauling laundry back and forth from the hospital.

One common mistake that hydrocephalus patients make is not having the proper clothing to wear home from the hospital when they are discharged.

> When I went in for my first revision, I was totally unprepared. The only clothing I had with me was what I wore to the hospital when I was admitted. Big mistake. My parents had to run home and bring me a pair of sweat pants and a flannel shirt because I couldn't get into my jeans or pull my sweater over my head.

Since shunt placement and revision operations involve an operation on your head, it's recommended that you bring along shirts that have loose collars, or ones that button or zip in the front. Pulling a T-shirt, sweatshirt, or sweater over your head can be awkward.

If you are having a VA shunt placed, it is advisable to refrain from wearing shirts with tight collars for at least two weeks following surgery so that the collar doesn't interfere with the sutures on your neck.

If you are having a VP shunt placed or revised, it is advisable to bring along a pair of sweat pants or loose-fitting pants to wear when you are discharged from the hospital. The incision in your abdomen will probably be tender for at least a week or two following surgery. Loose-fitting clothes will prevent pressure over or near the sutures.

Additional clothing items that you could bring include:

- Underwear.
- Pajamas.
- Bathrobe.

- Socks.
- Slippers.
- Shoes.

Preparing children

If your child is going in for neurosurgery, you will want to talk with him and prepare him before admission to the hospital. Pick a time when both parents can be present. Sit with your child, tell him what's happening, and let him ask questions about why he is going into the hospital. Note his questions and answer them as best as you can, one by one.

You will also want to sit down, all together, with other children in the family, to tell them what will be happening to their sibling, when you will be gone, and who will take care of them. Give them a chance to ask questions. Sharing strengthens the family, allowing all members to face the crisis together.

Sample dialog

With the family gathered around, explain to your children what will happen in age-appropriate terms. Before you begin, make sure you have a drawing pad and some markers available so you can make any diagrams or drawings that you think will help illustrate and answer questions your children may have. Make sure that your family is in a room where everyone can get comfortable, and that there are tissues available in case any of the children (or parents) start to cry.

You might begin, for example:

> Kids, you may have noticed that your brother Max hasn't been feeling very well lately. We have been taking him to see some special doctors who have decided that Max needs an operation to make him feel better.

Pause after each statement and allow your children an opportunity to ask questions. If they do not respond or ask questions, you can continue.

> The doctors are going to place (or replace) a small pump, called a shunt, in Max's head. This pump will allow water from his brain to drain into another part of his body, probably his tummy.

This might be a good time to start drawing a simple picture of where the shunt will be placed.

To do this, Max will need to be in the hospital for a few days after the operation until he feels better and the doctor says he can come home.

Chances are that both parents will be at the hospital while your child is being operated on. Let your children know who will be taking care of them while you are away.

Your Aunt Sue will stay here with you and bring you to the hospital to visit Max later in the day. Daddy will come home to sleep here with you every night, but while Max is in the hospital, I'm going to stay there with him to keep him company.

It is important for siblings to know that their brother or sister is going to be okay, and if they will be able to visit him or her in the hospital. If you take a tour of the hospital prior to the operation, take the whole family along so your children can see where their brother or sister will be.

Your mom and I have checked with Max's doctors and the people at the hospital about how soon you can see him after he has his operation. His doctor said that Max will need to rest right after his operation, but we can take you up to see him later in the day.

Your children may be upset that they won't be able to play with their brother or sister, or see one of their parents for a few days. Reassure your children that everything will be okay, and that whoever is going into the hospital will be in good hands.

Max has one of the best special doctors in our town, and she plans on taking very good care of him while he is at the hospital. The nurses who will be taking care of Max while he's in the hospital will make sure Max is okay, and that he has everything he needs to get better fast. And before you know it, Max will be home, and all of you will be able to play together again.

Let your children ask questions of you and of the child who is going into the hospital (if he is old enough to talk). Answer their questions in simple terms that they can comprehend.

Taking a tour of the hospital

Hospitals can be scary places, especially for a child. To a small child, hospitals are full of commotion and big people who are all strangers. Here, she is out of her "safe zone," and needs to be reassured that she will be in good hands.

One way you can prepare your child for being in the hospital, if time permits, is to visit the hospital ahead of time. Taking a tour can be an excellent way to familiarize your child with the hospital prior to admission.

By taking a tour, your child will be able to see and meet some of the doctors and nurses who will be taking care of her during her stay. Children are less afraid of adults they know; and doctors and nurses often form attachments to children they have met in a more social, rather than medical, situation.

To arrange for a tour, contact someone in the community relations department of your hospital. The tour might include a look at the operating room, an explanation of anesthesia, and an opportunity to talk with other patients who have undergone a similar operation.

It also helps to tell your child some of the positive things about going to the hospital.

- She will not have to make her bed, do her chores, or wash the dishes.
- She will probably get her own telephone, television, and remote control.
- She will have buttons to push that make the bed go up and down.

Show your child that all beds in the hospital—even beds for adults—have rails on the sides. Let your child know that this is for safety purposes, to keep them from falling out bed when they are sleeping.

You might also make the tour part of an educational experience. If your child will return to school shortly after the hospitalization, your child can talk to her teacher about letting her do a report or research project on some aspect of hospital life. Asking questions and becoming something of a hospital expert may help your child feel more informed and in control of the situation.

Who's who in the hospital

In large hospitals, a steady parade of anonymous faces passes through the life of the patient.

For children, the constant stream of strangers in white coats can be confusing and a little scary. As a parent, you can help your child understand who all of the people are by getting to know the hospital's hierarchy and sorting out who is responsible for your child's care.

I had many surgeries at a university hospital. I detested rounds. Hordes of people came in and stared at me, and said inappropriate things. Often, I was treated like a specimen instead of a young patient. It was very emotionally upsetting for me. These medical students would present my case right in front of me and say things that were very upsetting. I think many doctors think that children cannot comprehend what they are saying—they are wrong!

The doctors

As with any other profession, doctors have many different specialties, temperaments, and skill levels. Your treatment will be greatly enhanced if you trust and communicate well with your doctor. The majority of discussions and decisions will be made by your neurosurgeon. Your neurosurgeon is in charge of your needs during your hospitalization. She will be the most familiar with your situation and is the best person to seek out if you have any questions about treatment.

- **Neurosurgeon.** While in the hospital, your neurosurgeon will be responsible for your care and treatment. When you are hospitalized, your neurosurgeon will check in on you frequently. She should answer any questions and address any concerns you have about your treatment.

- **Primary care physician (PCP).** Your family doctor or pediatrician may be involved in your medical care. Your PCP may visit, receive reports from your neurosurgeon, and check in on you in the hospital.

Along with the doctors you choose, you may see many other doctors if you are in a teaching hospital.

- **Medical student.** A medical student is a college graduate who is attending medical school. Medical students wear white coats, but do not have MD on their name tags.

- **Intern.** An intern is a doctor who is in her first year of postgraduate training.

- **Resident.** A resident is a doctor who is in her second to seventh year of postgraduate training.

- **Fellow.** A fellow is a doctor who has completed four years of medical school, the requisite years of residency, and is taking additional specialty training.

- **Attending physician.** An attending physician (sometimes simply called the "attending") is the doctor who is responsible for your care, usually the neurosurgeon.

The nurses

The nursing staff is an essential part of the hospital hierarchy. Several nurses with different levels of training may play a role in your treatment and recovery.

- **Nurse assistant or aide.** A nurse assistant can take vital signs (heart rate, breathing rate, blood pressure), perform hygiene care, or help with your mobility.

- **Licensed practical nurse (LPN).** An LPN has completed a vocational training program and has a narrow scope of practice. LPNs take vital signs, give medications, and perform general care under the direct supervision of a registered nurse.

- **Registered nurse (RN).** An RN receives a bachelor's or associate's degree in nursing, then takes a licensing examination. These medical professionals give medicines, take vital signs, start and monitor IVs, communicate changes in your condition to doctors, change bandages, and care for patients in hospitals, clinics, and doctor's offices.

- **Nurse practitioner or clinical nurse specialist.** A nurse practitioner is a registered nurse who has completed an educational program that covers advanced skills. In some hospitals and clinics, nurse practitioners perform procedures, such as spinal taps (lumbar punctures).

- **Head nurse or charge nurse.** A head nurse supervises all the nurses on the floor for one shift.

- **Clinical nurse manager.** A clinical nurse manager is the administrator for an entire floor for one shift.

Working closely with nurses is the unit secretary. The unit secretary has many duties, including answering call buttons and relaying requests to nurses, answering the telephone, and transcribing all doctors' orders.

Child-life specialists

In children's hospitals, child-life specialists are trained to integrate play therapy and activities into your child's care. The playroom is a colorful retreat where your child can watch TV, play games with other patients if the doctor permits, and take a break from the hospital routine. Many hospitals are also staffed with specially trained playroom volunteers who will watch the patients there while parents take a little break for a shower, coffee, or to make phone calls.

My son was having many CT scans in a short period of time and the sedation was no longer working. Our child-life specialist arranged for our son to be brought down to the CT scanner to look around and ask questions. She also brought a tape player with a storybook tape of his favorite characters for him to listen to while he lay there. He was so comfortable listening to the tape that he never needed sedation again.

Hospital admissions

Depending on when the operation is scheduled, you will be admitted to the hospital either the night before or the day of your operation. If you are having an emergency shunt placement or revision, chances are you'll be admitted to the hospital thirty minutes to an hour prior to your operation. Either way, hospital admissions can be hectic and stressful if you don't know what to expect.

Upon reaching the admissions desk, you will be asked some simple questions and asked to complete a variety of questionnaires and insurance forms. The admissions clerk will make sure you have medical insurance or have some way of ensuring the bill will be paid.

The worst and most humiliating experience we had with the hospital was being hassled by their "financial counselor," who asked for a $7,000 cashier's check on the morning of my son's operation. (We were in dispute with our insurance company about what they would or wouldn't cover.) Meanwhile, a parade of other patients went by without being asked for a dime. Handing over my American Express card for a $7,000 deposit in order to get my child admitted was definitely a low point in my life.

Being told by the cashier, "You cannot charge $7,000!" was uncalled-for, especially when our card was approved and I was able to admit our son. The fact that we had to charge a huge deposit on our credit card was treated like a joke, and my son's life was anything but a joke.

Your insurance company will be contacted by the admissions clerk to ensure that they will pay for your bills. It's always best to have approval from your insurance company prior to the time that you are admitted to the hospital. Ask the neurosurgeon's office to contact your insurance provider at least a day or two prior to surgery to get precertification. Many insurance companies levy penalties if you fail to notify them 48 hours prior to nonemergency surgery.

In the United States, you cannot be denied care by a hospital in an emergency, regardless of your ability to pay for the hospitalization or operation. If you find yourself at the admitting desk for an emergency shunt placement or revision and are being held up because of a glitch with your insurance company, remind the admitting clerk that they cannot refuse your need for emergent care. If your insurance company requires additional information about the procedure or its necessity prior to approving your admission, the admissions clerk should refer them to your neurosurgeon's office immediately.

Forms are a big part of admissions. Some of them are similar to those you're required to fill out at your doctor's office—asking you general information (i.e., name, address, Social Security number, etc.), questions about medical history, and why you are being admitted.

> My mother is a nurse, so I have the utmost respect for them and their duties. I tried to make it easy on them prior to admission by writing down our son's medical history ahead of time and just handing the admissions clerk the information.

As soon as the information has been entered into the hospital's computer system and your insurance has been approved, you will have an ID bracelet placed around your wrist. Information on the ID bracelet includes your name, the name of your attending physician (in this case, the name of your neurosurgeon), and the date you were admitted. If you are allergic to any type of medication, you will also receive a red bracelet that alerts hospital staff to medical allergies and lists the medications you are allergic to.

In some hospitals, the parents of an infant or small child will also be given an ID bracelet to identify them as parents or legal guardians of a child. This is to ensure that your child does not pass through security or leave the hospital without his identification being checked against yours. If your child's hospital doesn't offer you an ID bracelet at the time your child is admitted, you should ask what their security policy is with ID bracelets, and if they check the child's ID bracelet against the ID of the person taking him from the hospital.

If you are being admitted to the hospital on the evening prior to surgery, you will be escorted to your hospital room, usually by an orderly. Once assigned a bed, you will be asked to change out of your clothes into a hospital gown. Most hospital rooms have a small closet or locker where you can place your belongings during your hospital stay. It's highly recommended that you give your wallet, purse, and any other valuable items to a friend or family member for safekeeping. Although hospitals are supposed to be safe places, there are still people who are waiting to take advantage of unsecured valuables.

If you are being admitted to the hospital on the day of surgery, you will be taken to a preop ward where you can change into the hospital gown. Since you probably won't have a room assigned to you until after your operation, the hospital will provide you with a plastic bag or other temporary storage where you can place your clothing. You can also give your belongings to a family member or friend to hold until you get assigned to a room.

As soon as possible after admission, ask for a tour of the floor. Find out if a microwave and refrigerator are available, learn what the approved parent sleeping arrangements are, and ask about showers or bathtubs for both patients and parents. Obtain a hospital handbook if one is available. These booklets often include information about billing, parking, discounts, and other helpful items.

Shift changes

Learn about the shift changes on your floor as soon as you can. These generally occur every eight or twelve hours. Resentments can begin when patients or parents don't understand what happens during a shift change.

> After the operation, Kaylee had a difficult time going to the bathroom. Because of this, she was catheterized for a couple of days. One day, they decided to remove the urinary catheter to try and make her go on her own—but she couldn't, no matter how hard she tried. It just so happened that she really needed to go when a shift change occurred. Kaylee kept screaming, "Mommy, mommy, I have to pee," and the nurses kept ignoring us when we rang the buzzer. I finally had to get up and grab one of the nurses to help Kaylee.

Shift changes are a necessary and sometimes hectic time. During this time, the nurses need to plan how to best deliver care for the next eight to twelve hours. During a shift change, the outgoing staff will meet with the incoming staff to report on the status of all the patients on the floor. They will discuss:

- A brief history of each patient.

- A summary of major events from the last two shifts, such as, "She vomited after each dose of morphine, so her doctor switched the meds to Tylenol® with codeine and she feels much better."

- What needs to be done, for example, "The lab work hasn't been done yet, and Dr. Doe is waiting for the results."

- Family information, such as, "Her mother went home for the night shortly after her daughter fell asleep. She asked to be called as soon as possible after her daughter wakes up in the morning or if there is an emergency. Their home telephone number is on a sticky note on her bedside."

After hearing a report on all the patients, the nurses will decide how to assign patients to incoming nurses to keep the workload even. Next, each nurse spends a few minutes organizing and prioritizing what he needs to do for each of his patients.

If at all possible, try not to call a nurse during the shift-change hour (thirty minutes before and after the hour) with any nonurgent questions, comments, or requests. If you press the call button, the unit secretary will tell you it may be a while before a nurse comes because, "They are in report." Of course, the nurses will respond to things that cannot wait, for instance if your child is vomiting or in severe pain.

Befriending the staff

There are many wonderful—and some not-so-wonderful—people on staff at the hospital. The attitudes and demeanor of nurses and residents can vary greatly. Don't take it personally.

> I had a lot of fears, but the nurses were superb! I found the pediatric neurosurgery residents to be the worst, until we got to a different hospital. In our previous hospital, we had many issues with the residents. It was frustrating to have roommates that had not undergone neurosurgery, with differing recovery and activity levels . . . .
>
> But all in all, my husband and I made our son Mike's hospital stays very calming to him. I have made it my business to make friends with the

nursing staff and make sure that he receives the best care available. I also call in a patient representative whenever I have any issues with tests or staff.

Nurses appreciate any assistance family members can give that lightens their workload. For instance, if you help change your child's soiled bedding, take out food trays, and give baths, you will free overworked nurses to take care of medicines and IVs. By working together with the nursing staff, you will help form a friendly relationship with the nurses who are caring for you or your child.

I did my son's diapering, which the nursing staff really appreciated. I try to be open and friendly, and don't interfere with their routine.

· · · · ·

I stay with my son at all times and do all of his care except medication preparation, and will never ask for anything that is not needed. We understand that our son is not always the sickest child on the floor, so that when he is, I expect the nurse to treat him as such. I feel that there is mutual respect with the nurses that goes both ways. I always leave bagels or some thank-you treats upon discharge.

Some things that parents or family members can do to help strengthen the relationship with the nurses on the floor are:

- Engage them in conversation when they're showing signs of stress or attitude problems. Most nurses are overworked and can get cranky, just like anyone else. It's rare that anyone will ask them how their day is going, or how they are doing. Take the time to get to know the nurses who are helping you, and you'll win them over.

- During slow times, invite them to converse with you. Sometimes, this will create a much needed break from their workday (or night), and will give you a chance to get to know each other better.

  It was a slow afternoon in the ICU and our daughter was sleeping, so instead of taking a walk around the hospital grounds, I asked the nurses if they wanted to play a game. We got to know each other pretty well over a few hands of euchre.

- Bring the nurses a treat.

When my wife had her shunt revised, I won over the nursing staff in ICU by bringing in a pan of home-baked cinnamon rolls—for all three shifts. I wanted to show them that I appreciated how well they were taking care of her during the day when I had to be at work.

Hospital food

Hospitals are not known for gourmet food. Hospitals do, however, hire nutritionists who carefully plan meals that are high in nutrients to help patients recover and that meet dietary requirements. Still, the timing is sometimes off.

The first meal that I can remember getting after my shunt revision almost made me ill. When I lifted the cover off the tray, all I could see was a withered pork chop with mashed potatoes and gravy. The smell turned my stomach. It was hard for me to look at food for a few days. All I wanted to do was drink juice and sleep.

Following surgery, patients are normally placed on fluids rather than on solid foods for a day or two, until the neurosurgeon says they can have solid foods. Your throat may be sore from the tube placed in your throat during surgery, so eating solid foods and swallowing may be difficult for a day or two. Because of this, the first thing you will be allowed to drink usually comes in the form of ice chips.

After every surgery I have ever had, I have always been given ice chips for quite a while after surgery. My throat is sore and dry, and I cannot take a drink of anything without it hurting. Although the ice chips help to ease my sore throat at the time, I have grown to hate them!

Another reason to delay solid foods is that your body has been through a traumatic experience and takes some time to recover. You will be given liquids to drink and liquid-based foods such as Jell-O, and receive necessary nutrients through intravenous lines that supply liquids.

If you are staying with your child, buying meals in the hospital cafeteria can get expensive. Check to see if the floor has a refrigerator for parents' food and stock it from home.

I used to take pudding cups to the hospital when I would visit. I always brought enough to share them with the nurses—especially since they were letting me keep them in their refrigerator.

Remember to put your name in a prominent place on your containers. Many hospitals have cooking facilities for families where you can cook or microwave meals brought from home. Ask family and friends to bring food when they visit, and consider ordering extra items to come up on your child's tray.

Parking

Parking at a hospital can sometimes be expensive. Just locating a parking spot can consume a lot of time.

For parents or other visitors who will be spending a lot of time at the hospital, an early goal should be to learn about short- and long-term parking arrangements. Ask other parents or members of the nursing staff if parking passes are available, or where the best place to park is located.

> I had no idea that the hospital gave out free parking passes to their frequent customers. Now I tell every new parent to check as soon as possible to see if they can get a parking pass. It will save them lots of money that they would have spent on meters and parking tickets, and save time they would have spent running out to move their car or to plunk coins in a meter.

Most nurses will be able to tell you where you can park for free. It may be on a neighborhood street or at a store parking lot a few blocks away, but if you don't mind the walk, it could save you a bundle.

Visitors

If you've ever stayed in the hospital, you know how much visitors can brighten up the day. Since patients who have hydrocephalus are normally in the hospital for a few days, and possibly one or two weeks, visitors play an important part of recovery.

Before telling friends and relatives they can visit, learn the hospital rules for visitors: who, how many, and when. Sometimes these rules depend on what ward or unit of the hospital you are in.

Hospital guidelines about visitors that you might encounter include:

- Sometimes young children are not permitted to visit.

When my son Mike was first shunted he didn't have any siblings. On the first revision I was three weeks away from my due date with my second child. By the time Mike had his third operation three months later, I had a 3-month-old and of course he was not brought to the hospital to visit.

Two years ago Mike had three revisions in a five-week period and Christopher (my other son) did come to visit Mike in the hospital. Siblings were allowed on Sundays, so Chris came and played with Mike. It did Mike good to have Chris come, as they are always together. It perked both of them up.

- Two or three visitors are normally permitted at a time, and normally only one at a time in an intensive care unit (ICU).

- In the ICU, visitors are usually restricted to spending 15 to 30 minutes, however, this policy is often not followed strictly. When the patient is a child or infant, parents are given more access. Many parents stay with their child 24 hours a day to reassure him, play with him, and be his advocate.

- Visiting hours are usually set around times when patients are most likely to be awake, active, and not in therapy, such as when meals are being served. For example, hospital visiting hours may be: Monday through Friday, 11 a.m. to 1 p.m. and 5 to 8 p.m., and Saturday and Sunday, 11 a.m. to 8 p.m.

Tell visitors what to expect when they come to see you or your child. After neurosurgery, patients:

- Will have their head shaved, bandaged, and perhaps wrapped to protect the incision.

- Will get fluids intravenously. Patients might also get medications through the IVs, as needed, such as antibiotics or medications to control nausea.

- Will normally sleep quite a bit following surgery.

- May still be hooked up to an EKG machine to monitor heart rate. In ICU, the information from the EKG machine is normally relayed to a central nurses' station where vital signs are monitored and recorded.

- May have a catheter in the bladder to collect urine. Catheters are usually removed within 24 to 48 hours after surgery.

Monitoring after surgery

Nurses will closely monitor your medical condition after neurosurgery, checking blood pressure, pulse, and respiration, as well as sensation and mobility of extremities. Temperatures will be taken to check for postsurgical infections.

Nurses will also ask questions to evaluate brain function, such as:

- What is your name?
- Do you know where you are?
- Do you know why you are here?
- What day (month, or year) is it?
- What are the names of your parents (brother, sister, spouse)?

The nurses will also check sensation and mobility of the extremities to look for a possible change in neurological condition. The nurse will ask you to move your arms and legs up and down and to wiggle your fingers and toes. Any loss in sensation could indicate to the neurosurgeon that there could be a problem.

Recovery

It is always difficult for family and friends to see a loved one lying in a hospital bed. On the first visit following surgery, the patient might still be a little groggy.

> When my daughter was first taken to the pediatric intensive care unit (PICU), she kept going in and out of consciousness. My husband and I were really scared, but the nurse assured us that this was common and was caused by the anesthesia. She suggested that we just wait out in the hall, and when Emily was finally alert enough, the nurse came out and got us.

Recovering in the hospital

Initially, patients usually are weak and sleep a lot in order to recover and allow the body to heal. As your condition improves, you will be allowed to do more on your own, but with close supervision by the nurses on the floor. Solid foods will be introduced, and you will be allowed to get out of bed and go to the bathroom without any assistance. Soon after surgery, you will be asked to get up and move about. Getting your blood circulating and activating the muscles again after an operation aid in speeding up your recovery.

As your condition continues to improve, you will be moved to a step-down unit prior to being discharged from the hospital. A step-down unit is a regular hospital ward where patients are allowed more frequent visitors and more freedom of movement. When your neurosurgeon feels that your neurological and physical condition has improved significantly, he will discharge you from the hospital.

> *I ended up having eight shunt surgeries and had paralysis on my left side. After about three weeks in the hospital, I was sent to a rehabilitation hospital. Unable to walk or speak clearly, I started a rehabilitation program. It was a very difficult time both emotionally and physically.*

Recovering at home

After release from the hospital, you will still need to rest quite a bit to aid recovery. Moderate activity during recovery is also important to build up physical strength again. It could be weeks before you are capable of returning to school or work.

Prior to being discharged from the hospital, check with your neurosurgeon to see if there are any restrictions or physical limitations. Knowing the limitations, and not pushing them, can help lead to a healthy and speedy recovery after surgery.

> *As a parent I was afraid to let my son do anything for a while. The neurosurgeon stressed to get him back to normal activity as soon as possible. The only restrictions he had were standing on his head, wrestling, and hanging upside down.*

Many insurance companies will cover the cost of short-term, in-home nursing care visits to check on patients after discharge. Nurses can handle any special requirements, such as administering intravenous antibiotics and monitoring vital signs and neurological status. In-home nursing care can be arranged by the hospital's discharge planner, a specially trained nurse who coordinates discharge from the hospital.

> *When the doctor was ready to discharge my son, he needed to go home on IV medications. At first, I felt overwhelmed at the thought of*

being responsible for all of his care. The discharge planner on the floor talked to my husband and me to detail the care Shaun would be needing at home.

She arranged for a nursing company to come to our house and teach us how to administer the antibiotics. They were fabulous. They came twice a week to check on us, and were only a phone call away whenever I needed them. Having them available allowed us to take Shaun home earlier, and to get our family back together sooner.

Follow-up visits

Once you are discharged from the hospital, your neurosurgeon will ask you to contact her office to schedule the first postop visit. Normally, she will want to see you in her office within one to two weeks after surgery.

Depending on the requirements of your neurosurgeon, you may or may not need to have another CT or MRI scan done prior to the first postop visit. Your neurosurgeon may want to compare pre- and postop films to see if the shunt is working properly. The scans also allow her to see if there are any problems developing, such as a shunt overdraining.

Your neurosurgeon may take out any stitches or staples that remain in the incision areas. Next, she will give you a neurological examination to see how recovery is progressing.

When you visit your neurosurgeon for follow-up visits, come prepared with any questions or concerns you may have regarding recovery. If something is bothering you or if you don't feel right, make sure your neurosurgeon is aware of this. It is her responsibility to provide you with the best care possible, and if you don't convey to her that you're not doing well, she probably won't know.

If everything goes well at the first follow-up visit, the next one probably won't be for another two to three months. Again, depending on your neurosurgeon, you may or may not need to have another CT or MRI series. Many neurosurgeons schedule bimonthly follow-up visits until you have gone a full year postop without complications. After that, your neurosurgeon usually needs to see you only once every year or if there are signs of a complication with the shunt.

CHAPTER 6

Shunt Revisions

For inherent technical reasons, it is probable
that a "shunt forever" is an impossible dream,
but delaying shunt malfunctions as long as
possible is a realistic goal.

—Drs. James M. Drake and
Christian Sainte-Rose
The Shunt Book

SHUNTS HELP TO STABILIZE intracranial pressure and reduce the risk of damage to the central nervous system (CNS) by draining cerebrospinal fluid (CSF) away from the brain. Unfortunately, as noted by Drs. Drake and Sainte-Rose, shunts are only a temporary solution for a permanent condition.

Shunts fail or need to be replaced for a variety of reasons. Patients and families can protect themselves by remaining alert—looking for the telltale warning signs of a possible shunt malfunction.

Careful planning allows problems to be caught early and helps prevent emergency surgery. Shunt revisions under optimal conditions can minimize future problems, lessen emotional stress, and possibly even save a life.

In this chapter, we explore some of the problems that accompany shunt systems, and discuss some of the factors that cause them to fail, such as infections, obstructions, and mechanical problems. We look at how these problems are treated, and what you and your neurosurgeon can do to keep them from recurring. At the end of this chapter, we discuss how the experience of the neurosurgeon treating your hydrocephalus affects the rate of complications associated with shunt malfunction and infection.

What is a shunt revision?

When a shunt system needs to be replaced, the operation is referred to as a revision. Revision simply means *to change or modify*. When a shunt is first put in place, it is the dream of every neurosurgeon (as well as the patient and family) that the shunt system will last forever. However, shunts do not last forever, and it is unrealistic to think they ever will.

Shunts are susceptible to failures and malfunctions, just like any other mechanical device. For instance, a valve rated by the manufacturer for one pressure may in fact be a different pressure, since some manufacturers don't test all of the valves they produce. And for reasons yet unknown, the shunt valve can simply fail to work properly, which can leave the patient with a system that either drains too much, too little, or not at all. Reasons why a shunt may need to be revised include:

- Mechanical failures.
- Use of the wrong type of shunt valve.
- Infections.
- Obstructions.
- Need to lengthen or replace the distal catheter.
- Need to replace a catheter that has slipped out of place, has been disconnected, or is disintegrating.

> In May of 1984, when I was 11, it became apparent that my shunt had come apart at the neck (I had almost constant headaches). When the neurosurgeon performed a revision, he discovered that my skull had grown completely around my shunt. When he finally got the shunt free of the cranium, he said that spinal fluid "went spurting across the operating room." He completely replaced the shunt. During the surgery, I became paralyzed on my left side. Over the next few months, I regained left side mobility and entered junior high school. I had four more revisions (including infections) in the fall of 1987, and again in the fall of 1988.

Signs of possible complications

When a shunt system fails to operate properly or becomes infected or obstructed, the patient's life and cognitive faculties are placed at risk, often requiring the shunt to be revised under emergency conditions. All patients, families, and close friends need to be aware of the signs of increased intracranial pressure (ICP), which could indicate there is a problem with the shunt.

> For eight years, hydrocephalus was a non-factor. I completed high school and went to college, living life like a normal college student with little sleep and some parties. Oh yeah, I even had time to study. Then at the end of my first semester of my senior year, I thought that my work, class schedule, and lack of sleep were catching up with me. It turned out that it was my shunt.

> I remember my roommates bursting into my classroom to get me. My neurosurgeon got the results of my CT scan from the previous day and wanted to see me immediately. Well, to say the least, I was not very happy about this. In fact, I was petrified. I was babbling the entire way to the hospital and into the preop.

> When I finally awoke and realized what happened I was shocked. During two weeks in the hospital, I had three surgeries. I don't remember any of it. I had the easy part. My family and friends had the anxious moments and worrying. Fortunately, it all took place just before my semester break and I resumed college a month later to complete my undergraduate degree.

Most of the signs and symptoms are identical to those at diagnosis. Other symptoms may relate to a particular type of shunt placement, i.e., ventriculoatrial (VA), ventriculoperitoneal (VP), ventriculopleural (VPl), etc.

> My family and I were originally told that a shunt was needed, but not how long it would last. I also wasn't told about symptoms that would happen when I needed a new shunt. I had to learn about those by experience.

Signs and symptoms include:

- Loss of appetite.
- Nausea and vomiting.
- Abdominal pain or cramps.
- Behavioral changes, irritability.
- Frequent or persistent headaches with increased severity.

After recovering from surgery, and returning to my normal activi-
ties, headaches started cropping up again. They weren't just run-of-the-
mill headaches, but shunt headaches.

- Gait difficulties such as frequent loss of balance or mobility, stumbling, or drifting to one side or the other while walking.

- Loss of sensation or numbness to one side of the body and extremities.

- Muscle tension, particularly of the neck and shoulders.

- Lethargy, defined as a sudden loss of energy, complaining all the time of being tired, or having an extremely difficult time waking.

- Reduced or impaired cognitive ability.

I was on my way to work and could not drive anymore. I somehow
parked my car and stumbled to a pay phone. I don't remember anything
after that. I ended up having eight shunt revisions.

- Inability to process thoughts or perform routine tasks without getting disoriented.

- Loss of memory or signs of dementia.

- Vision problems, including impaired or double vision, and crossed or wandering eyes.

- Loss of upward gaze (sunsetting of the eyes).

- Increased sensitivity to light and/or sound.

- Impaired or slurred speech.

- A persistent low-grade fever (usually greater than 100°F or 38°C), or a high-grade fever (102-104°F or 39-40°C) if the infection is more aggressive.

- Redness or swelling along the shunt tract.

- Tenderness in the areas surrounding the shunt system, including the abdomen (particularly with VP shunts).

- Coma.

- Difficulty in breathing (with VPl shunts).

- Cardiac arrhythmia (abnormal heart rate).

Symptoms should be taken seriously, especially if you notice two or more at the same time. Neurological status can deteriorate slowly (over a few months) or quite rapidly (over a few hours or days). Therefore, when symptoms of a possible problem with a shunt begin to show, it is imperative that you seek medical attention immediately.

> *I had noticed over the past couple of days that Shaun's behavior was getting more extreme. He was crying over things that never bothered him before, and he was nasty to his brothers and me. I had taken him to the pediatrician to check for an ear infection or sore throat, anything that could have been causing this change of behavior, but the pediatrician couldn't find anything wrong. He sent us for a CT scan, which showed a change in his ventricles. This was our first experience with a revision, and I had no idea that he could present in this way.*

If you cannot get an appointment with your doctor or neurosurgeon, go to a hospital emergency room as soon as possible for testing and evaluation. Delaying the diagnosis of shunt failure can result in permanent damage to the brain and possibly death.

Shunt lengthening procedures

Some shunt systems may need to be upgraded by lengthening the distal catheter. Lengthening procedures are more commonly performed on infants and small children who were first shunted at birth or soon thereafter. As your child grows, the distal catheter may pull out of the area where it was originally placed (e.g., the right atrium of the heart, the peritoneal cavity, etc.).

Although the operation is often called a lengthening procedure, the entire distal catheter (in most practices) will be replaced. The procedure is referred to as a *lengthening* procedure because the neurosurgeon is essentially increasing the overall length of the shunt system. Most lengthening procedures require your child to be admitted to the hospital and to stay overnight for observation.

Most neurosurgeons prefer initially to place VP shunts in infants and small children because the procedure for lengthening the distal catheter of a VA shunt is more difficult and risky. Ventriculoperitoneal shunts also allow your child's neurosurgeon to place more catheter distally than with a VA shunt, significantly reducing the necessity of shunt lengthening procedures.

With VP shunts, your child's neurosurgeon can put in all the tubing that is necessary to reach adult size—even in a premature newborn. With a VA shunt, it is necessary to lengthen the shunt when the end comes out of the atrium to reside in the superior vena cava. Another option is to convert a VA to a VP or VPl rather than place the distal catheter back in the right atrium.

Testing for shunt problems

Your neurosurgeon can order a variety of tests and procedures to determine if there is a problem with the shunt system.

Initially, your neurosurgeon will order a CT or MRI series to see if the ventricles are enlarged or if there is any type of cyst or tumor growth which might be obstructing the flow of CSF. If the imaging series is inconclusive, your neurosurgeon can perform other tests—such as a radionuclide shuntogram, shunt tap, or intracranial pressure monitoring—to evaluate the shunt and check for increased ICP.

These three tests are described below. They can all be used on either children or adults with hydrocephalus.

Radionuclide shuntogram

A radionuclide shuntogram determines if the shunt system has been obstructed or if there is a degradation of the shunt catheters. Shuntograms allow neurosurgeons accurately to diagnose shunt-related problems that cannot be detected by normal CT or MRI scans.

Unlike traditional imaging methods that rely on external radiation, such as with computed tomography (CT) or X-ray machines, shuntograms use a radioactive isotope and a gamma camera to take pictures of the shunt system. The gamma camera photographs the radioactive material as it moves through the shunt system. Shuntograms can also be imaged using a single-photon computed tomography (or SPECT) machine, the next generation of gamma imaging devices.

You will be admitted into a hospital or imaging center on an outpatient basis for a shuntogram. You will be asked to lie down on the bed under the gamma camera or SPECT machine for approximately 15 minutes prior to the beginning of the test. This allows CSF within the ventricles and shunt system to balance out before the test starts.

Next, your neurosurgeon or a nuclear radiologist (a radiologist who is trained in nuclear medicine) will inject a small amount (approximately 0.5 to 1 milliliters) of a radioisotope into the bulb reservoir of the shunt valve. Because the imaging agent is injected directly into the shunt valve, the material should flow from the shunt valve back into the ventricles of the brain. If the agent does not reflux into the ventricles, this could indicate that the proximal catheter is obstructed, possibly by the choroid plexus.

The shuntogram will take about 30 minutes or more to perform, which should be enough time for the CSF and the imaging agent to flow from the ventricles through the shunt valve and out of the distal catheter. Your neurosurgeon and the nuclear radiologist will carefully follow the flow of the imaging agent through the shunt system to see if the CSF is flowing out of the distal catheter without any problems.

During the shuntogram, the neurosurgeon and nuclear radiologist will look for signs of a disconnected or cracked catheter. If your shunt system has become disconnected, or if the catheters have become cracked, CSF will flow out of the shunt system and into surrounding tissues. The images may clearly show CSF and the imaging agent flowing out of the part of the shunt system that has been compromised.

Shunt tap

Neurosurgeons can test ICP by performing a shunt tap. Most shunt valves have a bulb reservoir (or dome) over the shunt valve system. This is where CSF collects before being drained out of the shunt valve to the distal catheter.

When you have a shunt tap, you will be asked to lie down on an examination table with your head turned to the side to expose the area where the shunt is placed. Your neurosurgeon will ensure that the area around the bulb reservoir is sterile to reduce the risk of introducing an infection into the valve system. To do this, your neurosurgeon will either shave a small area of the scalp to expose the shunt reservoir, or he will tape the hair out of the way to give him direct access to the area. He will swab the area with an alcohol preparation and then with an iodine/alcohol-based solution, such as Betadine.

Your neurosurgeon will insert a small-gauged needle through the scalp into the bulb reservoir of the ventricular catheter or the shunt valve. He will connect the hub (the opposite end) of the needle to a manometer to measure ICP. A manometer is a small U-shaped tube that contains water.

Once connected to the hub of the needle, the fluid within the manometer should fall rather quickly to indicate the closing pressure of the shunt system. If the fluid does not fall, your neurosurgeon can assume there is a distal obstruction within the shunt system. If the fluid falls slowly, a partial obstruction can be assumed. If he is unable to obtain fluid from the reservoir, this would indicate an obstruction within the ventricles, requiring the shunt to be revised.

After taking a pressure reading and determining whether or not there is a shunt obstruction, your neurosurgeon will disconnect the manometer and attach a syringe to withdraw a small amount of CSF that will be sent to the lab for analysis of the fluid, to look for any signs of infection.

When the procedure is completed, your neurosurgeon will remove the needle and place a small Band-Aid over the area where it was inserted. The average amount of time it takes to do a shunt tap is about 15 to 20 minutes. Following the shunt tap, you will be asked to lie on your side for up to an hour or more. The reason for this is that you might be light-headed following the procedure, due to CSF being removed from the shunt.

Intracranial pressure monitoring

Another technique used for evaluating ICP is to temporarily implant an intracranial monitoring device (a small fiber-optic cable). Hospitalization is required to perform this test. The ICP monitoring cable is implanted through a burr hole that is made behind the hairline in the right frontal region. The cable, which transmits pressure readings to a monitoring device, is inserted through the dura. The ICP monitor is usually left in place for 24 hours and sometimes longer, depending on the preference of your neurosurgeon.

> Kathie was monitored for five days. She was able to play in the playroom, was encouraged to run in the hall, and to bend over and pick up a ball and roll it to me. The doctors wanted her to do anything that could safely mimic her normal behavior at home to check for changes in her pressure.

Staying in the hospital allows ICP to be monitored while you are awake and asleep, as well as while you are lying down, sitting, and standing. Based on data received from the monitoring device, your neurosurgeon will make a decision, usually the next day, on whether or not he needs to place or revise your shunt.

Another technique used by some neurosurgeons is to place a ventriculostomy catheter within the ventricles and directly measure your ICP. Some neurosurgeons have found this to be more accurate than the use of the fiberoptic cable.

Obstructions

One of the most common shunt complications is an obstruction of either the proximal (ventricular) or distal catheter.

Proximal catheter obstructions

The proximal catheter is the most likely to be obstructed. When CSF is drawn into the shunt system, the catheter creates a suction effect within the ventricle, similar to that of the drain in a bathtub. This suction could possibly draw the choroid plexus, blood, and debris toward the holes at the end of the catheter and contribute to obstruction.

Obstructions of the proximal catheter can be caused by a variety of factors, including:

- In-growth by the choroid plexus.

- Collapsed ventricles, which occlude (block) the holes at the end of the ventricular catheter.

- Blood clots resulting from hemorrhaging during placement or removal of the ventricular catheter.

- Buildup of tissue debris.

When the proximal catheter is inserted into the ventricles, brain matter can sometimes get caught in the holes of the catheter. In some cases, bleeding may occur when the ventricles are catheterized. When this happens, blood and/or brain matter can get sucked into the catheter along with CSF. If the matter is too large, it can block one or more of the holes of the catheter or get pulled into the catheter and cause a complete obstruction.

In some cases, such as obstruction of the proximal catheter by the choroid plexus, your neurosurgeon may decide it is safer to leave the existing catheter in place rather than removing it, to eliminate the risk of causing an intraventricular hemorrhage. Your neurosurgeon will be able to tell if the catheter has been obstructed by the choroid plexus or other adhesions if the catheter resists being removed when it is pulled.

> *When the neurosurgeon came out of the operating room to talk to us, he told us that they had to leave the end of the catheter in Brian's ventricle. It had become so clogged with the choroid plexus that it would not come out easily. This has happened many times. Now his CT scans show many "shunt artifacts" in his ventricles, and they cannot be removed safely.*

If a hemorrhage does occur, your neurosurgeon will flush your ventricles with Ringers lactate to stop the bleeding before reinserting a new proximal catheter. A slight degree of bleeding is not uncommon, and usually results in no consequences. However, in cases where the bleeding is severe, the patient might experience some form of neurological deficit as a result of the intracranial hemorrhage. The true extent of the damage may only be determined after recovery from the operation.

> *When my shunt was originally placed in 1972, I was in the hospital for 47 days. The only complication during that procedure was an intraventricular hemorrhage. I became paralyzed and had to learn how to walk and use my right hand all over again. I also had problems remembering who I was.*

Distal catheter obstructions

Distal catheter obstructions are less common than proximal catheter obstructions, but they do occur.

The distal catheter for VP shunts can be obstructed if debris in the peritoneal cavity accumulates around the tip of the catheter. This is more common in distal catheters that have slit valves rather than an open end to allow CSF to flow out of the system. Loss of absorptive ability by the peritoneal cavity or the growth of peritoneal pseudocysts also contribute to distal catheter obstructions.

Ventriculoatrial shunts can become obstructed when the distal catheter migrates out of the right atrium of the heart and lies against the wall of the superior vena cava (one of two main veins that deliver blood to the right atrium of the heart). If the tip of the distal catheter resides outside the heart, it is also at risk of clotting.

Subdural hematomas

A subdural hematoma (SDH) is an accumulation of blood (hematoma) between the dura mater and the arachnoid layers of the meninges. This area is known as the subdural space. In Figure 6-1, the SDHs can be seen as the darkened areas near the frontal lobes, left and right, where the arrows point.

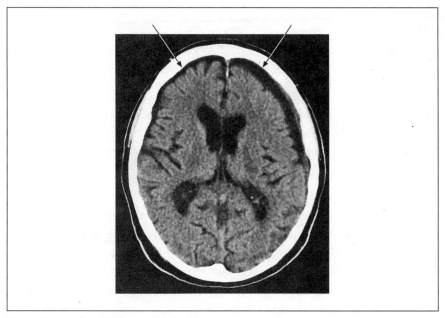

Figure 6-1. Chronic bilateral subdural hematomas

When a proximal catheter is inserted into the ventricles and a working shunt system is attached to drain the excess CSF, the ventricles can deflate fairly rapidly, and the surrounding brain matter will move inward to assume a smaller form. However, if the ventricles deflate too quickly, the veins that bridge between the brain and dura can be stretched and torn, resulting in an accumulation of blood in the subdural space.

Subdural hematomas can also be caused by trauma to the head (e.g., getting hit in the head with a fast-moving baseball). In these instances, the hematoma results from an intracranial hemorrhage.

Detecting subdural hematomas

Subdural hematomas have the same symptoms as a malfunctioning shunt system, particularly lethargy, gait disturbances, headaches, numbness or loss of sensation to one side of the body, and reduced mental faculties.

An SDH is detected with imaging equipment, usually ultrasound for infants and small children, and CT or MRI in older children and adults. Once detected, your neurosurgeon will determine the proper course of action to treat the SDH.

Treatment

Treatment for SDHs requires hospitalization to relieve the hematoma. If the SDH is caused by a faulty or improper shunt valve, the entire system may be revised.

There are many schools of thought on how to treat SDHs. The long-standing debate revolves about whether to evacuate (or drain) the SDH by creating a burr hole or to perform a craniotomy directly over the area of the subdural accumulation of blood.

The burr hole operation is performed by drilling a hole through the cranium directly over the deepest area of the SDH. Your neurosurgeon will create a small hole in the dura layer to relieve the pressure of the hematoma. Interoperative CT scans may be taken at this time to determine if additional drainage of the hematoma is required. Upon completion of the procedure, the burr hole will be capped and the incisions will be cleansed and closed, either with sutures or surgical staples.

> Mike had two subdural hematomas drained externally during a revision. Postop I was told how Mike could not be allowed to move—yeah, he is 18 months old and he certainly will agree to lie flat on his back now that he is feeling free of headache! I was also told how the drains had to be a specific amount of inches off the floor, etc. The nurses and doctors kept checking it over and over again, then checking the fluid that flowed into the two bags hanging on the side of the bed.

A craniotomy is more complex than a burr hole operation, requiring your neurosurgeon to remove temporarily a small section of the skull to access the hematoma. This allows him to access a larger area of the dura in order to treat the hematoma. To relieve the SDH, your neurosurgeon will create a small hole in the dura layer. Once drainage is complete, the section of skull will be put back into place, where it will fuse together with the surrounding skull.

In both types of operations, additional drainage of the hematoma may be required. This is done by inserting a drainage tube through the dura layer into the hematoma to suction out additional fluid.

Most neurosurgeons perform burr hole operations to relieve SDHs, since craniotomies are more invasive and require longer hospitalization.

Shunt infections

Shunt infections are the most serious complication related to the treatment of hydrocephalus. They most commonly occur within one to two months following a placement or revision procedure. Although a shunt system can develop an infection many months or years after insertion, these cases are extremely rare.

Symptoms of shunt infections

Symptoms of a shunt infection include:

- A persistent low-grade fever (usually greater than 100°F or 38°C), or a high-grade fever (102-104°F or 39-40°C) if the infection is more aggressive.

- Irritability and changes in mood or personality.

- Changes in cognitive ability.

- Redness and/or tenderness along the shunt tract.

- Swelling or tenderness of the abdomen (with VP shunts).

- Sudden, frequent vomiting or persistent nausea.

- Headaches.

- Soreness of the neck and/or shoulder muscles.

Any of the above symptoms, especially in combination with a high fever, could indicate the possibility that something is wrong. If you suspect a shunt infection, contact your primary care physician or neurosurgeon immediately.

Shaun had had a revision the week before and he began to have a low-grade fever with some general aches and pains. I thought it was a flu

that maybe he had picked up in the hospital, but he began to look sicker
as the day went on. He did not respond to Tylenol and actually looked
very sick, even though his fever was low. We went to the emergency room
and they found out he had a shunt infection.

What causes shunt infections?

Shunt infections can be caused by a number of various factors, including:

- Bacteria being introduced to one of the incisions during surgery.
- Placement of an improperly sterilized shunt valve or catheter.
- Meningitis.
- An infection near the distal end of the shunt system, such as peritonitis for VP shunt placements. An infection near the distal end is also termed a pseudocyst, which is a collection of infected fluid that forms a cyst around the tip of the distal catheter.
- Length of time the shunt procedure takes. The longer the shunt procedure is, the greater the risk of infection.

The most common types of infections in shunts are Staphylococcus aureus (65 percent) and Gram-negative bacteria (GNB, 19-22 percent). Shunt infections occur in approximately 2 to 10 percent of all newly placed systems, including revisions (J. K. Stamos, "Ventriculoperitoneal shunt infections with Gram-negative bacteria," *Neurosurgery* 33, no. 5, 1993: 858-62).

Treating shunt infections

Treatment of shunt infections can be a long and arduous process that requires hospitalization. If you have a shunt infection, you will be placed on high doses of intravenous antibiotics to fight off the infection. Removal of the entire shunt system—including the ventricular catheter—is necessary to prevent any possibility of reintroducing the infection to your body.

After removal of the shunt system, CSF is drained through an external ventricle drainage (EVD) system. An EVD consists of a ventricular catheter, a shunt valve, and a bag which collects CSF at the distal end. With the EVD in place, you will continue to receive intravenous antibiotics until further tests of CSF indicate that the infection has been cured. This could take anywhere from two to fourteen days. If ventricular CSF cultures continue to show signs of infection, antibiotics can be injected into the ventricles through the EVD. After the CSF has been proven to be sterile for seven to ten days, your neurosurgeon will insert a new shunt system.

> *Our 13-year-old son was born premature, and was shunted for hydrocephalus at 13 months. He is doing absolutely great! He has had three revisions.*

> *At the age of 5, his tube became clogged with tissue at the valve, and required a revision (#1). They placed the tube in the wrong spot, and had to go through another operation that evening (revision #2).*

> *Then last year, at the age of 12, he developed an infection in his stomach that put him in the hospital for emergency surgery. They externalized his shunt and fought the infection with antibiotics for 10 days. His neurosurgeon replaced the shunt (revision #3) and sent him home on an IV to continue the antibiotics.*

How to avoid shunt infections

Most shunt infections occur at the time the shunt is inserted or revised and make their presence known within the first month following placement. These infections were probably introduced to the shunt system or the incisions during or immediately following the operation.

Following surgery, you can help reduce the risk of contracting a shunt infection by:

- Not scratching or picking at the area around the incisions (or not allowing your child to do so). Although the incisions may itch, scratching them before they have healed properly could possibly introduce bacteria, which may cause an infection.

- If the area surrounding the incisions starts to redden, swell, or ooze, contact your doctor immediately.

- Since bacteria travel through the body in the blood, some neurosurgeons recommend that patients with VA shunts take antibiotics at least 24 hours prior to visiting their dentist. This is not necessary for people with VP shunts since the catheters are outside the bloodstream. Your dentist can prescribe the antibiotics for you.

Silicone allergies

Almost all hydrocephalus shunts today are made from silicone. Silicone is a synthetic plastic polymer material that is rigid, yet flexible enough to allow it to bend without kinking.

Silicone allergies are extremely rare, but because of their nature, they need to be taken seriously. Silicone allergies are very serious, as the patient can develop anaphylactic shock within hours after the shunt is implanted. Symptoms that indicate an allergic reaction include:

- Difficulty breathing.
- Convulsions or seizures.
- Reddening, swelling, and sometimes blistering of the area surrounding the shunt catheters.
- Elevated temperature.

The neurosurgeon will need to remove the shunt system immediately and connect an external ventricular drainage (EVD) system using a catheter made of polyurethane rather than silicone. Once your condition improves, usually after 24 to 48 hours, he will assess your condition and decide whether or not to implant a shunt system made from polyurethane.

Shunt complications

In addition to shunt failures, infections, and obstructions, shunts are subject to other problems that sometimes require them to be revised.

Cracked catheters

The longer a shunt system remains in place, the more prone it is to some form of structural degradation. In shunt systems placed in infants and small children, the catheters will be stretched as the child grows. Over time, the catheters may crack, resulting in shunt malfunction.

One way to determine if a shunt catheter is cracked is by taking an X-ray of the body where the shunt is placed. In some instances, however, the crack may not show up on an X-ray, particularly if the crack is very small. Another method of testing for a cracked catheter is by performing a radionuclide shuntogram. By tracking the flow of CSF through the shunt system, your neurosurgeon will be able to determine where the catheter has been compromised. Your neurosurgeon will then make a decision whether to revise the entire shunt (if the proximal catheter is cracked) or to replace the distal catheter alone.

While many one-piece shunts (e.g., the Codman Uni-Shunt) don't have the inherent risks of the catheters becoming disconnected, their catheters are susceptible to cracking and fracturing, just like any other shunt catheter.

Disconnected catheters

Most shunt systems are made up of three parts: the proximal catheter, the distal catheter, and the shunt valve. The proximal and distal catheters are connected to the shunt valve and secured in place with sutures. Over time, it is possible for one of the catheters to become disconnected from the shunt valve—for example, it might be pulled out of place as your child grows.

When a shunt catheter becomes disconnected, the patient might start to show signs of a shunt malfunction. Since the catheters will be disconnected at the shunt valve, another sign that the neurosurgeon can look for is a subcutaneous buildup of CSF near the shunt valve. A small pocket of fluid may begin to balloon beneath the scalp as CSF tries to enter or exit from the shunt valve or elsewhere along the shunt. As long as the shunt valve is still working properly and the catheters are in good shape, your neurosurgeon may be able just to reconnect the shunt catheter to the valve with a simple operation. However, if either the shunt valve or catheters are compromised, the entire shunt system may need to be revised.

If the distal catheter gets disconnected and migrates into the peritoneal cavity, the catheter can be removed by laparoscopic surgery. The primary concern is that the distal catheter could wander around in the abdomen and possibly damage vital organs.

> I had a catheter disconnect and slip into my pelvis, where it wrapped around my uterus. I was lucky; an OB/GYN was called in to perform laparoscopic surgery in order to retrieve the wayward catheter. The end of the catheter had been stabbing me in the pelvis for about two months. It didn't cause any damage to my reproductive organs, but I know another woman who wasn't as lucky. In her case, the catheter damaged her uterus, causing her to need a hysterectomy.

A laparoscope is an illuminated surgical tube used by surgeons to view the internal organs of the abdomen. A small incision is made through the abdominal wall, and the laparoscope is inserted into the peritoneal cavity. The neurosurgeon can use tiny forceps to grab onto the catheter and remove it through the laparoscope. However, if no sign of infection is present and the catheter doesn't appear to be tethered around any vital organs, your neurosurgeon may decide just to leave the catheter in the peritoneal cavity.

Loculated ventricles

Ventricles can become compartmentalized (loculated) when scar tissue builds a wall between the different areas of the ventricular system. When this happens, CSF gets trapped inside the different compartments, making management of hydrocephalus even more difficult.

In the past, neurosurgeons would place ventricular catheters into each of the loculated sections and connect them either to one main shunt valve or to their own valve. By connecting the various catheters to their own valves, your neurosurgeon will be able to check each catheter individually should problems arise.

Some neurosurgeons have begun to use neuroendoscopy to puncture holes through the walls of the loculated ventricles, allowing CSF to flow freely between the ventricles. The primary risk from this procedure is creating debris that could obstruct an existing catheter or valve.

Peritoneal pseudocysts

Peritoneal pseudocysts are a rare side effect of having a VP shunt. Pseudocysts are cysts, made up of CSF and other debris, that can form in the peritoneal cavity near the distal catheter. Pseudocysts can block the tip of the distal catheter, either reducing the flow of CSF through the shunt system or completely obstructing the distal end.

Pseudocysts may be a sign of a low-grade shunt infection. Your neurosurgeon may obtain a sample of CSF to rule out the possibility of an infection. Signs of peritoneal pseudocysts are swelling or pain of the abdomen. Pseudocysts can be detected with X-rays or by ultrasound.

If pseudocysts are detected, your neurosurgeon will need to revise your shunt system and remove the cysts from your peritoneal cavity. Since you will be at an increased risk of getting pseudocysts again if the distal catheter is placed in the peritoneal cavity, your shunt may be revised to a ventriculoatrial or ventriculopleural path.

Slit ventricle syndrome (SVS)

Slit ventricle syndrome is commonly associated with shunt-dependency. The syndrome is diagnosed by CT or MRI, revealing very narrow or almost non-existing ventricles. When the ventricles are narrow, they can occlude (obstruct) the holes of the proximal catheter, causing the shunt to malfunction intermittently. The problem is alleviated by replacing the partially blocked ventricular catheter. Slit ventricle syndrome is usually seen after the shunt has been in place for several years, and is characterized by chronic or recurring headaches.

The initial step in evaluating SVS is to ensure that the shunt system is operating properly. This is done by testing the system with a shuntogram. If the shunt is obstructed, a revision will be performed. If the shunt is functional, the patient's intracranial pressure is monitored using a shunt tap or with an intracranial monitoring device.

> When our son's ventricles became "slit," the treatment of his hydrocephalus became more difficult. Normal CT scans could no longer be trusted solely to show if he was having pressure fluctuations, as his ventricles never changed size. A more invasive procedure, ICP monitoring, was needed to detect our son's pressure fluctuations. This test proved to be monumental in his treatment as it showed us large fluctuations in pressure were happening that were not being shown on the scans.

Experience of the surgeon

Chapter 3, *Selecting a Neurosurgeon,* explains that it is important that the neurosurgeon who performs the shunt placement or revision is familiar with the treatment of hydrocephalus and all its complexities. Most surgeons won't openly admit that they aren't qualified to perform a shunt placement procedure. However, many neurosurgeons simply don't perform enough shunt procedures to remain proficient.

In a study by doctors in Norway to investigate the risk factors in shunt surgery, two of the findings were:

- Residents performed a higher number of inadequate operations than specialists did.

- The infection rate was higher among patients operated on by residents (M. Lund-Johansen et al., "Shunt failures and complications in adults as related to shunt type, diagnosis, and the experience of the surgeon," *Neurosurgery*, 35, no. 5, 1994: 839).

In many teaching hospitals (such as university medical centers), operations are routinely performed by surgical residents with the attending surgeon observing and instructing throughout the procedure. It is also not uncommon for more than one resident to perform a different part of the operation (e.g., one resident operates on the cranium, while another inserts the distal catheter into the peritoneal cavity).

As a patient, you have the right to know who will perform your operation. Prior to signing the consent form for your operation, ask your neurosurgeon whether she or someone else will be performing the shunt procedure. If she responds that a neurosurgical resident will be performing the operation, you have the right to at least meet the surgeon prior to the operation. If you do not feel comfortable having a surgical resident perform the operation, you can request that your neurosurgeon be the person who performs the procedure and that the resident only be permitted to observe. On your consent form, fill in your neurosurgeon's name and cross out the section that gives permission to her colleagues. Make sure you discuss this with your doctor and show her the amended consent.

This doesn't mean that everyone should run out and tell their neurosurgeon they don't want a resident to perform their operation. After all, even the neurosurgical specialists in this study were not infallible. Operations in which the surgeon is present and instructing have much lower rates of problems than those in which residents perform the operation on their own. The purpose of surgical residencies are to allow future surgeons the opportunity to perform operations on live patients under the direction of skilled surgical specialists. You, however, have the right to choose the surgeon who will be operating, and have a legal right to have your choice respected.

When shunt problems become chronic

Shunt revisions, as with any other type of surgical procedure, can be stressful for everyone. It is not uncommon to hear stories from patients who have had numerous shunt revisions in a year. This can be part of the harsh reality of living with hydrocephalus.

> I received my first shunt when I was 13 years old. I'm 29 now, and have had 20 revisions in 16 years—including five in the last year alone.

Some neurosurgeons explain the likelihood of problems with the shunt, while others do not. Some doctors feel that a frank discussion will cause undue alarm and create additional stress. Discuss with your doctor the risks associated with your particular system, and remain alert for signs and symptoms of problems.

> Before my shunt was revised, my neurosurgeon made it perfectly clear to me about the possible need to have the valve revised in the future. He explained to me that, "No shunt will last forever," and that it could last six weeks, six months or twenty years. "Nobody knows how long these things will last," he said. And he was right. Six months later, almost to the day, I found myself needing another revision caused by a subdural hematoma. All I could think was, "Here we go again," but I was thankful that my neurosurgeon warned me of the possibility of this happening.

Patients and their families need to know that there is no guarantee that a shunt valve or catheter will last a lifetime. Somewhere, sometime, you will probably need to have your shunt replaced. If you find yourself in need of emotional support in this very stressful time, contact and rely on your friends, family, church members, and other hydrocephalus patients who have been through a similar situation (see Chapter 8, *Finding Support*).

> It was our son's third shunt revision that year that threw us for a loop. The fact that it was only two months after the last revision made my wife and me want to give up all hope. But we trusted our son's neurosurgeon. He was well respected around the hospital, an excellent communicator, and was truly sympathetic to our situation. He referred us to a local support group for children with chronic illnesses. All along, we thought we were the only couple riding in this boat, but that couldn't be further from the truth.

CHAPTER 7

Side Effects

*Prosperity is not without many fears and
distastes; and adversity is not without
comforts and hopes.*

—Francis Bacon
On Adversity

NOW THAT WE'VE TALKED ABOUT the diagnosis of hydrocephalus, how it is treated, and some of the complications that accompany shunts, it's time we turn our attention to the dark side of hydrocephalus—side effects.

The side effects of hydrocephalus—some of which are visual problems, seizures, precocious puberty, and learning disorders—vary greatly from patient to patient, depending on the condition that causes fluid to collect in the brain and on individual response to brain surgery.

We examine these side effects and hear firsthand stories from patients and parents about how they deal with problems that often last a lifetime. We also discuss the importance of neuropsychological testing and rehabilitation therapies for children and adults who have learning or attention deficit disorders.

Common complaints

Most patients with hydrocephalus experience side effects and have some common complaints. How hydrocephalus affects you depends greatly on how your brain and body have reacted to a shunt-related operation.

Hydrocephalus and its treatment can cause a range of common side effects:

- Intellectual (confusion, forgetfulness, or short-term memory problems).

- Visual (eye misalignments or loss of vision).

- Physical (headaches, nausea, or tenderness around incision sites).

- Neurological (seizures or problems coordinating motor skills).

- Endocrinologic (precocious puberty or diabetes insipidus).

Although side effects may be caused by increased intracranial pressure (ICP) or an operation, your neurosurgeon usually won't handle them. Since her job is to operate on the brain and help control hydrocephalus, she may not be trained to handle its side effects. While a majority of neurosurgeons are very proactive about their patients' care, others may be dismissive of complaints of side effects.

> My daughter's neurosurgeon is great. She listens to our concerns, calls us out of the blue to check up on her, months after she's had a revision. She's a real sweetheart.

· · · · ·

> I had been having headaches in the evening for about two weeks straight, and it seemed like nothing would make them go away. I finally called my neurosurgeon to ask if it could be a problem with my shunt, but he was quick to write the headaches off as being stress-related. Well, another two weeks went by, and the headaches were still there, and they seemed to be getting worse, too. Rather than call the neurosurgeon and probably be ignored again, I went to the emergency room, where they did a CT, which showed that my ventricles were enlarged.

When side effects arise, you will need to see another specialist such as a neurologist, neuropsychologist, endrocrinologist, neuro-ophthalmologist, or rehabilitation specialist to determine what is wrong and what can be done about it. If your neurosurgeon deals with a lot of hydrocephalus patients, chances are that she will have the names and phone numbers for the best specialists in your area, and can also provide you with a referral.

Neuropsychological testing

Approximately one third of patients who are treated for hydrocephalus will attain a normal intelligence level (i.e., a mean score of between 80 and 100 points on an IQ test) or higher. These patients are more apt to be self-sufficient and capable of leading a normal life. They may, however, have other mental difficulties, including:

- Poor spatial relations.

- Short-term memory problems.

- Difficulty in concentration.
- Non-verbal learning disorder (NVLD).
- Problems with social skills.
- Difficulty processing complex language.
- Learning disabilities.
- Physical limitations and problems with coordination.

Long-term side effects can be caused by the condition itself or as a result of one or many operations on the brain. The sad thing is that many patients and their families aren't told about these side effects.

If you have a neuropsychological examination (neuro-psych exam, for short), the neuropsychologist can identify specific neurological deficits and learning or social disorders. Then, based on the results of the testing and examination, she can identify ways for you to relearn how to perform specific tasks to help make your daily life easier.

Although performed on both children and adults, neuro-psych exams are more commonly given to children. A neuro-psych exam can be given as a baseline, and then if there are difficulties after subsequent shunt revisions, the child can be retested and the scores compared with those of the baseline exam. Armed with the information from these tests, parents and educators can know when to make or change an individualized education plan.

Paying for the exam

Just getting in to see a neuropsychologist can be a battle in itself. A thorough neuropsychological examination can cost up to $2,000, particularly if the findings are reviewed with you afterwards. What an insurance company sees when a referral request for a neuro-psych exam is received is usually the word "psychologist." This makes claims reviewers think that the exam is to study the patient's psychological or mental health, which is untrue. Because most insurance companies don't recognize neuropsychological examinations as a form of treatment for hydrocephalus patients, the approval process may be very difficult.

> Our daughter's neurosurgeon recommended that she have a neuro-psychological exam following her last shunt revision. At first, the insurance company flat-out refused to cover the cost of the testing. It's been

four months now, and we're still going through the appeals process with them, but we're standing our ground because the outcome of the test could have a dramatic impact on Emily's future. If push comes to shove, we'll pay for it ourselves, but the way we look at it, if the neurosurgeon recommends a test, or series of tests, to help Emily recover from her surgery, then the insurance company should agree with the recommendation instead of playing games with our daughter's health.

Before making an appointment with a neuropsychologist, contact your insurance company and ask if your policy will cover the cost of the testing. If your medical insurance company refuses to pay for the neuro-psych exam, remind them that this is a medical evaluation specifically related to surgical problems, and not an exam of the patient's psychological or mental health. If they continue to deny you access to the examination, you could:

- Have your primary care physician (PCP), neurologist, and/or neurosurgeon contact your insurance company stating their reasons for recommending the exam.

- Write a letter of appeal. In your letter, ask them to reexamine their denial for treatment, and give valid reasons why this examination is important to long-term care. (See the section at the end of Chapter 10, *Insurance,* for sample appeal letters.)

Remember, neuropsychological testing should be included as a part of the care and treatment for hydrocephalus. Be firm with your insurance company about them covering the cost of the examination, and encourage your doctors to take part in the appeal process if one becomes necessary.

How do you benefit from the exam?

The results of a neuro-psych exam pinpoint the specific areas in which you have problems. Results can then be used:

- To help you develop strategies to maximize performance of various tasks.

- To help make you more conscious about the condition and its effects.

- For parents, to provide you with ammunition to deal with schools when developing an individualized education program for your child and to help in making realistic decisions regarding your child's educational needs.

- For adults, to help in making realistic career decisions.

Selecting a neuropsychologist

Time spent selecting a neuropsychologist is an investment in the future. Your neuropsychologist will help identify any deficits resulting from the condition or surgeries and will make specific, practical recommendations on how to address them. The neuro-psych exam will help you chart a course through life based on a clear understanding of strengths and weaknesses. For example, the report will be the basis on which you plan your child's education.

Before starting the neuro-psych exam, meet with or phone prospective neuropsychologists to ask the following questions:

- Are you licensed by the state? If so, what is your license number?
- Are you registered with the American Board of Professional Neuropsychology (ABPN) or the American Board of Clinical Neuropsychology?
- How long have you been in practice?
- Do you prefer to work with children or adults?
- How many hydrocephalus patients have you evaluated?
- How do you determine which tests to give the patient?
- After the testing has been completed, how will your findings be presented to us? Will we receive a written report? Will there be a follow-up session where we can go over your findings and recommendations?

Look for a neuropsychologist who has excellent credentials, an excellent reputation in your community, and experience in evaluating and examining the needs of people with hydrocephalus. At the end of the examinations, and after the neuropsychologist has had a chance to evaluate the data, you should receive:

- A written report or have the opportunity to talk with the neuropsychologist regarding the test results.
- A summary or a full report that details the findings of the neuropsychologist's recommendations.
- A review of that report at length.

What is a neuro-psych examination?

A neuro-psych exam involves a series of tests administered by a licensed neuropsychologist. Neuropsychology is a branch of psychology that focuses on the relationship between brain functioning and behavior. Testing is done to assess brain function, to predict outcomes, and to provide strategies to modify the outcome as needed.

The neuropsychological examination includes different phases. The exam usually begins with a thorough screening of medical records. The neuropsychologist will become familiar with the medical history, including:

- The types of operations performed.

- Complications that may have occurred during surgery.

- Any short- and long-term side effects specifically related to various operations and hydrocephalus.

- Physical problems which are attributable to hydrocephalus, including a lack of coordination, gait disorder, visual impairments, difficulty interpreting speech, and problems with hearing.

- Any medications used for other conditions such as seizures.

- Any other medical conditions.

Once the neuropsychologist has had an opportunity to review all the medical records, the next step is to meet with the family. During this consultation, the neuropsychologist will ask about some of the difficulties experienced on a day-to-day basis.

Results of the neuropsychological examination

Based on the results compiled from the tests, the neuropsychologist can make recommendations for rehabilitation. Some typical recommendations may include:

- Speech therapy to improve written, oral, and audible language comprehension.

- Physical therapy to help rehabilitate motor problems and improve coordination. Physical therapists can help patients by retraining them to coordinate the use of muscles and limbs which may have been weakened or have reduced functionality as a result of damage to the brain.

- Occupational therapy to help train or retrain patients in how to perform certain tasks to maximize independence in daily life.

- Social skills training to help patients learn how interact with other children and adults.

- Social support to help families cope with any short- and long-term care needs.

Believe it or not, it can be better to suffer brain damage as a child than later in life as an adult. This is because the neurons in the brain of a child can assume functions from damaged areas more easily than in an adult because the child's brain is still growing.

Eye and visual problems

Hydrocephalus can weaken the nerves that control eye muscles and visual responses, resulting in eye misalignments and loss of vision. Adults may experience double vision. Children may see double at first, but later develop a "lazy" eye if a prompt diagnosis and treatment isn't made. Additionally, eye and visual problems can occur slowly as ICP increases, and can also occur after a sudden decrease in ICP following a shunt placement or revision.

How the brain sees

Although the eyes are located in the front of the head, the part of the brain that interprets the images—the occipital lobe—is located at the back of the head. The images come in through the eyes, and the information travels along the optic nerves, through the brain, and into the occipital lobe. The occipital lobe translates information sent from the eyes so you know what you are looking at.

Four cranial nerves control eyesight and movements:

- **The optic nerve.** Also known as the second cranial nerve, the optic nerve is responsible for transmitting visual images from the eyes to the brain. The optic nerve is made up of approximately one million tiny fibers which receive information from the rod and cone cells of the retina.

- **The oculomotor nerve.** Also known as the third cranial nerve, the oculomotor nerve is responsible for controlling four of the six main muscles of the eye, as well as those of the upper eyelid. The fibers of the oculomotor nerve help control eye movements and reactions of the pupils to light. The oculomotor nerve is rarely affected by hydrocephalus alone, unless there are other problems within the central nervous system.

- **The trochlear nerve.** Also known as the fourth cranial nerve, the trochlear nerve is responsible for rotating the eyeball while at the same time turning it downward and from side to side.

- **The abducens nerve.** Also known as the sixth cranial nerve, the abducens nerve is responsible for controlling the lateral rectus muscle of each eye, which turns the eye outward, away from the nose.

These four nerves affect vision in different ways: controlling eye movements, helping to adjust pupil reactions, moving the eyelids, and transmitting the images to the occipital lobe. The way these four nerves are affected by hydrocephalus, however, is the same.

Each of these nerves must travel from the back of the eyeball, through the meninges, and into the brain. When ICP increases, the pressure can be transmitted to the eye nerves, causing visual and eye problems. The problem can be traced back to the individual or group of nerves that supply the eyes.

Symptoms

If left untreated for an extended period of time, visual impairment (including blindness) can be permanent, and eye misalignments become more complex to treat. Therefore, it is important to watch for symptoms associated with increased ICP which affect the eyes. These include:

- Grayed-out or fuzzy vision.
- Double vision (diplopia).
- A reduced field or loss of peripheral vision.
- Misaligned, lazy, or wandering eyes.
- Unstable, shaking eyes.
- Eyes in a downward gaze (mainly found in infants).

If you detect any of these signs and symptoms, contact an ophthalmologist or pediatric ophthalmologist as soon as possible.

Ophthalmologists

An ophthalmologist is a physician who specializes in the diagnosis and treatment of eye diseases and abnormalities. A neuro-ophthalmologist is an ophthalmologist who has additional training in neurology and specializes in treating visual problems that are caused by neurological conditions. Finding a neuro-ophthalmologist may necessitate a call to one of the larger teaching institutions, as the subspecialty is not found at every hospital center.

All patients who have hydrocephalus should have an annual examination by an ophthalmologist to monitor any changes in vision and to diagnose and treat them promptly.

Children who have hydrocephalus should be examined by a pediatric ophthalmologist. Pediatric ophthalmologists, like pediatricians, are specially trained to work with children and infants.

> *We were having an unusual eye involvement issue after a series of revisions. Shaun's eyelid would droop down whenever he had a headache. Our neurologist suggested we see a neuro-ophthalmologist. He was able to pinpoint that his droop, or ptosis, of the lid was due to a third nerve palsy that would just become more defined when he was not feeling well.*

Pediatric ophthalmologists use specialized methods to diagnose problems. For example, younger children are best tested using picture vision tests or by observing tracking behavior for small toys.

The ophthalmologist will look for the following when examining the eyes:

- Swelling of the optic nerve (papilledema).

- Eye misalignments (strabismus).

- Crossed eyes (esotropia) is the most common form of eye misalignments.

- Lazy eye (amblyopia). Amblyopia causes a reduction in vision but is reversible by patching the good eye to improve the lazy eye's condition.

- A reduction of color vision.

- Reduced or loss of peripheral vision (vision to one or both sides).

- Abnormal pupil reaction to light.

- Vision that is less than 20/20.

A reduction in vision is not always the earliest sign of hydrocephalus affecting the eye. Other parts of the eye exam are more sensitive in identifying early eye problems caused by hydrocephalus. Of particular importance to the ophthalmologist is the appearance of the optic nerve. The appearance of the optic nerve is evaluated with a three-dimensional view to look for any swelling or paleness, which would indicate that the optic nerve is damaged as a result of increased ICP.

If papilledema is present, it is a sure sign that the ICP is elevated. However, the absence of papilledema does not mean that the ICP is normal. Most patients with elevated ICP do not have papilledema.

Eye misalignments

Some children with hydrocephalus develop eye misalignments, or strabismus. Strabismus can force your child to assume a head posture with a tilt or turn in one direction to bring her other eye into focus with the misaligned eye. If she is learning to walk, she may be hindered by turning her chin downward or turning her head to the side to reduce double vision. To treat strabismus, your child's ophthalmologist will prescribe patching in an alternating fashion to eliminate double vision. If her eyes fail to realign following a shunt placement or revision, her ophthalmologist may need to perform surgery on the eye muscles to improve the alignment.

A reversible cause of poor vision called amblyopia can occur in children who are less than eight years old when one eye is favored due to strabismus or another cause. The ophthalmologist will try patching the good eye in an effort to get the brain to use the amblyopic eye.

A problem seen in some infants with hydrocephalus is that the eyes are turned downward, restricting the child from gazing upward ("sunsetting" of the eyes). Sunsetting of the eyes normally occurs before children are properly diagnosed and treated for hydrocephalus. A sudden reoccurrence of sunsetting may indicate that the shunt is not working properly.

Impaired vision

Trouble with seeing small items or objects in the peripheral field of view indicates that ICP is probably rising. Visit your ophthalmologist immediately so she can check out your current vision and compare it to the results from previous examinations. In these situations, prior baseline results enable the doctor to note subtle changes in vision or the early stages of increasing ICP.

Perceptual defects

It is fairly common for children with hydrocephalus to have difficulty naming objects, reading, or calculating math problems. An early step in evaluating perceptual defects in your child should include visual and hearing examinations. Your doctor can advise you about additional testing, including formal educational and developmental assessments offered through school or by a medical facility. Many hospitals provide developmental assessments or neuropsychological testing through their department of neurology or psychology.

Perceptual defects can add to a child's frustration at school or an adult's frustration in the workplace. Social situations can become awkward as well. However, these perceptual difficulties can be assessed, and strategies can be learned to compensate for them.

Seizures

When people hear the word "seizure," the first thing that usually comes to mind is a person lying on the ground, writhing with convulsions. However, seizure activity can range from staring off into space for a few seconds to loss of consciousness with convulsions. Numerous medical conditions cause seizures, and treatments exist to control or eliminate them.

What causes a seizure?

Some of the causes of seizures in persons with hydrocephalus are:

- Reaction to a drug.
- Buildup of scar tissue in the brain from operations and shunt revisions.
- Infections such as meningitis or encephalitis.
- Brain abnormalities.
- Increased ICP.
- Subdural hematoma (SDH).
- Brain tumors or cysts.

- Metabolic conditions, such as hypoglycemia (a deficiency of sugar in the bloodstream), hyperglycemia (too much sugar in the bloodstream), electrolyte imbalances, uremia (excessive amounts of urea, waste products produced by the kidneys, in the bloodstream), and fluid overloads.

Children and adults with hydrocephalus are at increased risk of seizures, particularly if there has been a complication (such as an intracranial hemorrhage) during a shunt placement or revision procedure. Whatever the cause of the seizures, they should be taken seriously—seek immediate medical attention.

Phases of a seizure

Although the causes of seizures vary, seizures themselves tend to follow a general pattern.

There are essentially four phases to a seizure:

- **The aura phase** indicates the onset of a seizure. During the aura phase, the patient may fall into sudden unconsciousness, experience localized muscle spasms (including involuntary jerking or shaking of one hand, forced turning of the head, etc.), a sense of fear, false sense of smell, or a feeling of déjà vu. The patient may or may not experience all of these sensations. Most people have identical auras before each seizure, helping them predict when a seizure is imminent.

- **The tonic phase** is when all of the muscles in the body become tense or rigid. Patients often make noises—grunts or a shrill cry—prior to losing consciousness. The tonic phase usually lasts from a few seconds to a few minutes.

- **The clonic phase**, which may or may not follow the tonic phase, is associated with loss of consciousness, convulsions, loss of bowel and bladder control, salivation or drooling, and irregular breathing and heart activity. The clonic phase of a seizure can last from 1 or 2 minutes to 30 minutes or more.

- **The postictal phase** follows a seizure. The patient may or may not regain consciousness during the postictal phase. If he regains consciousness, he will most likely be tired, confused, and unaware of what happened or where he is.

Seizures do not always include the four phases mentioned here. For instance, your child may experience only the aura phase followed by the postictal. Or she may go from aura to tonic or clonic (one or the other), and then to postictal.

Types of seizures: partial and generalized

There are two main types of seizures: partial and generalized. Partial seizures are caused by specific areas of the brain. With partial seizures, the physical response directly corresponds to a region in the brain where the problem lies. The right side of the brain affects the left side of the body, and vice versa, so if muscle spasms are on the right side of the body, the problem will lie in the left side of the brain. It is rare that a person who is having partial seizures will lose consciousness, although he may feel dazed or confused following the episode.

Partial seizures are further categorized as:

- Simple-partial. The person does not lose consciousness during the seizure.

- Complex-partial. The person will lose consciousness.

- Secondary-generalized. The onset of the seizure can be directly attributed to one part of the brain, which then triggers a generalized seizure.

Generalized seizures are more severe and involve both sides of the brain. They are accompanied by convulsions, muscle activity on both sides of the body, and loss of consciousness.

Symptoms associated with partial and generalized seizures

Symptoms	Type of Seizure	
	Partial	Generalized
Interference with motor activity (i.e., muscle spasms, shaking hands, etc.)	✓	✓
Confusion	✓	✓
Unfocused attention	✓	✓
Loss of consciousness		✓
Salivation or drooling		✓
Muscle constriction or tenseness (tonic phase)		✓
Bilateral convulsions (clonic phase)		✓

Symptoms associated with partial and generalized seizures (continued)

	Type of Seizure	
Symptoms	Partial	Generalized
Loss of bowel or bladder control		✓
Temporary amnesia (postictal phase)		✓

Diagnosis

Since seizures may indicate a deteriorating neurological condition, the condition should be evaluated immediately to determine the cause. Your doctor will try to find out what is causing the seizures and then determine a course of action for treating them. Tests that may be performed to determine the cause of seizures include:

- Blood tests check for hormone imbalances, hypoglycemia, or hyperglycemia.

- CT and MRI scans look for any intracranial abnormalities. These could include increased ventricular size, SDH, or tumor or cyst growth.

- A lumbar puncture (LP) or shunt tap looks for signs of infection, an increased white blood cell count, or decreased glucose (sugar) levels in the cerebrospinal fluid (CSF).

- An electroencephalogram (EEG) monitors brain waves to determine the area of the brain where the seizure is originating.

- ICP monitoring checks for elevations or fluctuations of ICP that could trigger the seizures.

Monitoring seizure activity

It is a good idea to keep a log book or record of your seizures to help your doctor properly diagnose and treat them. Information that you can include in a seizure log includes:

- Date and time of the seizure.

- Duration, or how long the seizure lasted.

- Notes about what happened during the seizure. This could include details about the aura, loss of consciousness, convulsions, temporary amnesia, and how you felt afterwards.

- Notes written by people present at the time of the seizure.

This information helps your neurologist determine the frequency and type of seizures and obtain a full picture of your seizure activity.

Treating seizures

Seizures are treated with drugs and, on rare occasions, surgery. Doctors can choose from a large arsenal of antiseizure medications for initial treatment of seizures. Surgery is reserved for unusually severe, intractable seizures or for those patients whose seizures do not respond to medication.

Questions to ask before taking antiseizure medication

Before you take any drug for seizures or give any to your child, ask the doctor for basic information, including:

- What is the dosage? How many times a day should it be given?
- What are the common and rare side effects?
- What should I do if any of the side effects occur?
- Will the drug interact with any over-the-counter drugs (e.g., Tylenol) or vitamins?
- What should I do if I forget a dose?
- What are both the trade and generic names for the medication?
- Should I buy the generic version?

Common side effects

Each of the antiseizure medications in this section have a long list of possible side effects. The following side effects are commonly found with these medications:

- Constipation.
- Diarrhea.
- Difficulty concentrating or processing thoughts.
- Dizziness.
- Drowsiness.
- Jaundice (yellowing of the eyes and skin).

- Lack of coordination.

- Loss of appetite.

- Nausea and/or vomiting.

- Skin abnormalities, including flaking, scaling, dryness, or the occurrence of red, blotchy spots which could indicate possible liver damage.

- Temporary hair loss.

- Weight loss or gain.

Check with your doctor and pharmacist for a complete list of side effects associated with any medication you are taking to control seizures. You can also look up side effects in the PDR (*Physician's Desk Reference*), located in the reference section of your local library. Online, the OnHealth site (*http://www.onhealth.com/*) has a pharmacy section that lists comprehensive information on more than 8,000 drugs.

Antiseizure medications

There are a variety of antiseizure medications on the market for treating seizures. Based on the test results and the type of seizures, your neurologist will determine the best drug or drug combination to help reduce the frequency of seizures. This section lists some of the common antiseizure medications, including information about possible drug interactions and side effects.

As with any medication, it is very important to take antiseizure medication as directed by your doctor. Contact your doctor immediately at the onset of any adverse symptoms from the medication. Be sure to ask your doctor what to do if you should forget to take a dose of your medication. Doubling up on the next dose can be harmful. If you forget to take more than one dose in a day, contact your doctor before taking the next scheduled dosage.

The following list tells you the commercial names of antiseizure medications if you know them by their generic names. After this list, specific information about each drug is given, with the drugs arranged alphabetically by their commercial names.

Generic	Commercial
acetazolamide	Diamox
carbamazepine	Tegretol (also Atretol, Epitol, Tegretol-XR)
clonazepam	Klonopin

Generic	Commercial
diazepam	Valium
ethosuximide	Zarontin
gabapentin	Neurontin
lamotrigine	Lamictal
phenobarbital	Phenobarbital (also Luminal, Solfoton)
phenytoin sodium	Dilantin
primidone	Mysoline
valproic acid	Depakene, Depakote

Depakene (dep-UH-keen); Depakote (dep-UH-coat)

Also called: Valproic acid.

How given: Tablets, taken with food if stomach irritation occurs.

Precaution: Liver damage is a possible risk of taking this medication. If you develop yellowing of the skin and eyes, loss of appetite, dizziness, drowsiness, weakness, and a general feeling of ill health, contact your doctor immediately.

> *The one side effect I had while taking Depakote is that I was losing my hair left and right. I was taking eight 500 mg tablets a day—at one time! But now I'm down to taking only two tablets a day and I'm not losing as much hair.*

· · · · ·

> *Depakote made Chris tired and moody. He gained a lot of weight as he ate more. He was so scrawny that this aspect was good. He's on Zarontin now, which seems to be much better—no side effects that we've noticed.*

Diamox (DYE-uh-mocks)

Also called: Acetazolamide.

How given: Tablets or capsules, taken orally.

Precaution: Diamox is a sulfur-based medication that can sometimes cause an allergic reaction, including development of a rash, bruises, sore throat, or fever. If these symptoms occur, continue taking your medication as prescribed and contact your doctor immediately.

Dilantin (dye-LAN-tin)

Also called: Phenytoin sodium.

How given: Tablets, capsules, or syrup taken orally.

Precaution: If you have been taking Dilantin on a regular basis, you should not stop taking this medication abruptly. Doing so can initiate a condition called *status epilepticus*—repeated or prolonged seizures with no recovery of consciousness between them. If not treated promptly, status epilepticus can be fatal. Another possible side effect of Dilantin is an overgrowth of gum tissues (known as gum hyperplasia).

> *The only antiseizure medication that gave me adverse side effects was Dilantin. Dilantin was the first seizure medicine I was on and it made my gums bleed. My dentist ordered that I be taken off it immediately.*

Klonopin (KLON-uh-pin)

Also called: Clonazepam.

How given: Tablets taken orally.

Lamictal (LAM-ic-tal)

Also called: Lamotrigine.

How given: Tablets taken orally.

Precaution: A rash may begin to form within the first 4 to 6 weeks of taking Lamictal, especially if taken in combination with Depakene. You should notify your doctor immediately if you begin to develop a rash.

Mysoline (MY-soh-leen)

Also called: Primidone.

How given: Tablets or syrup taken orally.

Precaution: Mysoline should not be taken if you are allergic to phenobarbital or if you have porphyria, a rare metabolic disorder that breaks down the red blood pigment hemoglobin.

Neurontin (NUHR-on-tin)

Also called: Gabapentin.

How given: Capsules taken orally.

Phenobarbital (fee-no-BAR-bi-tal)

Also called: Luminal, Solfoton.

How given: Tablets taken orally, or injection.

Precaution: Phenobarbital is a barbiturate, and can be addictive. Your body may become tolerant of the medication, requiring more of the drug to accomplish the same effect.

> *The way I reacted to the phenobarbital was just the opposite of how one is supposed to react to it. Instead of it calming me down, it made me really hyper.*

• • • • •

> *I was on phenobarbital from the time I was one week old until three or four years ago. The main side effect I had while on phenobarbital was drowsiness and a lack of concentration. As my body became accustomed to the dosage, those side effects wore off. During that time (from age 10 to 19), I had noticed an increased body odor. It didn't matter how much deodorant I wore, it was never enough to rid myself of the odor caused by the phenobarbital.*

Tegretol (TEG-re-tawl)

Also called: Carbamazepine; Atretol, Epitol, Tegretol-XR.

How given: Tablets or syrup taken orally with food.

Precautions: Tegretol should never be taken on an empty stomach. Tegretol increases the risk of liver and kidney disorders. Symptoms include fever, sore throat, dry mouth, reddish or purplish spots on the skin, and bruises. If any of these symptoms appear, contact your doctor immediately.

I was placed on Tegretol for a few years. Slowly but surely it adversely affected me. One Saturday we were at a large mall and I started walking like a drunk and started showing the first signs of a shunt malfunction.

Later that day, my husband convinced me to go to the emergency room. By the time they got around to doing an MRI and a real live doctor came to see me, the medication had worn off and I was doing a lot better. However, my neurosurgeon would not let me quit taking the medication— which both my husband and I knew was the cause of all the problems.

While on Tegretol, I got lost (more than usual). I couldn't concentrate, I had bad headaches, nausea—you name the side effect, I had it. My neurosurgeon finally switched me to Depakote, and all the bad things went away.

I have no ill effects (although I know it is very hard on your liver, so my blood is checked every three months). The one thing I have noticed is that it helps with the partial seizures and keeps my mind intact. I just wish it could help me regain some of my short-term memory.

Valium (VAL-ee-um)

Also called: Diazepam.

How given: Tablets taken orally.

Precaution: Valium is addictive. When taken as an antiseizure medication, Valium must be taken at the same time every day.

Zarontin (zar-ON-tin)

Also called: Ethosuximide.

How given: Capsules or syrup, taken orally.

Surgery

Surgery is reserved for unusually severe seizures that do not respond to medication. On occasion, seizures may be caused by a tumor or cyst. In those instances, surgery would be performed to remove the mass. Once treated, the patient will be closely monitored following surgery to see if removal of the mass has stopped the seizures from occurring.

Other surgical procedures are used as a last resort for treating seizures that are not responsive to drugs. For example, temporal resection surgery removes a portion of the temporal lobe to treat patients who have focal seizures (seizures restricted to a particular region of the brain).

First aid for seizures

Most people don't know what to do to help when someone near them has a seizure. The myth that someone having a seizure may "swallow his tongue" is physically impossible. Because of this myth, people tend to do more harm than good by trying to force something in the mouth of the person having a seizure to hold his tongue down.

The following are some dos and don'ts for helping a person who is having seizures. (You might want to photocopy this list for people who are likely to be nearby when a seizure occurs, such as neighbors or baby-sitters.)

What you should do

- If you do not know the medical history of the person having the seizure, check for an emergency medical identification bracelet or necklace.

- If you know the person and know they haven't had seizures before, send someone to call for emergency medical assistance (911).

- Make note of the time the seizure begins and how long it lasts. This information should be given to emergency medical professionals or the person's doctor.

- Try to protect the person from falling down if he loses consciousness. When he first starts to notice the aura, have the person lie or sit down on the floor in an area that is safe.

- Move any hard or sharp objects away from the person having the seizure.

- Surround the person with pillows, blankets, or cushions, if available. If possible, try to place some type of padding beneath the person's head to protect him from injury.

- Try to loosen any tight clothing the person may be wearing, including belts, ties, and shirt collars.

What you shouldn't do

- Do not attempt to place anything between the person's teeth or in his mouth during the seizure—especially your fingers or anything metallic. The person having the seizure might clench his teeth or bite down unexpectedly, causing harm not only to himself, but to you as well.

- Don't hold the person down or try to restrain him during the seizure. This could place both you and the person having the seizure at risk of injury.

- Do not attempt to move the person, unless he is near something immovable that could cause harm or injury to him.

- Do not yell at or get angry with the person having the seizure. Understand that he has no control over what his body is doing; getting upset with him will only make him feel worse afterward.

When to call for help

Since most seizures last for only one to two minutes, it isn't necessary to call for emergency medical services (EMS) personnel immediately. However, if the seizure lasts more than a few minutes, or if the person has one seizure after another, you should send someone to call EMS (911 in most states and provinces) immediately.

You should also call EMS:

- If the person has been injured.
- If the person is pregnant or suspected to be pregnant.
- If the person has diabetes.
- If the person is an infant or child.
- If the person fails to resume consciousness following the seizure.

Precocious puberty

Precocious, or early, puberty is a disorder that causes some children to go into puberty prematurely. Although precocious puberty is rare in the general population, it can be fairly common in children between the ages of 5 and 13 years old who have hydrocephalus, myelomeningoceles, cerebral palsy, and microcephaly. It affects both males and females, but occurs more often in girls than boys.

> Linda started developing at about five years old. She is nine years old now, and she is showing signs of hormones—PMS. When it first started to happen I thought she was going through shunt malfunction. I believe that it also affects her shunt. She also has hair (pubic and under her arms) coming in, and her breasts are developing now. She has not, however, gotten her period.

What causes precocious puberty?

Precocious puberty is presumed to be caused by ICP. This increase in pressure can cause damage to the hypothalamus and the pituitary gland, which are responsible for timing the release of gonadotropins and sex hormones into the bloodstream.

Precocious puberty has been linked to the number of shunt revisions a child has prior to reaching the normal age of puberty (10 to 15 years old for girls and 12 to 18 years old for boys). Young children are at greater risk of experiencing precocious puberty if they have had numerous shunt revisions related to increased ICP.

Symptoms

The symptoms of precocious puberty are easy for parents to recognize, as children will begin to develop sexually at an age much earlier than their peers. Girls experience early breast development, menstruation, growth of pubic and body hair, an increase in weight caused by muscle development, and an increase in hip size. Boys experience growth of facial, body, and pubic hair, development of the penis and testes, deepening of the voice, and an increase in weight caused by muscle development.

If you begin to notice these changes in your child, you should make an appointment with your primary care physician (PCP). After examination by your PCP, your child should be referred to see a pediatric endocrinologist, who will order blood tests to check for increased hormone levels in the bloodstream.

Precocious puberty is also responsible for shutting down the growth plates of the bones, causing short stature. The pediatric endocrinologist may order an X-ray of your child's hand to see if your child's bones are aging too quickly.

If caught early enough, precocious puberty can be suppressed by treating the condition with hormone suppressants.

Diabetes insipidus

Diabetes insipidus is an extremely rare form of diabetes that is unrelated to diabetes mellitus (commonly known as "sugar diabetes"). Diabetes insipidus is caused when the secretion of the hormone vasopressin is inadequate, or when the kidneys don't respond to stimulation by the hormone. Vasopressin (also known as the antidiuretic hormone, or ADH) is the hormone that regulates fluid reabsorption by the kidneys.

Many of the same conditions that cause or accompany hydrocephalus can also cause damage to the hypothalamus or the pituitary gland, which produces the hormone vasopressin. Those causes include:

- Meningitis.
- Head trauma.
- Brain tumors.
- Increased ICP.

Symptoms and tests

People who have diabetes insipidus often complain of constant thirst (polydypsia), and frequent urination (polyuria), particularly at night.

> I have always gotten up in the middle of the night to go pee, but since my last shunt revision, it was getting much worse—as frequent as six or

seven times a night. My sleep was getting disrupted and I always seemed to be tired throughout the day.

Another common symptom for diabetes insipidus is abdominal bloating. People with diabetes insipidus often complain of having a swollen abdomen at night before bedtime, which disappears by morning.

> *It was awful. I do about 100 sit-ups a day, and I always seem to be bloated. There were some nights where I would look like I was three or four months pregnant before going to bed. Then by morning, I'd have a flat tummy again! I would notice that by midday my tummy would start bloating again. It was embarrassing.*

Additional symptoms include dry hands and constipation.

Your doctor or endocrinologist has several methods to diagnose diabetes insipidus. A CT or MRI scan of the head is done to evaluate the pituitary gland. A simple blood test can identify the level of vasopressin in your bloodstream. Another test that can be performed is a water-deprivation test. You will be asked to drink a normal amount of water throughout the day, then medical staff will weigh you frequently over several hours to check on water retention. Any urine you produce will be tested. During the test, your blood will be drawn every hour for several hours to check the vasopressin levels in your bloodstream.

Treatment

If you are diagnosed with diabetes insipidus, your endocrinologist will prescribe desmopressin, a drug more commonly referred to by its trade name, DDAVP. DDAVP is usually prescribed as a nasal spray, but is also available as nose drops and in tablet form. The nasal spray is sprayed into each nostril prior to going to bed and, if needed, in the morning as well. As with all medications, check with your doctor or pharmacist about the proper use and dosage, and be sure to ask if there are any possible drug interactions.

DDAVP

Also called: Desmopressin acetate.

How given: Nasal spray, nose drops, or tablets.

How it works: Prevents or controls frequent urination or loss of water associated with diabetes insipidus by supplementing ADH.

Common side effects: Headache, nausea, mild abdominal cramps, stuffiness or irritation to the nose, flushing.

Infrequent side effects: Nosebleeds, sore throat or cough, upper respiratory infection, cold symptoms (runny nose, chills, etc.), conjunctivitis (pinkeye), depression, dizziness, an inability to produce tears, development of a rash on the legs, swelling around the eyes, and weakness or fatigue.

Possible drug interactions:

- Any drug used to increase blood pressure.
- Clofibrate (Atromid-S).
- Glyburide (Micronase).
- Epinephrine (EpiPen).

CHAPTER 8

Finding Support

For all loss, you have an equal opportunity to
gain: closer relationships, more poignant
appreciations, clarified values. [By choosing]
how we experience illness, we can become
more than victims.

—Arthur W. Frank
At the Will of the Body

THE EMOTIONAL STRAIN OF LIVING WITH HYDROCEPHALUS can be immense and at times devastating. The financial burden in itself can be a crushing responsibility. Dealing with uncertainty and stress—from arranging transportation to finding someone who understands—can be a major hardship.

Support during an illness can come from many different resources: friends and family, church members, the neurosurgical team, support groups, and books. These support systems can help you cope with disruptions in your daily life. You are not alone. There is always someone to whom you can turn for emotional support.

In this chapter, we talk about various sources of support, including support groups for parents and children, support organizations, counselors, hydrocephalus conventions, and online support groups. We also provide tips on how to organize a support group if one cannot be found in your area.

Why support is needed

You will probably need support more during times of increased stress—a new diagnosis, changes in your life, medical emergencies, or chronic shunt revisions. Emotions that people with hydrocephalus, or their family and friends, might feel are many:

- Disbelief at a condition that came out of the blue, or perhaps when a healthy birth or simple illness was expected.

- Guilt because you feel maybe it is your fault that your child has hydrocephalus even though you know you're not to blame.

- Anger because you are tired, you've had no sleep for days, you're not getting answers from the medical team, and all you want is for your loved one to get better.

- Isolation, feeling like you are the only one going through this right now, and not knowing where to turn for help.

- Shock when you learn that hydrocephalus has no cure and is a lifelong condition that you will need to cope with forever.

- Despair because you are worn out and feel you just can't go on any more.

- Frustration because you've just experienced three shunt revisions in less than two months and you just want to get on with your life.

- Resentment because you see other people leading a "normal" life, and want to do the same, but feel that you can't.

- Fear because you don't know what the future may hold.

Hydrocephalus is a condition that can place great demands on people who love the patient:

- Parents are constantly on "heightened alert," not letting themselves relax, watching for possible complications with a shunt that could malfunction at any time.

- Brothers and sisters are separated from their parents, and they see their sibling having difficulty trying to lead a normal life while going in and out of the hospital; siblings may wonder if the next time they might not return.

- Friends who were once close may pull away for fear of what may happen, and only after they know all is well do they emerge again.

> *I found that I have good friends who stay by us and support us through all of this. There are some friends who do shy away, but I think it is out of fear of outcome or unknown outcome. I rely on my good friends and don't worry about the others.*

Sometimes you might feel all alone.

I feel like I went through finding out about my daughter's condition and her surgeries (four in five weeks!) all on my own. My husband didn't handle it well, looking at her in the lethargic state (she is only one year old) when she was previously so active. My parents wanted to pretend that it wasn't that bad. That is, until they saw her and totally lost it. My friends—even my best ones—couldn't even talk about it. They said they were too scared about what was going on.

I remember crying alone in my room and wishing there was someone there to tell me it was going to be okay rather than me telling everyone else she would be fine. My husband and I did nothing but fight. From the lack of support, I felt my whole mental state was becoming numb to anyone who made a remark about Michaela's progress or lack of it. It wasn't until Christmas time that people started expressing how strong a person I was—how did I handle all that? I had no choice—everyone else was afraid to handle it and then who would be there for Michaela?

But the experience was good for me internally. It made me think about what is really important in life and not to take a minute for granted. It also taught me that I am much stronger than I ever gave myself credit for, and that it is okay to cry by yourself. You are the only one who can heal yourself. In my short life (I am 25 years old) I think I have experienced more than many do in a lifetime. I am not angry for the way people handle their emotions. And now I know I can do anything!

When things go bad—for yourself, your child or spouse, or a close friend or family member—you need to know there is a place you can turn to for support. No matter how you deal with stress, having sources of support is key. Support comes in many forms. It's okay to admit that you need help, and when you do, to go out and find it.

Sources of support

Usually the people closest to you can offer the best support. Support can be emotional—being there to talk, or lending a shoulder to cry on—or physical—taking care of things like grocery shopping or walking your dog. If you can rely on people you know—family, friends, and coworkers—to take on one task each, your life will be a little less stressful. Others will gain comfort in knowing that they've helped you when you needed it the most.

Friends and family

Friends and family members are usually eager to offer assistance. It is important to let them help you. Allowing family members or friends to run errands gives you a chance to rest or recuperate. For example, when you are overwhelmed by the stresses of your child's condition, friends and family might help by:

- Baby-sitting your other children whenever you take your child to a doctor's appointment, the emergency room, or during prolonged hospital stays.

- Helping out with household chores, such as cleaning, cooking meals, doing laundry, and taking care of pets.

- Taking care of your other children by taking them to the park, a sporting event, or a movie; inviting them over for meals; helping them with homework; driving them to lessons, games, or school.

It's important to have caring individuals around you. They can help care for you as well as have true compassion for what you are going through.

> I am fortunate that I have a very supportive family that lives close to us. When Shaun is in the hospital, I feel torn. I need to be with him and I need to be at home with our two other boys. My husband and I have large families and between them, someone is always there to care for the boys at home. They have continued to support us unconditionally for six years now, and without them, this struggle with hydrocephalus would be so much more difficult.

· · · · ·

> I knew that something was wrong with Mike when I hadn't heard from him in a few days. When he answered the phone, his voice was shaky, and it was obvious that he was under a great deal of stress. Immediately, I thought that there was trouble in paradise, but when he told me that his fiancée had been admitted to the hospital two days earlier for another shunt revision, I told him to stay where he was, and that I'd be right over.

*When I got to his place, I could see that he hadn't slept in a while,
and that his place needed to be cleaned up. I told him to get some rest,
and then got busy washing dishes and straightening up around the place.
By the time he woke up, he looked rested, and relieved that he didn't have
to clean up before going to the hospital to see Katie.*

Neighbors

When a crisis strikes, your neighbors can help out by taking care of your
children, pets, or everyday household chores.

*Aside from family, our greatest source of support was our neighbors.
They all knew that Emily had hydrocephalus and helped keep an eye on
her when she would play with their children. When she needed a revision
last year, our neighbors pitched in by helping out with yard work, like
mowing the lawn and tending to our garden, as well as making sure that
we never had to cook a meal.*

• • • • •

*Our next door neighbors were very helpful with taking our other
children to school and to soccer. They let their kids take turns walking our
dog and feeding our fish. But the best thing they did was simply to be
there for us to talk to when we weren't at the hospital.*

Coworkers

Most people can usually count on at least one person at work to be a source
of support.

*When the doctors thought Jonathan was having trouble with his
shunt, I was anywhere but at work. Between running him around for tests
at one hospital, to an imaging center at another, and then to the neurosurgeon, neuro-ophthalmologist, and back to the neurosurgeon again, I had
little time for work. I knew my work was piling up, but when I went into
work, everyone in my department had pitched in to take care of things for
me. I went to my supervisor to thank her for taking care of this for me,
and she said that she had nothing to do with it; everyone else jumped in
and picked up my slack without a word being said or anyone being asked.
I was really touched by their generosity.*

Hospital social workers

While the need for skilled pediatric social workers is widely recognized, shrinking hospital budgets often prevent adequate staffing. If you bring your child to a children's hospital that's well staffed with social workers, child-life specialists, and psychologists, consider yourself lucky. Sadly, millions of dollars are spent on technology, while programs that help people cope emotionally are often the first to be discarded. If your pediatric center doesn't offer support, explore other methods to get help in dealing with the emotional stresses that hydrocephalus often brings.

Pediatric social workers usually have a master's degree in social work with additional training in neuropsychology and pediatrics. They serve as guides through unfamiliar territory by mediating between doctors and families, helping with emotional or financial problems, locating resources, and easing patients back into their daily routines. Many social workers form close, long-lasting bonds with families and children, and continue to answer questions and provide support long after treatment ends.

In addition to social workers, some hospitals have on-staff child-life specialists, psychiatric nurses, psychiatrists, psychiatric residents, and psychologists who can help families deal with problems during hospitalization.

Even if you have had hydrocephalus for years, support can still be needed.

> *Part of my daily recovery while in the hospital was to talk with a psychologist about my anxieties and how to deal with them. I know it sounds vain, but I was really concerned about what people at work would think of me when I returned with a partially shaved head. I was afraid they would make fun of me, just like the kids did when I was in elementary school. Meeting with the on-staff psychologist helped me work through this issue and others.*

Support groups

Support groups counter the social isolation often experienced by people with hydrocephalus. The sense of joining with others who struggle with the same problems is also a therapeutic tool. Support groups should not be misconstrued as a substitute for medical treatment, but rather as a complement to medical treatment.

Families often join support groups to talk with other people who share the same problems and concerns. Having a base of people who are in a similar situation is a great source of comfort. In many cases, support groups offer a safe place where you can let down your guard with other people who understand what you are going through.

Support groups for parents

Support groups fill the void left by withdrawal or misunderstanding of family or friends. Parents in similar circumstances can share practical information learned through personal experience, provide emotional support, give hope for the future, and truly listen to your concerns. Coping with hydrocephalus requires perspective—the ability to accept the gravity of the situation while not blowing it out of proportion. In support groups, many families find this frame of reference, for there are always those with more severe problems than yours, as well as families whose children are thriving. Just meeting people who are living with the same condition is profoundly reassuring. Many people find comfort in formal support groups, while others get support from informal groups.

> *This experience with hydrocephalus has been very difficult and emotionally draining. When my husband and I joined a local support group for hydrocephalus we suddenly realized we were not alone. Like us, others were going through the same ups and downs, motions and emotions that we were. I truly believe out of everything that we perceive as bad comes something good. We've made some special friends through the group. One couple lives just a few miles from us and we get together now on a regular basis. Their child has hydrocephalus too, and the kids love to play together.*

Hydrocephalus can be a very isolating experience. When you or your child is in the hospital for a shunt placement or revision, there probably won't be another person in the same facility undergoing the same operation. In times like these, you may feel as if you have nowhere to turn, but there are always options. Look around you. In the hospital, many people are having critical operations every day. The operations may not be the same operation your daughter just had, but chances are, other people are also looking for someone they can talk to.

If you do find someone else who is dealing with hydrocephalus, either in or out of the hospital, you will probably have much to talk about. You can compare notes about the procedure being performed, and offer and receive advice and support from someone who knows what you are going through. You will be able to understand each other's feelings and emotions because you will be sharing the same experience. The understanding of a mother, father, spouse, or sibling of a patient with hydrocephalus cuts across all social, economic, and racial barriers.

Greg Tocco, executive director of the Hydrocephalus Foundation, explains how HyFI came to be:

> Approximately eight months after getting out of the rehabilitation hospital, I embarked on creating the Hydrocephalus Foundation, Inc., (HyFI) as a way to "give back" the support and resources to others with hydrocephalus. During 1995, I underwent eight surgical procedures and made my recovery in a rehabilitation hospital. It was a lot of hard work to get back to the physical and cognitive level that I am at now and it could never have been done without my family and friends.
>
> HyFI has been a tremendous support mechanism for both others and myself. It has definitely expanded my family and friends. Born out of the firsthand knowledge of the ramifications of being hydrocephalic, HyFI was created out of love, persistence, and the desire to assist others with hydrocephalus.

In addition to national support organizations like the Hydrocephalus Association and the Hydrocephalus Foundation, Inc. (HyFI), there are dozens of different types of support groups, ranging from those with hundreds of members and formal bylaws, to three moms who meet once a week for coffee. Some groups deal only with the emotional aspects of hydrocephalus, while others may focus on education, advocacy, social opportunities, or crisis intervention. Some groups are facilitated by trained mental health professionals, while others are self-help groups made up of a few families who get together for outings. And, naturally, as older members drop out and new families join, the needs and interests of the group may shift.

> Our support group grew from four parents and two children, to nearly thirty people over the span of a couple years. The age of people in the group with hydrocephalus ranged from newborns to adults in their mid-30s. As time passed, some people left the group for various reasons.

New people would join because they heard of us through the children's hospital or through their neurosurgeons. The way we look at it, it's not the number of people in your group that counts, but the fact that everyone is joining together to share information and comfort each other.

Support groups for children

Many pediatric or children's hospitals have ongoing support groups for children with a range of life-threatening conditions. Often, these are run by experienced pediatric social workers, who know how to balance fun with sharing feelings. For many children, these groups are the only place where they feel completely accepted—where most of the other kids have shaved heads or are in the hospital for critical care needs such as cancer. The group is a place where children or adolescents can say how they really feel without worrying if they are causing their parents more pain. Many children form wonderful and lasting friendships in peer groups.

Check with your neurosurgeon, pediatrician, or a hospital social worker to see what groups are available in your area. There are also organizations that hold workshops or have other programs in which children communicate with each other.

For example, the Center for Attitudinal Healing (CAH), located just north of San Francisco, is a nonprofit, nonsectarian group, founded by a child psychiatrist, that sponsors a program for children with catastrophic or life-threatening diseases and conditions. Siblings are also welcome. They use music and art in a loving, supportive program to help children ages 6 to 16 share their feelings about their situations. CAH also sponsors local and national workshops, and publishes several excellent books. Should you desire further information, contact:

The Center for Attitudinal Healing
Diane Cirincione, Outreach Consultant
33 Buchanan Drive
Sausalito, CA 94965
Phone: (415) 331-6161
Fax: (415) 331-4545
Email: *cah@well.com*
http://www.healingcenter.org/

For children who are too ill or shy to join a group, there are alternatives. They can use computers to contact and chat with other kids in similar situations. See "Support on the Internet" later in this chapter for a listing of some of the more popular hydrocephalus groups.

Another way for children to communicate with other children in similar circumstances is to contact:

Children's Hopes and Dreams Foundation
280 Rt. 46
Dover, NJ 07801
Phone: (800) I-DREAM-2 (437-3262), or (201) 361-7366
Fax: (201) 361-6627
http://www.thefamilyplace.org/hopes.html

Children's Hopes and Dreams Foundation has been fulfilling "dreams" for children with life-threatening illness since 1983. The program provides dreams throughout the United States, as well in 37 foreign countries. There are no residence or illness boundaries when fulfilling a dream. This organization operates a free, worldwide pen-pal program for children ages 5 to 17 with disabilities and chronic or life-threatening illnesses. They will gladly send free enrollment cards to parents, social workers, teachers, nurses, or any other interested person.

If you would like your child to receive letters and gifts to provide emotional support, contact:

Love Letters, Inc.
P.O. Box 416875
Chicago, IL 60641
Phone: (630) 620-1970
Email: lletters01@aol.com
http://www.loveletters.org/

Founded in 1984, Love Letters provides emotional support to children dealing with long-term or catastrophic illness. Love Letters is a free, confidential service started by a mother whose son died of cancer. It is not a pen-pal organization; confidentiality is guaranteed. It is run by a group of volunteers who wish to bring some happiness into the lives of ill children by sending them letters, cards, and gifts. They send out 4,000 pieces of mail monthly.

Support groups for siblings

Many hospitals have reacted to the growing awareness of siblings' natural concerns and worries by creating hospital visiting days for them. This not only allows one-on-one parent time for brothers and sisters, but also gives them the opportunity to explore and become familiar with the hospital environment. Sibling days allow interaction with staff, a time to have questions answered and concerns addressed. Some hospital staffs have expanded these one-day programs into ongoing support groups, aimed not just at siblings who are having "problems," but also at improving communication, education, and support for all siblings.

Parent-to-parent programs

Some pediatric hospitals, in conjunction with parent support groups, have developed parent-to-parent visitation programs. The purpose of these visits is for veteran parents to provide one-on-one support for newly diagnosed families. The services provided by the veteran parent can be informational, emotional, or logistical. The visiting parent can:

- Empathize with the parents of a newly diagnosed child.

- Help notify family and friends of the situation at hand and explain any details about the condition to them.

- Help overcome loneliness.

- Ease feelings of isolation.

- Provide tours of the hospital and introduce the parents to some of the nurses and hospital staff.

- Write down parents' questions for the medical team.

- Advise parents on sources for financial assistance.

- Explain unfamiliar medical terms and procedures in terms that are easy to comprehend.

- Be available by phone or email for any problems that arise.

- Supply lots of smiles, hugs, and, most of all, hope.

If your child is newly diagnosed, ask if your hospital has a parent-to-parent program. If not, ask to speak to the parent leader of the local support group. Often, this person will ask a veteran parent to visit you at the hospital. Many veteran parents are more than willing to visit, as they know only too well what those first weeks in the hospital are like. They are often accompanied by their child, who may have recently recovered from a shunt placement or revision procedure, full of energy and a beacon of hope.

Our son was diagnosed in utero as having hydrocephalus. Before my obstetrician said that word to me, I'd never heard it before. Fortunately, he knew of another couple in the area whose daughter was diagnosed in utero as well, only two years earlier. My obstetrician called them on our behalf and shortly thereafter, they called us and we met. As first-time parents, it was good to meet someone else who experienced a similar situation, and to see their beautiful daughter laugh and play. That meeting gave us great hope for our son's future.

Clergy

Religion is a source of strength for many people. Many parents and children find that their faith is strengthened by their ordeal with hydrocephalus, while some begin to question their beliefs. Others who have not relied on religion in the past sometimes turn to it now.

My parents aren't very religious people, but when they learned that our daughter was in the hospital again for another revision, they went to the Catholic church closest to their home and asked for our daughter to be placed on their prayer list. When they told us this, we began to cry because we thought at first that meant they were losing hope for their granddaughter. But that wasn't the case. They felt that pulling the community together to pray for our daughter would help us all in this time of need—and it did.

Many hospitals have staff chaplains who are available for counseling, religious services, prayer, and other types of spiritual guidance. Often, the chaplain visits families soon after diagnosis and is available on an on-call basis. As with any mental health encounter, some approaches that work well with one family are not welcome with others.

After my wife had her shunt revised, she was comatose for nearly four days. One morning, after I had fallen asleep in the ICU next to her bed, the hospital chaplain came into the room and wanted to speak to me about what had happened to her. I was drained emotionally and physically, and the only people I had been speaking to were close friends and family. Everyone was concerned that she might die or never come out of her coma. But the chaplain helped to give me hope that I thought didn't exist.

Parents who were members of a church or a synagogue prior to the diagnosis of their child's hydrocephalus often draw great comfort from the clergy and members of their home church. Members of the congregation usually rally around the family, providing meals, child care, prayers, and support. Regular visits from the priest, minister, or rabbi provide spiritual sustenance throughout the initial crisis and subsequent years of treatment.

Support organizations

There are a number of national and international support organizations for hydrocephalus. These organizations can offer you and your family access to many things, including:

- Contact information for hydrocephalus support groups in your area.

- Basic information about hydrocephalus and how it is treated.

- Updates on new technological advances or treatments.

- Names, addresses, phone/fax, and sometimes email addresses for adult and pediatric neurosurgeons in your area.

- Information about emotional and financial support.

- Monthly or quarterly newsletters with information about hydrocephalus.

Some organizations that provide information and support for families are listed below. Contact information for the groups, including phone, fax, email, and web addresses (where available), is listed in Appendix B, *Associations and Organizations*.

- **Association for Spina Bifida and Hydrocephalus (ASBAH)**. ASBAH was formed in 1966 and serves England, Wales, and Northern Ireland. Through a network of professional advisers backed up by specialists in mobility, continence management, education, and medical matters, ASBAH provides advice and practical support to people with these disabilities, their families, and their care providers. ASBAH aims to improve services for people with spina bifida and/or hydrocephalus, to work with them to extend their choices, and to maximize opportunities for independence and achievement.

- **The Brain Tumor Society (TBTS)**. The Brain Tumor Society exists to find a cure for brain tumors. It strives to improve the quality of life of brain tumor patients and their families. It disseminates educational information and provides access to psychosocial support. It raises funds to advance carefully selected scientific research projects, improve clinical care, and find a cure.

- **Hydrocephalus Association**. The Hydrocephalus Association is a non-profit organization founded in 1983 that provides support, education, and advocacy to individuals, families, and professionals. They publish and distribute a wealth of resource materials, including *About Hydrocephalus: A Book for Parents; About Normal Pressure Hydrocephalus: A Book for Adults and Their Families; Directories of Pediatric Neurosurgeons and Neurosurgeons for Adult Onset Hydrocephalus;* and more than a dozen fact sheets on a variety of topics, including *Primary Care Needs of Children with Hydrocephalus, Learning Disabilities in Children with Hydrocephalus, Eye Problems Associated with Hydrocephalus, Headaches and Hydrocephalus,* and others. Their services include one-to-one support by trained parents; LINK Program, a nationwide network of individuals and families listed in directory format; a college scholarship awarded annually to a young adult with hydrocephalus; and a biannual National Conference for families and professionals.

- **Hydrocephalus Foundation, Inc. (HyFI)**. The Hydrocephalus Foundation was established to assist patients and their families during the transition from their diagnosis to a resumption of their normal lifestyles. The primary focus of HyFI is to contribute emotional support to patients of hydrocephalus and their families. The foundation promotes and encourages research that assists in the comprehensive treatment of people with hydrocephalus, and training of competent professionals.

- **Hydrocephalus Support Group, Inc. (HSG)**. The Hydrocephalus Support Group, Inc., is a 501(c)3 tax-exempt, nonprofit organization that was founded in 1987 by Deborah Buffa, mother of two daughters with hydrocephalus, and Diane Williams, R.N., M.S.N. A quarterly newsletter is provided, parent referrals are offered, and they maintain a library of more than 200 articles and tapes. The group also sponsors an annual conference on hydrocephalus in St. Louis. Goals of the group are education, information, and support.

- **International Federation for Hydrocephalus and Spina Bifida (if)**. The International Federation for Hydrocephalus and Spina Bifida is the worldwide umbrella organization for these two disabilities and has a contact on the Internet on every continent. Its members are national organizations for spina bifida and hydrocephalus in more than 30 countries that support people with spina bifida and hydrocephalus in their daily lives.

- National Hydrocephalus Foundation (NHF). The National Hydrocephalus Foundation was incorporated in 1980 as a voluntary, nonprofit, 501(c)3, public service organization. The objectives of NHF are to assemble and disseminate information pertaining to hydrocephalus, its treatments, and outcomes; to establish and facilitate a communication network among affected families and individuals; to help others gain a deeper understanding of those areas affected by hydrocephalus, such as education, insurance, tax and estate planning, employment, and family; to increase public awareness and knowledge of hydrocephalus; and to promote and support research on the causes, treatment, and prevention of hydrocephalus.

  In addition to providing the public with informational pamphlets, NHF maintains a reference library and videos on hydrocephalus, promotes and helps support groups, and offers parent-to-parent and adult-to-adult referrals. NHF also issues a quarterly newsletter, *Life-Line.*

Individual and family counseling

When hydrocephalus is initially diagnosed or problems with an existing shunt are detected, the condition can create a crisis of major proportions in even the strongest of families. You do not need to face this crisis alone and unassisted. Many find it helpful to seek out sensitive, objective, mental health care professionals to explore the difficult feelings—fear, anger, depression, anxiety, resentment, guilt, isolation—that hydrocephalus arouses. Family responsibilities and authority undergo profound changes when a child or spouse is initially diagnosed with hydrocephalus or is in need of a shunt revision. Sometimes members of the family have difficulty adjusting to the changes. While some families discuss the uncomfortable changes and feelings openly and agree on how to proceed, many need help.

Seeking professional counseling is a sign of strength, not weakness. In dealing with hydrocephalus, problems often become too complex for families to deal with on their own. Seeking advice sends children a message that the parents care about what is happening to them and want to help face it together.

One of the first questions that arises is, "Who should we talk to?" There are a number of resource people in the community who can make referrals and valuable recommendations, including:

- Your neurosurgeon or neurologist.

- Your pediatrician.

- A nurse practitioner.

- A clinical social worker.

- Your school psychologist or counselor.

- A health department social worker.

- Other parents who have sought counseling.

- Human resources representatives at work.

Ask each of the above for a short list of mental health professionals who have experience working with your issues. Generally, the names of the most well-respected clinicians in the community will appear on several of the lists.

In making your decision, it helps to understand the different levels of training and education of the various types of mental health professionals. You will be able to choose from individuals trained in one of these four related areas:

- Psychology (Ed.D., M.A., Ph.D., Psy.D.). Marriage and family psychotherapists have a master's degree, clinical and research psychologists have a doctorate (in some states, the use of the title "psychologist" may also be allowed for those with only a master's degree).

- Social work (M.S.W., D.S.W., Ph.D.). Clinical social workers have either a master's degree or a doctorate in a clinically emphasized program.

- Pastoral Care (M.A., M.Div., D.Min., Ph.D., D.Div.). Laymen or members of the clergy who receive specialized training in counseling.

- Medicine (M.D., R.N.). Psychiatrists are medical doctors (and only they are able to prescribe medications). In addition, some nurses obtain postgraduate training in psychotherapy.

The designations L.C.S.W. (Licensed Clinical Social Worker), L.M.F.C.C. (Licensed Marriage and Family Child Counselor), L.P.C. (Licensed Professional Counselor), L.M.F.T. (Licensed Marriage and Family Therapist) refer to licensure by state professional boards, not academic degrees. These initials usually follow others that indicate an academic degree (e.g., Jane Doe, Ph.D., L.M.F.C.C.). If they don't, you should inquire about the therapist's academic training to find out what type of degree they have, and where it was obtained.

You may also hear all of the above professionals referred to as counselors or therapists. Currently, 37 states require licensure or certification in order for professionals to practice independently; unlicensed professionals are allowed to practice only under the supervision of a licensed professional (typically as an intern or assistant in a clinic or licensed professional's private practice).

When you are seeking a good counselor for yourself or your family, ask the professional how long he has been in practice. A licensed marriage and family therapist who has been seeing patients for ten years or more may be a much better choice for your needs than a licensed psychiatrist in his first year of practice.

Another method of finding a suitable counselor is to contact:

The American Association for Marriage and Family Therapy (AAMFT)
1133 15th Street, N.W., Suite 300
Washington, DC 20005-2710
Phone: (202) 452-0109
Fax: (202) 223-2329
Email: *central@aamft.org*
http://www.aamft.org/

This is a national professional organization of licensed/certified marriage and family therapists. It has more than 23,000 members in the U.S., Canada, and abroad. Its membership is made up of licensed clinical social workers, pastoral counselors (who are M.F.C.C./L.M.F.T.s), psychologists, and psychiatrists. The AAMFT also publishes the *Journal of Marital and Family Therapy* for scholarly research and a newsletter, *Practice Strategies,* for behavioral health care providers.

To find a therapist, a good first step is to call two or three therapists who appear on several of your lists of recommendations. During your telephone interview, the following are some suggested questions to ask:

* Are you accepting new clients?

* Do you charge for an initial consultation?

* What training and experience do you have working with ill or traumatized children?

* How many years have you been working with families?

- What is your approach to resolving the problems people develop from trauma? Do you use a brief or long-term approach?

- What evaluation and assessment procedures will be used to define the problem?

- How and when will treatment goals be set?

- How will both parents be involved in the treatment?

- What are your fees?

- Will my insurance company be billed directly?

The next step should be to make an appointment with one or two of the therapists you think might be able to address your needs. Be honest about the fact that you are interviewing more than one therapist prior to making a decision on who you will eventually see. The purpose of the introductory meeting is to see if you feel comfortable with the therapist. After all, credentials do not guarantee that a given therapist will work for you. Compatibility, trust, and a feeling of genuine caring are essential. It is worth the effort to continue your search until you find a good match.

> *Three years after my last round of revisions, I started to feel like our marriage was falling apart. My husband was virtually living on the edge. He was constantly worried about me, and anytime we talked about my hydrocephalus, he would either get angry or upset and would never tell me why. I knew we would be in trouble if we didn't get help. We went through two different marriage counselors before we finally settled on a third. The first two didn't have any experience dealing with couples who had been through a traumatic experience. But the third time was the charm.*

Children need to be prepared for psychological intervention as for any unknown procedure. The following are several parents' suggestions on how to prepare your child:

- Explain who the therapist is, and what you hope to accomplish. For instance, you might be taking the whole family to improve communication or resolve conflicts. If you are bringing your child in for therapy, explain why you think talking to an objective person might benefit her.

- Older children should be involved in the process of choosing a counselor. Younger children's likes and dislikes should be respected, too. If your young child does not get along well with one counselor, you should look elsewhere for another.

- Make the experience as positive as possible, rather than threatening or intimidating.

- Reassure young children that the visit is for talking, drawing, or playing games, not for anything that is physically painful.

- Ask the therapist to explain the rules of confidentiality to both you and your child. Do not quiz your child after a visit to the therapist, as that may only break his trust with the therapist and you.

- Make sure that your child does not think he is being punished; instead assure him that therapists help both adults and children understand and deal with their feelings.

- Go for counseling yourself or to support group meetings to model the fact that all ages and types of people need help from time to time.

Employee assistance programs (EAPs)

One benefit that some companies offer is an employee assistance program, or EAP. EAPs consist of a group of licensed counselors (psychologists, psychiatrists, family and marital counselors, etc.) in your area who can be called upon in time of need.

When you call the phone number for your participating EAP, you will go through an initial screening process over the telephone to evaluate your situation and to determine if there is any need for immediate crisis intervention. You will receive a confidential referral to a participating doctor under their plan, whom you can call to schedule an initial consultation.

If you are not sure if your employer offers an EAP, check with your human resources department at work.

Conferences on hydrocephalus

There are a number of groups who hold small conferences around the world on hydrocephalus. Unfortunately, not all of these conferences are intended for or promoted to the patients who have the condition; many are for researchers or neurosurgeons only. However, as neurosurgeons begin to understand patients' need for information and willingness to learn more about how to deal with the condition, more conferences on hydrocephalus are beginning to include the patients.

In North America, some of the best conferences available for sharing information are those hosted by the Hydrocephalus Association. The biannual conference of the Hydrocephalus Association is geared specifically toward patient education, advocacy, and learning. You will find a broad range of people:

- Parents whose child has only been recently diagnosed with hydrocephalus, desperately searching for information about the condition.

- Children and adults with hydrocephalus who are willing to talk about their condition and how it has affected them or their families.

- Neurosurgeons and medical professionals making presentations about hydrocephalus and its associated problems.

- Shunt manufacturers demonstrating their latest products.

It is truly a healing experience to go to one of these conferences. You will have the opportunity to absorb a great deal of information from a variety of sources and walk away feeling much more knowledgeable. Most attendees enjoy the opportunity to network with other parents or patients in an environment where everyone has something in common—hydrocephalus.

Everyone is welcome, and people are encouraged to express how they feel and to talk about their situation. During two short days, you will make many new friends and contacts. You will probably do a lot of crying and hugging. You will do a lot of learning. But most importantly, you will leave knowing that you are not alone. You are not the only parent who worries day and night that your child might go into seizures, or if anything can be done to improve your brother's vision problems. The expense of going to a conference is a very small price to pay for the amount of information you will acquire.

A list of all known conferences and workshops on hydrocephalus, including dates, locations, and registration information, is maintained on the Hydro-Central web site: *http://www.hydrocephalus.org.*

Support on the Internet

To some, the Internet might seem like a cold place to find support, but that couldn't be further from the truth. The Internet can be a way to find and communicate with others in similar situations through mailing lists (email lists that you subscribe to and receive messages from; also called listservs), chat rooms, and newsgroups.

Hydrocephalus mailing list

The hydrocephalus mailing list (HYCEPH-L) has more than 500 subscribers. Subscribers to the listserv are parents, patients, friends, and family members who have a connection to hydrocephalus. The number of messages received from the list can range from 20 to more than 100 messages daily.

> When I joined HYCEPH-L, I was not sure what I would find. I knew there were other families out there dealing with hydrocephalus, but would they be having the same problems? Would they share my ideals, hopes, and desires for my child?
>
> On the list I have found a wide range of patients, parents, grandparents, caregivers, children, teachers, and professionals who represent all walks of life. Their unique perspectives and honest display of their own situations have helped me deal with my own struggle with my son's hydrocephalus. Together, we on the list represent hydrocephalus and the wide range of people it affects. When we share our stories, emotions, trials, and tribulations with each other, we are spreading the word about this condition. We see just how not alone we really are.

To subscribe to HYCEPH-L, you will need an Internet connection with an Internet service provider and an email account. The directions for subscribing to the list are as follows:

- Send an email message to: *listserv@listserv.utoronto.ca*.
- Leave the subject line blank. In the first line of the body of your message, place the following: SUBSCRIBE HYCEPH-L *yourname*.

After sending the message, you will receive a notification that your request has been received, and you will be asked to reply to that message with a code included in the notification message. Reply to the message and put the code into the body of your reply, with no other text. Upon receipt of your message, you will receive confirmation from HYCEPH-L that you are now subscribed to the list. You will also receive additional messages from the list manager that will explain the rules of the list and how you can change your list preferences. The address for posting messages to the list is *hyceph-l@list-serv.utoronto.ca*, but first you need to be a subscriber.

Other mailing lists

Since hydrocephalus is caused by other conditions and has other problems associated with it, some people might be interested in subscribing to a list-serv that also applies to the causative condition.

- **Brain tumors**. To subscribe to the brain tumor mailing list, send your message to: *braintmr-request@mitvma.mit.edu*. In the first line of the body of your message, type the following: subscribe braintmr.

- **Cerebral palsy**. To subscribe to the cerebral palsy listserv, send your message to: *listserv@sjuvm.stjohns.edu*. In the first line of the body of your message, place the following: subscribe c-palsy *yourname*.

- **Epilepsy**. To subscribe to the epilepsy listserv, send your message to: *list-serv@home.ease.lsoft.com*. Leave the subject line of your message blank, and place the following in the body of your message: subscribe Epi-lepsy-L *firstname lastname*.

HydroHaven

HydroHaven (*http://www.geocities.com/Heartland/6950/HydroHav.html*) is a web-based chat area where people with hydrocephalus can go to talk with others about their condition, share experiences, and find support. The web site is managed by Don Cook, an active member of HYCEPH-L and a patient with hydrocephalus.

Usenet newsgroups

Usenet newsgroups are free discussion areas on the Internet that are open for anyone to post messages to without being subscribed. You can access news-groups by using a news program, such as NewsWatcher (Macintosh) or WinVN (Windows), or by using your regular web browser (Netscape Communicator or Microsoft Internet Explorer). Both Communicator and Internet Explorer have built-in features that allow you to read and post messages to newsgroups.

Some newsgroups of particular interest to parents or patients include:

- Attention deficit disorders (ADD): *alt.support.attn-deficit.*
- Epilepsy: *alt.support.epilepsy.*
- Disorders of migraine/headache ailments: *alt.support.headaches.migraine.*
- Traumatic brain injury (TBI): *bit.listserv.tbi-support.*

Starting a local support group

Many parents have taken it upon themselves to start up a hydrocephalus support group to share information and support other families in their area. Hydrocephalus support groups vary in format and size, from several parents who get together for coffee once in a while, to a formal group with regular meetings and agendas. Before you start, take into consideration:

- What do you want your group to accomplish?
- Should your group be affiliated and/or registered with one (or all) of the national organizations?
- How large do you want your group to get?
- How will you recruit new members?
- How will you promote your group?
- How will you fund your group?

Getting started

If the time comes when you decide to form your own support group, there are some things you can do to get organized. Make a list of the goals for your support group, including the following:

- How many times a week/month do you want to meet?
- Where will you hold your meetings?
- Will your meetings be structured (i.e., will there be an agenda?), or will people be invited to come in and just talk openly?

Finding members and promoting your group

Make a list of neurosurgeons, neurologists, neuropsychologists, imaging centers, and hospitals in your area with whom you can promote your group. Talk with the nurses in the intensive care units at local hospitals and let them know of your group, as most patients who are having a shunt operation will spend time in an ICU. Since these people are likely to treat patients with hydrocephalus, they're your best bet for finding new members.

Other ways you can promote your hydrocephalus support group include:

- Have your group listed with one or all of the national hydrocephalus organizations. People call these larger organizations from time to time looking for information about hydrocephalus and support resources near them. The national organizations can also supply you with information materials that you can hand out to new members.

- Have your group listed with other organizations, such as the American Association of Neurological Surgeons (AANS), The Brain Tumor Society (TBTS), and the National Head Injury Foundation (NHIF).

- Post notices in hospital waiting rooms (if permitted), libraries, and doctors' offices.

- Submit press releases about your group to local newspapers and radio and television stations. If you are affiliated with a nonprofit organization, radio and television stations can run a 30-second public service announcement (PSA) about your group. A PSA should be submitted as a double-spaced, typewritten document, and should include information about hydrocephalus, when your group meets (including the time and location), and a name and phone number that people can contact for more information.

- Work with your local media to produce a human interest story about hydrocephalus.

Securing a meeting location

To begin with, meetings can probably be held in one of the members' house. But eventually word will get out about your group, and you might find yourself in need of another place to meet. When your group starts to outgrow the space available, one of the following may work as an alternate meeting site:

- Schools.

- Churches.

- Libraries.
- A meeting room or auditorium at the local hospital.

Inviting speakers

When your group begins to grow in size, you may want to think about inviting guest speakers to give presentations on different aspects of hydrocephalus. Your initial contacts in the medical community will come in handy when searching for speakers. Although very busy people, most medical professionals (neurosurgeons, neurologists, nurses, etc.) welcome the opportunity to meet and talk with patients and their families to help them better understand the condition. Make an extra effort to promote the meetings that feature speakers.

Taking field trips

Every once in a while, it's good to break up the usual routine of meeting at someone's house or the library. If you have a good rapport with your local hospital, you should try to arrange field trips and tours that all family members can attend, including small children. Your members and their families will have an opportunity to take a behind-the-scenes look at an emergency room, CT or MR imaging center, operating room, and ICU. By planning the tour ahead of time, you can also try to have the hospital's public affairs coordinator arrange for people in each department to meet your group and talk with them about that particular area of the hospital.

Some groups also like to plan one or two outings each year, such as a picnic in the summertime. Here children and parents can meet more informally and have some fun.

Membership

Keep in mind that the size of your support group will ebb and flow. Once people learn about your group, you may see an initial influx of new families, which may taper off over time. And as time passes, people may decide that your group isn't right for them, or that they've received enough information to help them deal with hydrocephalus. When people want to leave your support group, they usually have a good reason. Let them know that you understand their needs and that they are always welcome back at any time.

CHAPTER 9

School

A child miseducated is a child lost.

—John F. Kennedy
State of the Union Address, Jan. 11, 1962

CHILDREN WITH HYDROCEPHALUS have many challenges to face in life, particularly when it comes to school and their education. When a child's condition turns chronic, with frequent shunt revisions or associated medical problems and disabilities, a child can not only miss out on receiving a proper education, but also the social interaction with his peers. By being absent from school for prolonged periods of time, a child can become isolated in the adult world of dealing with doctors and nurses instead of being able to romp and play with his friends.

In this chapter, we examine some things you can do as a parent to help your child's classmates understand what is happening, and how to involve them in supporting your child. We discuss how to work with your child's teachers and the school nurse to help educate other children about your child's condition.

Then we turn our attention to the specialized education needs of children with hydrocephalus. Here, we examine the 1997 Amendments to the Individuals with Disabilities Education Act (IDEA). IDEA guarantees specialized education to all children with disabilities, ensuring that your child will receive the same educational opportunities as children without disabilities.

The goal of this chapter is to help you find your way through school bureaucracy, and to provide you with information and resources you need to ensure that your child receives the education he deserves.

Absences from school

Children who grow up with hydrocephalus will probably experience at least one disruption in education as a result of having a shunt placed or revised. Shunt placements and revisions require your child to be away from school from as little as one week to as long as a month or more, not counting the many doctor visits and tests conducted during weekdays. Absence from school can create another level of stress for the parents if left unplanned, but there are some steps you can take to help alleviate the stress and potential problems that could arise when your child is away from school.

Informing your child's teacher and school

Upon learning that your child needs to have a shunt operation, contact the school as soon as possible. If you have time before the operation, one or both parents should try to meet with the child's teacher and a member of the school administration to inform them of your child's pending absence. At this meeting, you can inform them about your child's condition, what type of surgery will be done, and any special attention that needs to be paid to your child upon return to class.

Parents should also find someone who can act on their behalf as a liaison or advocate between the family, school, home, and the hospital. You might think that you're fully capable of handling this task alone, but between work, maintaining family life, and visiting your child in the hospital, be prepared to have very little time for anything else. A possible candidate to act as your liaison would be the parent of one of your child's friends or classmates. Or, if you don't feel comfortable asking a friend, you could try asking a hospital social worker or the nurse at your child's school.

The most important qualifications for this role are good communication skills, knowledge of education programs and procedures, comfort in dealing with school issues, and organizational skills. Choose someone you trust to act fairly on your child's behalf. It is important that the person you select as your liaison be introduced to your child's teacher and the appropriate hospital staff as soon as possible. This is to ensure the staff are aware that this person is acting not only on your behalf, but in your child's best interest.

The first priority for the person you choose to be the liaison is to establish a line of communication with someone at the hospital and at the school. By doing so, the liaison can find out information about your child's condition from the hospital and relay any messages to the school to inform your child's classmates of how she is doing and when she is expected to return to class.

Parents should also talk with the school administrator and the child's teachers to ensure that the other children in her class know what is wrong with your child. Your child's classmates should know that she will be absent for a few days because she will need an operation to make her better and that she will be back in class as soon as possible.

Involving the teachers and classmates

Your child's well-being in the hospital depends, in part, on staying connected with his teacher, classmates, and friends. Since your child spends a majority of the day in class and playing with other children, he is likely to miss the daily interaction of school. To maintain that connection, have your liaison provide the teacher with regular updates about your child's condition, and relay any notes or messages to his classmates. Likewise, your liaison can obtain messages, notes, and cards from classmates and either bring them to you or directly to your child's room in the hospital. If your child is in middle or high school, it is important that all of your child's teachers receive the same updates about his condition.

Shaun has missed a lot of school. The lessons were sent home and done in the hospital or home. His teacher occasionally came to the hospital to check up on him, and to pick up and drop off lessons.

Some suggestions for keeping your child's class informed and up to date on his progress include:

- Initially, you or your liaison can provide updates on your child's condition to his teacher. These can be used as general information for the teacher and administration or can be passed along to the other students.

  The children at our son's school sent our son a massive get-well basket with cards, notes, pictures, and lots of junk food. They made sure he got all of the day's hand-outs and homework from teachers, which his older brother brought home for him.

- The classmates should be encouraged to make get-well cards or to sign a class poster that can be delivered to your child's hospital room.

Returning to school

After your child has been discharged from the hospital, it's quite possible that she will still need to recover from her surgery at home prior to returning to school. You should check with your child's neurosurgeon first to ensure that your child is well enough to return to the rigors of daily life in the classroom. The neurosurgeon can also provide you with a list of limitations and instructions, which can be passed on to your child's teacher and the school administration.

> Our son's classmates always send cards and gifts. They are always very supportive when he returns to school.

Before sending your child back to school, parents should contact the school nurse, administrator, and any of your child's teachers. Let them know that your child is okay, and what her condition is. Tell them that your child will be missing some hair on her head, and that she will probably be tired for the first little while. Some responses will be positive:

> The children were very happy to see him back at school. My son is still young, so his stitches were very cool to the other kids in his class.

Others may not be so positive:

> When my son returned to school, he was treated like a leper. The parents actually acted worse than the kids did. Nobody spoke to us, and they stared at the scar on my son's head. And when I tried to bring the subject up with anyone, they just rushed off.

And others can be mixed:

> The children at our son's school were mostly very supportive when he returned to class. A few kids teased him or fooled around with his hat, but most were very supportive and would stay with him during recess and lunch.

Parents should talk with the school administrator and the child's teachers to ensure that classmates know what is wrong with her and how to react to her when she returns to class. The school should also know whom to contact in case of an emergency. Of course, all that information should already be on file with the school, but it never hurts to make sure the correct information is right at their fingertips.

Learning disabilities

Some children with hydrocephalus are affected adversely when it comes to school. Birth defects, brain tumors, trauma, and increases or extreme fluctuations of intracranial pressure (ICP) can cause damage to sensitive areas of the brain that help us learn to speak, read, write, and reason, as well as to perform well in subjects such as math, science, and language development.

What may seem like a routine task to others may seem like an insurmountable task for your child. When a child is confused by what he is supposed to be learning, and is not receiving appropriate instruction to help him meet his educational needs and goals, he may lose interest in school very quickly.

Common learning disorders of children with hydrocephalus include:

- Attention deficit disorder (ADD).

- Nonverbal learning disorder (NVLD).

This section briefly examines these two learning disorders, how they can be diagnosed, and how they affect children and adults with hydrocephalus.

Attention deficit disorder (ADD)

Attention deficit disorder, or ADD, is a mental disorder that is primarily diagnosed in childhood. However, ADD can also be found in adults who probably had the disorder as a child, but it went unnoticed until later in life when it was clinically diagnosed. In children, ADD may also be referred to as attention deficit hyperactivity disorder, or ADHD. There really isn't much of a difference between the two labels; however, ADHD is more commonly used when referring to children who have more hyperactive character traits.

Characteristics of ADD and ADHD

Children and adults with ADD typically have an increased level of hyperactivity and a significantly reduced attention span. According to the American Psychiatric Association's *Diagnostic and Statistical Manual of Mental Disorders, Fourth Edition* (DSM-IV), the criteria for diagnosing someone with ADD or ADHD are as follows:

- **Inattention.** At least six of the following symptoms of inattention have persisted for at least six months to a degree that is maladaptive and inconsistent with developmental level:

— Often fails to give close attention to details or makes careless mistakes in schoolwork, work, or other activities.

— Often has difficulty sustaining attention in tasks or play activities.

— Often does not seem to listen to what is being said to them.

— Often does not follow through on instructions and fails to finish schoolwork, chores, or duties in the workplace (not due to oppositional behavior or failure to understand instructions).

— Often has difficulties organizing tasks and activities.

— Often avoids or strongly dislikes tasks (such as schoolwork or homework) that require sustained mental effort.

— Often loses things necessary for tasks or activities (e.g., school assignments, pencils, books, tools, or toys).

— Is often easily distracted by extraneous stimuli (such as peripheral noises or people walking by).

— Is often forgetful in daily activities.

- **Hyperactivity-Impulsivity.** At least four of the following symptoms of hyperactivity-impulsivity have persisted for at least six months to a degree that they are maladaptive and inconsistent with developmental level:

Hyperactivity:

— Often fidgets with hands or feet, or squirms in seat.

— Leaves seat in the classroom or in other situations in which remaining seated is expected.

— Often runs about or climbs excessively in situations where it is inappropriate (in adolescents or adults, may be limited to subjective feelings of restlessness).

— Often has difficulty playing or engaging in leisure activities quietly.

Impulsivity:

— Often blurts out answers to questions before the questions have been completed.

— Often has difficulty waiting in lines or awaiting his turn when playing games or in group situations.

Additional terms for properly diagnosing ADD/ADHD include:

- Onset must be no later than age seven.

- The above-mentioned symptoms must be present in two or more situations (e.g., at school, work, and at home).

- The disturbance causes clinically significant distress or impairment in social, academic, or occupational functioning.

- Symptoms do not occur exclusively during the course of pervasive personality disorder (PPD), schizophrenia, or other psychotic disorder, and are not better accounted for by mood, anxiety, dissociative, or personality disorder.

ADD/ADHD intervention

Once you or your child has been diagnosed as having ADD or ADHD by a trained psychologist or neuropsychologist, it is important to follow the course of treatment offered. Children and adults who have ADD/ADHD are also at risk for secondary problems. These include behavioral problems and learning disorders (verbal and nonverbal), as well as a variety of interpersonal and social problems as a result of their activities.

Treating ADD requires a variety of different approaches, including medication and psychosocial therapy to help manage abnormal behavioral patterns. The most common form of medication used for treating ADD is Ritalin. Ritalin is a mild stimulant that affects the central nervous system (CNS), and is usually prescribed as part of a comprehensive treatment program.

> I was shunted for hydrocephalus in 1956. I was also put on Ritalin in 1963 at the age of 7. My ADD was really out of control. My IQ was tested in the genius range, but I couldn't get any work done, couldn't even stay in my seat. That this might have been even partially attributable to hydrocephalus was not looked into at the time. There just weren't any resources available. Although my ability to organize and pay attention never got much better, I was able to attend a prestigious college and earn a degree.

Parents of children with ADD/ADHD will also need to be instructed on what to do to help change their child's behavioral problems. Additionally, some psychologists recommend family counseling to educate the entire family about what they can do to help the family member with ADD/ADHD.

> *Shannon's teachers first approached us when she was in kindergarten, saying they thought she had attention deficit disorder (ADD). We didn't really know that much about it, but had heard the term before. We took Shannon to see our family doctor, who recommended we take her to a local psychologist for evaluation. After some testing, the psychologist came back and told us that Shannon indeed had ADD. His first course of action was to place Shannon on Ritalin-SR (slow-release), and recommended some family counseling to help us help Shannon adjust her behavior. At first, we thought this was kind of odd, but it really helped in many different ways.*

Early intervention and treatment will ensure that children with ADD or ADHD can overcome many behavioral problems and go on to lead productive, successful lives.

Nonverbal learning disorder

Nonverbal learning disorder, or NVLD, is a type of learning disability that affects the child's academic progress, as well as social and emotional development. A nonverbal learning disorder means that the child has the ability to learn tasks that are explained to him verbally, but has difficulty visualizing complex problems that require intense concentration.

What causes NVLD?

Deficits in the function of the right hemisphere, which can be observed in children with NVLD, could emerge in a variety of ways. If there is any early interruption in the development of the central nervous system (CNS), the right hemisphere is more likely to be compromised than the left. Direct damage to the right hemisphere—through trauma, tumors, and/or seizures—can reduce the hemisphere's ability to function properly, creating a situation where the left side of the brain compensates for most of the learning functions that would normally be performed by the right.

As described in Chapter 1, *What Is Hydrocephalus?*, the right hemisphere of the brain receives sensory data (things you see, hear, smell, taste, and touch) and is capable of processing this information all at once. When someone talks to you, the right hemisphere not only processes the words that are spoken, but also cues in on any visual responses (such as facial expressions and hand gestures). The combination of words and visual messages gives the spoken words different meanings.

The role of the left hemisphere is for processing instructions and information. Children and adults with NVLD might have a hard time following instructions unless they are presented in a step-by-step manner. For example, your child may need to be told how to do something a few times, or even have detailed instructions written out for him to follow. However, once he has it down and committed to memory, the task can be recalled without him fully understanding the reason why he is doing something a certain way. This is commonly referred to as practiced and rote—if you were to ask your son to tell you how to do something, he can probably recall all of the steps from memory, but may not be able to tell you why each task was done a certain way or in a particular order.

Nonverbal learning disorders are caused by the conflict of message interpretation between the two sides of the brain. The right side of the brain manages the interpretation of visual (or nonverbal) information, while the left side of the brain tries to process the words that are heard. Instead of being able to interpret both the spoken word and visual responses, the right hemisphere cues in only on visual input, and leaves word interpretation to the left hemisphere. Since the left hemisphere isn't able to process visual input, the words heard often go without meaning since the brain has to interpret both speech and visual responses on the same side of the brain. Therefore, in children with NVLD, the right hemisphere becomes involved in understanding anything new or contradictory between the verbal and nonverbal messages.

Characteristics of NVLD

A valid diagnosis of NVLD includes a combined evaluation of learning, academic, social, and emotional issues. While most children with learning disabilities do not have significant problems with normal social and emotional development, others may not be so fortunate. Since some children with NVLD may have difficulties processing words and complex thoughts along with visual responses from the people they are talking to, they might tend to have a difficult time in social situations. Because the pattern of academic strengths and weaknesses may not show up early in life, and difficulties with social relations are not always apparent in very young children, it is often difficult to make a diagnosis of NVLD until the child is in middle to late elementary school (grades 3 to 6, or age 8 to 11).

Children with NVLD have difficulty with mechanical arithmetic, particularly more complex math involving columns, such as long division or complex multiplication problems.

> Brian always excelled when it came to English. He was always getting As for his creative writing. But when it came to math, the teachers just couldn't figure him out. Brian had no problem with simple math—adding, subtracting, and basic multiplication or division. This meant he was fine through first, second, and third grade. But when Brian hit fourth grade and started working on long division and multiplication with larger numbers, it was like his brain shut off. You could see it in his face when he was doing his homework. With some math problems, it would take 15 or 20 minutes to figure out the answer on what I saw as a simple multiplication problem. The worst, however, was long division, especially when decimals were involved.

Children with NVLD also have difficulty with word problems or math reasoning, being unable to read a math problem and know what operation to perform. Higher math skills that rely on spatial abilities or seeing the relation between concepts (as with geometry or algebra) are more difficult for children to learn.

> Brandon's teacher first thought he had NVLD when he began having difficulty understanding story problems in math class (where they give you a paragraph of information on which to perform mathematical computations). He could read the paragraph quite well and understood there were numbers involved, but couldn't see how to take a number mentioned in one part, multiply it by something in another sentence, and then divide it by a fractional amount of something mentioned in the last sentence.

· · · · ·

> I always did well with math through elementary school, and even junior high, but when I got into high school, everything changed. In ninth grade, I was required to take algebra. I know algebra is fairly complex, but I really bombed. It was the first time I got a D grade in math my entire life. My parents thought I was slacking off—spending too much time socializing instead of studying—but that wasn't the case. I spent

hours toiling over those equations and just couldn't get it. It took me sitting down with a math tutor, who explained everything step by step, before I started to get it. Unfortunately, by the time I got the math tutor, I'd already scored a D and a D+ in the first two quarters.

In addition to having difficulty with language comprehension and math, children with NVLD also have problems in learning and interpreting speech patterns. At first, some children may be slow to learn how to speak, but then show rapid progress, becoming quite verbose. This speech pattern is commonly referred to as "cocktail party syndrome," because although the children are quite talkative, there may be little substance or value to what is being said, and they may speak out of context or for no reason at all. Compared with other children their age, children with NVLD tend to rely more on language to engage and relate to other people, to gather information, and to relieve anxiety. For instance, when young, instead of picking up and manipulating an object new to them, they may instead question an adult about what it is, how it works, etc.

We always thought our daughter, Emily, was like a Chatty-Cathy Doll—just pull her string and let her natter away. When she was younger, we thought it was cute. But as she got older, we started to notice that she was saying things that were inappropriate, particularly when she was around a bunch of new people for the first time.

Humor or sarcasm can also be hard for children with NVLD to appreciate. Sarcasm, which is a mismatch of spoken messages, facial expressions, or tone of voice, requires the child to integrate types of sensory input. As such, they tend to miss the meaning of most jokes because they are missing the verbal and visual cues, and are paying too much attention to piecing together the words that are spoken.

Helping your child progress with NVLD

There are some things you as a parent, or your child's teachers, can do to help your child learn, regardless of the extent of NVLD:

- Children with NVLD do best with instruction that is verbal and descriptive in nature. Instead of showing your child how to work out a particular math problem, instruct him verbally on how to do it step by step.

*We started to notice that Brian's math skills improved when we care-
fully walked him through the math equations step by step. We made a
point of explaining each step of how the math problem should be worked
out, and why we were doing it that way.*

- Assess reading comprehension carefully because good oral reading can
hide the extent of weak comprehension. Teach strategies to aid comprehension, such as learning how to identify the topic of a sentence and
highlighting important information for later study or review. Tell your
child what specific facts he will need to know for a test rather than asking him to determine on his own what important information within the
text or lecture he should focus on.

*Amy's English teacher noticed she was having trouble with compre-
hension quizzes after reading almost anything. She worked with Amy
after class, showing her how to break the sentences of a paragraph apart
separately so she could glean the overall concept that was being discussed.*

- Because language concepts can be weak, children with NVLD need to
understand terms such as "same" versus "different," part-to-whole relationships (fractions), how to classify or categorize objects, and the difference between cause and effect. In expressive language instruction, they
should focus on staying on the topic, listening without interrupting, and
recognizing when someone has signaled the end of a conversation.

*Jake's biggest problem was not knowing when to shut up. If his
teacher or another child got him started on a topic, he would keep going,
then head off on a tangent. It was also difficult for anyone to get a word in
edgewise. We worked with Jake's teacher on teaching him the proper eti-
quette for holding a conversation or talking in a public setting, assuring
him that he wasn't being bad, just that it would be nice to allow the other
person to talk back to him.*

- The concept of spatial concepts and relations may also be difficult to
grasp for a child with NVLD. The child may need to learn verbal self-
instruction for analyzing and reproducing designs. Certain tasks, such as
map reading or learning the location of all the capital cities, should be
avoided altogether. If telling time on a clock with a face is difficult for your
child to learn, try teaching him first how to tell time using a digital clock.

Whenever my wife and I go on vacation, she's the driver and I'm the navigator. I'm the one who sits in the co-pilot's seat with the maps and tells her where and when to turn because maps are too confusing for her to look at. She says that she first noticed this problem when she was a Girl Scout and was trying to learn how to read maps before a camping and hiking trip.

- Written work can be extremely frustrating due to the combination of mechanical problems related to fine motor delays and poor visual spatial relations. Educators and parents alike should aim to reduce the quantity of writing expected and instead allow verbal expression of information. Additionally, by teaching your child computer keyboard skills at an early age, you can help him improve his motor skills.

Mike's IEP (individualized education plan) specifically states that he's to answer questions verbally, rather than in writing. His teacher has noted that this has significantly improved his test scores from before the IEP was implemented.

- Involve your child's school counselor or social worker to foster social development at school. Friendship groups that involve a small number of selected peers are one possible intervention. Teachers can identify which classmates would be most responsive to and supportive of your child. Specific and concrete instruction, such as teaching him how and when to initiate conversations with other children, when and when not to speak, how to make eye contact with the person he is speaking with, and pleasant facial expressions can be very beneficial.

Because Jake was so talkative, and his tangents so lengthy, some of the children in his class began to shy away from him. His teacher helped other kids in his class to understand Jake by first working on one-to-one conversation skills, and slowly bringing in more and more children. She noticed that as more children were added, at least at first, Jake would become more talkative—probably because he didn't feel comfortable in groups. But as they worked on group conversations, Jake started to realize that everything was okay, and he didn't need to blurt out the first thing that popped into his head while someone else was talking. This was a big step forward, and Jake seems to be more comfortable and confident in group situations now.

- Create a supportive environment where your child feels secure and successful. Try to minimize any demands that may highlight your child's weaknesses by being very clear and specific about what you expect. Observe your child carefully in new or complex situations to gain an appreciation of strengths and weaknesses, and set your expectations accordingly.

> *When playing games that involve the whole family, we like to choose something that won't make Amy feel uncomfortable. For instance, we play games like Pictionary rather than Scrabble, because she has an easier time picturing words in her head than piecing together words from tiles with different letters on them. Not only is she able to see the word, but she can also use her imagination and artistic ability.*

- Provide as much positive reinforcement as possible, rather than criticizing your child. Let him know when he is doing something correct or when he is acting appropriately in social situations, and help him make the necessary adjustments in a way that it doesn't hurt his self-esteem.

> *No matter how frustrating it felt to explain something over and over again to Ben, we would always keep our cool. We always made a point to let him know when he did something right, and corrected him in a constructive way so that he could learn by his mistakes without feeling bad about it.*

Nonverbal learning disorder is not widely recognized, and most school personnel may be unsure how to best serve your child's educational, social, and emotional needs. A comprehensive and thorough neuropsychological assessment, performed by a qualified clinician with regular follow-ups, is critical to assuring that appropriate strategies are in place to assist your child in realizing his full potential.

Individuals with Disabilities Education Act

In 1973, approximately 750,000 American children were not attending school. Many of these children were disabled.

The Individuals with Disabilities Education Act (IDEA) first saw light as the Education for All Handicapped Children Act (or EHA, known as public law 94-142) in 1975. The EHA was amended in 1990 and was renamed IDEA.

Additional amendments were made to IDEA in 1997; these are commonly referred to as IDEA '97.

IDEA guarantees that no child can be excluded from receiving specialized education services—including children who have hydrocephalus. IDEA is the only federal law that mandates education. Although most states have laws that regulate education, this is a federal law that has been upheld by the Supreme Court.

The purposes of the IDEA '97 are to clarify and strengthen IDEA by providing parents and educators with the tools to:

- Preserve the right of children with disabilities to a free, appropriate, public education.

- Promote improved educational results for children with disabilities through early intervention, preschool, and educational experiences that prepare them for later educational challenges and employment.

- Expand and promote opportunities for parents, special education, related services, regular education and early intervention service providers, and other personnel to work in new partnerships at both the state and local levels.

- Create incentives to enhance the capacity of schools and other community-based entities to work effectively with children with disabilities and their families, through targeted funding for personnel training, research, media technology, and the dissemination of technical assistance and best practices.

In the 23 years since EHA first became law, states have made excellent progress in identifying children with disabilities and providing them with access to special education. There are now approximately 5.5 million children with disabilities—10 percent of all American children aged 3 through 17—who are receiving specialized education under IDEA.

The term "special education" used to mean being segregated into a separate setting with limited educational demands. Now special education indicates that a properly trained teacher works with therapists, family, or administrative staff to develop an individual education plan, or IEP. It is at this point that parents and schools sometimes clash. Some parents opt instead for home schooling.

For all children, the quality of early education defines much about the quality of their future lives. For children with disabilities, their best chance for independence is equal access to education at all levels. Education remains one of the key issues for the disability community—and for the parents who are vocal and passionate advocates for their children.

Before we go any further into the details of IEPs as specified under IDEA, it is important to be familiar with the terminology used in the law and by educators:

- **Individualized education plan (IEP).** An IEP is a specialized education program designed to meet the needs of your child. An IEP should address academic development, social skills development, and any emotional needs. An IEP can also address any physical needs, such as needs for physical and/or occupational therapy to help your child function in a classroom environment. An IEP establishes short- and long-term goals. The school makes a placement recommendation, which could include a separate program or integration into a "normal" classroom.

- **Free appropriate public education (FAPE).** Parents of children with disabilities should not have to pay for any specialized education or therapy that the child receives through the school system. All schools in the U.S. receive tax dollars under IDEA to pay for specialized education. If your child's school district determines that your child needs to be educated at a private facility, the district pays for this, not you.

- **Least restrictive environment (LRE).** Children with disabilities must be educated with children who are not disabled, in an environment that accommodates the disability. Special classes, separate schooling, or other removal of children with disabilities from the regular educational environment occurs only when the nature or severity of the disability is such that education in regular classes with the use of special education and related services or supplementary aids and services cannot be achieved satisfactorily.

  Placement options available for the child should include instruction in regular classes, special classes, special schools, home instruction, and instruction in hospitals and institutions. When a disabled child is placed in a regular classroom, supplementary aids and services must also be provided. A least restrictive environment cannot place undue stress on the child. For example, your child needs schooling within a relatively close proximity to your home. Asking you to drive your child to another school district that is far from your home is certainly against the definition of a least restrictive environment.

- **Local education agency (LEA).** The LEA is the organization that oversees all school and classroom operations in your area or your local school district. One or more representatives from the LEA will be part of your child's IEP development team.

  In implementing its standards, IDEA requires that LEAs make an ongoing good-faith effort to recruit and hire appropriately and adequately trained individuals to provide specialized education to children with disabilities.

  The LEA must also employ these individuals in areas where they are needed. In other words, an LEA can hire what they consider an adequate number of special education teachers, but they must ensure they are assigned to the schools that need them. For example, it won't do you or your child any good if the nearest special education teacher is located 50 miles away. Asking you to take your child that far away to receive specialized education is a violation of the LRE clause (above); the LEA would be required by law to relocate a special education teacher closer to where your child attends school.

- **State education agency (SEA).** The SEA is responsible for overseeing all of the school districts in your state. Their job is to disseminates federal and state funds to the various school districts, as well as to oversee and approve school curricula.

- **Comprehensive system of personnel development (CSPD).** Under Section 612 of IDEA, the law requires that states establish a CSPD to ensure that an adequate supply of qualified teachers are hired to provide specialized education to children with disabilities. The CSPD is required by law to establish a set of procedures, whereby it acquires and disseminate knowledge obtained through educational research, and adopts promising practices, materials, and technology for educators within the state.

Developing your child's IEP

Developing an IEP that fits your child's needs can be a fairly long process. As easy as it is to get frustrated with the process, always keep in the back of your mind that the long-term goal of the IEP is to allow your child to lead a more productive life. Patience is necessary as you enter the IEP process. In this section, we examine some of the basic steps to setting up an IEP for your child, and provide you with some tips for things to do before, during, and after the IEP is developed.

Essentially, there are four steps in the IEP process. These are:

- Referral, either by the parents or school officials, to recommend specialized education for your child.

- Consent, granted by the parents, to enter into the IEP process.

- Assessment of your child by trained professionals and yourself to determine your child's needs.

- Development and implementation of the IEP.

Referral

Your child needs a referral to have an individualized education program. This can come from either parent, your child's teacher, or a school counselor. The referral starts the ball rolling in helping to determine the educational needs of your child.

Consent

If the referral for specialized education comes from someone other than the child's parents, the parents must be informed as soon as the referral is made to the principal of the school. The parents can refuse the referral. However, your refusal can be challenged by the court on behalf of the child's best interest.

Assessment

Once consent has been granted by the child's parents, the next step in the process is to assess the child in his least restrictive environment. The LRE assessment can be a combination of observing your child at home as well as at school.

During the assessment phase, educators will examine your child's reading, writing, math, and social skills through a combination of interdisciplinary or transdisciplinary exams. As part of the assessment, your child should be tested and observed in his regular school setting, rather than somewhere else. Some tips for parents regarding the testing of your child include:

- If assessment tests are mentioned in the IEP, ask the team members for details about the specific tests: what they are, how they will be used to track your child's progress, and how the results will be used to help your child.

- Take test results with a grain of salt. The scores for your child are traditionally compared against those for a broader base of children in his age group who don't have a disability or learning disorder.

- Know what the tests are for, and agree to them only if they are going to yield a direct result for your child. Again, make sure that you know how the test results will be used to help gear specific learning needs for your child. If the teachers want to conduct a certain test but can give you no substantial reason why, then refuse the test.

The people conducting the assessment (i.e., speech therapist, occupational therapist, neuropsychologist, etc.) need to be brought into the classroom to observe your child over a period of time to determine what he needs help with. For instance, an occupational therapist may be brought in to observe the way your child is holding a pencil or crayon to determine the type of therapy to offer.

The evaluators must also involve the parents as part of their assessment. As a parent, you have more information about your child to offer the evaluators. You see your child every day, and you know what he has a difficult time with and how he struggles to keep up with his classmates. The insight you can provide to the evaluators is invaluable to the data they collect by observing your child in the classroom setting. The evaluators should look to you for any missing links to help them determine the education needs for your child.

> Yesterday I went to review Mike's progress with his teachers and counselor. After two years of negativity on the part of the school, I was shocked to hear them suggest Mike not be afforded the "resource room" for math anymore—only for English. I voiced my concern that he will fall behind and that it was too early to suggest this. His regular classroom teacher backed me up in saying we have a good thing going here and if we took this action he might not stay on top of things. In the end, we decided the individual attention and quiet atmosphere of the resource room should be kept in Mike's routine at this time.

Next was the occupational therapy—his handwriting is average (according to the teacher), and they tried to take this therapy away too. I said, "No! Mike goes to occupational therapy twice each week and this will continue." However, I did agree that another child also receiving occupational therapy could join the session if Mike agreed to it.

Development and implementation of the IEP

Once all the assessment of your child has taken place, the next step involves the development and implementation of your child's personal IEP. The IEP needs to be specifically designed to meet the educational and developmental goals for *your* child, not adapted from one previously developed for another child.

We have been fortunate in all of our dealings with his school system. They have been very detailed and accommodating in his IEP and have made sure that both he and I are comfortable in his placement. They have made a personal aide available to Shaun to be with him every day in school to watch over him so that his teacher can focus on the other kids too. I am so comfortable dropping him off in the morning with the same person everyday who will watch him and be my eyes and ears while he is at school.

To develop an IEP for your child that will meet your goals and his needs, start by keeping a journal. Make a list of everything you want your child to learn and be able to do. Also make note of the things he can do. Take notes about the things your child has a difficult time with; note what he was attempting to do and how it affected him, as well as anything you or your spouse (or siblings) did to help him along. When you go in to meet with the IEP development team, bring your journal with you to help in the evaluation process.

The people who attend the IEP planning meeting should be looked upon as a team consisting of:

- You, the child's parents.
- Your child's teacher (or teachers, if your child has more than one teacher during the day).
- At least one special education teacher, preferably the special education teacher who will work with your child.

- Representatives from the LEA qualified to provide or supervise special education programs that meet the needs of children with disabilities. This person, or persons, should also be familiar with other local agencies in the area that can assist in meeting your child's needs.

- Someone who can interpret the results of the evaluation to help determine the needs of your child. This person may already be a member of the team, for example, a special education teacher or a representative from the LEA.

- Any other person you feel is qualified. For instance, this person could be someone who works with a local United Way chapter in providing care and services for children with disabilities. Such a person could also assist the school in obtaining any special equipment your child may require.

- And last, but certainly not least: your child. As the IEP will be specially designed to fit the needs of your child, he should be included as part of the team. Having your child there also helps other team members remember who they are developing the IEP for. If your child has any input about how a certain task is going, he can provide valuable information, firsthand, to the other members of the IEP team.

Throughout the development and implementation phase, parents should:

- Keep track of phone conversations and make notes about things said. Note the time of the call, who you spoke with, and what you talked about, especially if any derogatory comments are made.

- Not feel rushed. The IEP meeting should be more than just one simple meeting. Your child's education will span many years, so it's important that you don't feel pushed into signing the IEP if it doesn't meet your child's long-term needs and goals.

- Understand all terminology in the IEP. If you don't understand something that has been said or written, ask for a clarification.

- Ask questions about the plan and what the school administrators are talking about.

- Bring along an ally or a friend. This person can be there to take notes throughout the meetings and help you interpret things being said.

- If you are still unsure about something and want more clarification, contact the state attorney general and request a copy of the state's regulations on special education.

In order for any team to accomplish its goals, everyone on the team must view the others as equal and valuable members of that team. Keep in mind that everyone is working to help your child. Insist on a plan that will help your child succeed, but do so in a manner that is nonconfrontational. If everyone works together in a calm, professional manner, your child will be the winner.

What the IEP includes

Your child's IEP should be a detailed outline that states the results from the assessment tests, what your child is capable of right now, and what the intended goal is. The IEP should:

- Describe your child's present level of ability. For instance, what is your child capable of doing right now? Can he graph large to small, count from one to ten, and/or draw or determine shapes?

- Note whether certain tasks can be done at home and not at school, or vice versa. If your child is capable of doing something in one place but not the other, this could indicate some type of barrier that's preventing your child from performing the task equally in both places.

- Define what your child needs to learn. What are the skills and goals that your child needs to learn before moving on to the next step? For instance, the IEP should state that your child will need to learn how to read sentences of a certain word length (e.g., sentences that have eight words).

- State how the teaching and learning will be done. This should include the mechanism for evaluating your child's progress, materials to be used, and requirements for adaptations or modifications to your child's learning environment.

Only when you are absolutely positive that the IEP contains everything you want for your child should you sign it. Don't feel pressured to sign the IEP if you are unsure about something or if you feel that it is still lacking something your child needs. Your child's IEP is a legally binding document between the school district and you, the parent.

CHAPTER 10

Insurance

*The Constitution says that if you are charged
with a crime, you have a right to a lawyer.
But it's even more fundamental that if you're
sick, you should have the right to a doctor.*

—Harris Wofford, U.S. Senator
Time magazine

HYDROCEPHALUS IS A CONDITION that requires lifelong management. Though you or your child may be free of problems for months or years, complications can arise at any time. Finding your way through the insurance maze can be frustrating or overwhelming. Understanding your benefits and claims procedures can help get the bills paid without undue stress.

The chapter starts with a questionnaire about your current medical insurance plan—what it will or will not cover. If you don't know some of the answers, try to find out. We look at important terms of your policy: pre-existing condition clauses, co-payments, deductibles, lifetime caps on payments, and going outside a provider network for care. Then we describe different types of health care plans, including Medicaid and Medicare. Finally, we turn our attention to the expense side of medical coverage, discussing hospital billing, keeping financial records, working through billing problems, and appealing denied claims or services.

Evaluating your coverage

Just how well do you know your medical insurance plan? If you've been through a lot of medical treatments, chances are you know it quite well. Many people pay attention to their medical coverage only in a crisis, when it is often too late or when they can't afford the time to read through 100 pages of insurance company rhetoric. Take a moment to answer the following questions to see how much you know about your current policy:

- What type of plan do I have (fee-for-service, health maintenance organization, preferred provider organization, independent practice association)? How are doctors paid under the plan?

- Can I go to a doctor or specialist outside of the plan? If so, will I be required to pay any additional fees?

- Do I need prior authorization from the insurance company before going to see a specialist or to the hospital?

- Are second opinions covered under the plan?

- Is there a lifetime cap on the amount the insurance company will pay on my family's claims? Is the cap per person or per family?

- Is there a limitation on the number of doctor visits per year?

- Will my policy reimburse me for all or part of expenses incurred when traveling to see a specialist outside the plan area?

- Does my policy cover in-home nursing care and physical or occupational therapy? If so, how many visits will be covered annually?

- Does my policy cover mental health care? Are there yearly limits on the number of visits?

- Will my policy pay for experimental treatments, devices, drugs, or participation in clinical trials?

- Does my policy have a preexisting condition clause? If so, what is the waiting period before I will be covered under this policy? Can I appeal the waiting period?

- What deductibles do I need to meet? Is the deductible per person? Is there a maximum number of deductibles per family? Do I have a co-payment for doctor's visits?

- What is the most I should expect to pay per year for out-of-pocket expenses?

If you don't know the answer to these questions or have others regarding your medical insurance policy, write the questions down and contact your provider's customer service office. Let them know that you have some general questions regarding your policy, and ask for explanations in terms you can understand.

Maintaining coverage

Having health insurance should be your number one priority. Unfortunately, recent statistics show that nearly 16 percent of Americans (41.7 million people) have no health coverage.

In the past, many people lost coverage when changing jobs or relocating to a new area. Legislation passed by Congress in 1997 requires that employers offer medical coverage to former employees during this time of transition. The former employee is entitled to continue under the same plan with no interruption of service. Coverage remains the same, but monthly premiums increase.

There are good reasons for the old adage, "An ounce of prevention is worth a pound of cure." It is far easier to prevent insurance problems—especially in an ever-changing HMO environment—than to try to fix them. You can forestall problems by taking a few basic precautions:

- Don't ever let your coverage lapse.

    Knowing my wife's condition, making sure we have medical coverage has always been a high priority. When I recently accepted a new position, the first thing I did was contact the human resources manager to talk about their health coverage. She gave me the number for their insurance representative, basic information about the types of coverage they offered to employees, and offered to mail me their latest benefits booklet.

- If you are laid off, continue with your insurance plan or get private coverage. If you change jobs, stay on top of the transition to a new plan.

    I had gotten laid off from the hospital I worked at three days after I found out my daughter Michaela was diagnosed with hydrocephalus. My insurance was there for one month following the layoff; after that I had to switch to my husband's insurance.

    Originally his small company offered just Blue Cross, which had a preexisting clause (which I hear will be abolished this July!) and did not want to pick up Michaela because of it. So his boss got some people together that were interested in Keystone Health Plan East (which I was on and which is a part of Blue Cross), and we had no problem being covered. They have been wonderful! The referrals are a pain, but if you have understanding pediatricians they are not too bad.

- Pick the best plan for your particular situation. Know when you are eligible to switch plans (usually once a year). Stay up to date on your policy coverage.

Assessing coverage and costs

Understanding your medical insurance policy can be a daunting task. Take the time to read through your manual so you can learn the details of your health plan. Get a copy of the actual contract—the small-print one that governs the plan, not the glossy booklets sent to plan members, which provide few details. Make sure you have all supplemental materials.

> When it comes to insurance companies, it's a good idea to stay one step ahead of them. Know your policy backwards and forwards. Work all the angles. For example, our policy will not pay for physical therapy, but will pay for a chiropractor, so I found one who is also a licensed physiotherapist. Simply find ways around the system. It's important to be your own advocate and check things out for yourself.

Most Americans are insured through their employers. You may pay all premiums or your employer may pay a portion of the premiums. Usually the rates for group health insurance are less than the rate you can get as an individual.

When assessing coverage, evaluate what you can and cannot get through the plan, how much your physician can or cannot do, and how restrictive the plan is overall. Consider the possibility of multiple shunt revisions being needed in a given year as well as years when your family's health care requirements are minimal. What restrictions would the plans' coverage place on you in a bad or good year? Will you be able to have access to neurosurgeons, hospitals, and tests that you currently use or want to use?

> My company offers a choice of managed care plans. I'm always amazed by the people who choose a plan based only on which one costs less and/or has lower deductibles. Later, they find out that the plan is too restrictive or that the doctors are dropping out monthly. People need to consider much more than out-of-pocket expenses. Don't be penny-wise and pound-foolish.

When assessing costs, first look at the total costs if you have "normal" medical costs for a year (for example, add premiums and what you would pay out of pocket under the plan for preventive care such as checkups, screening tests, inoculations, a few mild illnesses or injuries, and prescriptions). Then look at costs if you also have one or more major events (for example, the above costs plus a shunt revision that includes a $50,000 bill for surgery and hospital bills, as well as therapy visits, six follow-up visits with the neurosurgeon, and four MRI scans in the course of a year).

The insurance company stays in business because the amount paid for your premiums—aggregated with the premiums for others in your group health plan or all others in the insurance pool—will be more than what the company pays out for your health care. Insurers limit what they pay by requiring waiting periods for preexisting conditions, co-payments for services used, deductibles, and lifetime caps on benefits. They may also restrict access to providers under contract with the plan and limit coverage or payments for certain care (e.g., physical therapy, psychiatric benefits, alcohol or drug treatment, elective surgery, eyeglasses, general physical exams, well-baby visits, etc.).

Preexisting conditions

A preexisting condition clause is a provision in a policy that excludes coverage for any physical or mental disability a person had before applying for insurance. If a subscriber currently undergoing expensive treatment subscribes to the plan, this clause gives insurers a way to exclude that treatment from coverage and limit financial liability.

> We eventually learned that there would be a six-month waiting period because Lee's hydrocephalus was considered a preexisting condition. However, if we could prove that she had medical insurance for the past twelve months, the waiting period would be waived. This was a huge relief for both of us.

. . . . .

> My insurance company did not think his condition of subdural hematomas and collapsed ventricles was life-threatening, in spite of the doctor saying the child may have brain damage or die. They argued that dying was only a possibility, and brain damage is not life-threatening, so they did not authorize a shunt revision for Michael when he was going on operation number three.

If your insurance provider has a waiting period before it will cover a preexisting condition, you can try to get it to waive or shorten this time by writing an appeal letter. In your appeal letter, state that you or your child needs medical coverage for hydrocephalus, as any complications that could arise would require specialized treatment you cannot afford. State arguments why the provider should make an exception for you, such as:

- The number of months since your last medical procedure/visit for hydrocephalus.

- A signed letter from your neurosurgeon stating that your or your child's condition is stable and shouldn't require treatment in the foreseeable future.

Usually there is a period of time, ranging from three to twelve months, during which a condition must be problem-free before the insurance company will begin to pay claims related to that condition or illness. If during the waiting period you need to have a test or operation related to hydrocephalus, the insurance company will refuse to pay for those medical expenses and will extend the waiting period an additional three to twelve months from the last date of service. When the waiting period is complete, the individual will be eligible for benefits.

> I had just started a new job in November of 1995. Our insurance was through Blue Cross/Blue Shield of Illinois. I was aware of their preexisting condition clause, but didn't think it pertained to our situation. The booklet made it sound like the clause only pertained to conditions that had been treated in the twelve months prior to the employee's hiring date, or if the person seeking coverage showed symptoms of the condition in the twelve months prior to the hiring date. My son Danny was eight years old, had had no surgery in four years and his last CT scan was in 1993. So I figured we didn't fall into that category.
>
> Unfortunately, in 1996, Danny's shunt did have a malfunction. He had a revision and was out of the hospital in no time. Ten days later, his shunt malfunctioned again and another surgery was required. Our insurer refused to pay for either surgery, stating that we were still in the one-year waiting period for coverage of preexisting conditions.
>
> I spoke to insurance representatives several times and wrote several letters. I would always get a different response. Eventually, it went to the appeal board and was denied again.

Our insurance covered absolutely nothing for those two surgeries. We are in debt to the neurosurgeon, anesthesiologist, radiologist, hospital, labs, etc.; the list is endless. We had to rework our monthly budget to make monthly payments. We are still $20,000 in debt.

I was paying my monthly premium to have coverage and when we needed them most they refused to pay. We felt like three little people fighting against a giant army. I've lost all respect for big insurance companies.

Co-payments

A co-payment is a flat fee that you will be required to pay for certain medical services. Co-payment fees are set by your insurance provider and normally apply to services such as doctor visits, lab work, and imaging studies. Most co-payments run between $10 and $20 for a doctor visit, while prescriptions might be around $3 to $10 per prescription.

Deductibles

A deductible is an amount that you must pay before the insurance company begins paying for eligible expenses. Most insurance policies have some form of deductible system built in, although deductibles vary from plan to plan. Two common types of deductibles are minor and major medical expense deductibles.

A minor medical deductible is one that is paid by the subscriber (you and your dependents) for day-to-day medical expenses, e.g., doctor visits, routine lab work, X-rays, etc. Traditionally, most insurance policies have an annual minor medical deductible that must be paid first before your insurance company will pay any additional charges. Generally, these deductibles range from $100 to $750.

With most plans, major medical expenses (e.g., inpatient or outpatient operations, hospitalization, etc.) are considered separate from day-to-day expenses and usually have their own deductible. Major medical deductibles tend to be higher than those for day-to-day care.

A sample plan might, for example, have a $100 deductible for minor medical expenses such as doctor visits and lab work. After you pay the first $100 of those expenses, other minor medical expenses are covered in full. For major medical expenses, there might be a deductible of $1,000. After the deductible is paid, major medical expenses will be covered at 80 percent until a limit of $5,000 is reached, after which the plan begins paying at 100 percent.

Here's how a typical major medical deductible might work. Your child is operated on for a shunt revision, and the total bill—including surgeon's fee and time spent in the hospital—comes to $50,000. Under your plan, you have a $2,500 per individual deductible for major medical expenses, after which your insurance company will pay 80 percent of the bill. Your cost for this procedure would be $12,000:

$50,000 (Total bill)	Amount Paid by You	Amount Paid by Insurer
−2,500 (your deductible)	$2,500	
$47,500 (balance)		
−38,000 (80% of 47,500)		$38,000
$ 9,500 (your balance)	$ 9,500	
	$12,000	$38,000

Some policies have a maximum amount for out-of-pocket expenses you will be asked to pay annually. With most policies, your maximum out-of-pocket expenses will be an amount that is three times the amount of your major medical deductible—including the deductible itself. For instance, you might have a $2,500 major medical deductible and a limit on out-of-pocket expenses of $7,500. You would then be responsible for paying $7,500, and the insurance company would pick up the rest of the tab.

$50,000 (Total bill)	Amount Paid by You	Amount Paid by Insurer
−2,500 (your deductible)	$2,500	
−5,000 ($7,500 - 2,500)k	$5,000	
$42,500		$42,500
	$7,500	$42,500

Check with your insurance provider or the benefits representative in your employer's human resources department for an explanation of the deductibles for your particular plan. When reading through the details of your plan, look to see if there is a point when your coverage increases to 100 percent.

What hospitals or doctors bill is not necessarily what insurance companies pay. Insurers negotiate with providers for a lower fee than the "list price." For example, if the hospital charges $5,000 for a service, the insurer may have an arrangement—as a volume customer with bargaining power—to pay only $3,700. When you get the explanation of benefits from your insurance company, you see the negotiated amount listed along with the original billed amount. Your deductible will be based (or should be) on the lower fee negotiated by your insurer.

Lifetime cap

Most health plans have a lifetime limit on the amount of benefits they will pay out for each individual subscribed to the plan. This is referred to as a lifetime cap. If your insurance provider has an unlimited cap, you probably won't have to worry much about paying for medical expenses that go beyond your standard deductibles. However, if your lifetime cap is relatively low (generally $1 million or less), it might be wise to look into obtaining a supplemental insurance policy to raise the ceiling.

Going outside the network

Typically, managed care plans have contracts with a select group of providers (i.e., physicians, hospitals, medical labs, imaging centers, etc.) in a particular region. When selecting participants for their plans, plan administrators look at the track records of physicians or facilities to see if they have consistent efficiency and scope of service, as well as a good reputation in the community.

Many managed care plans allow the customer to choose between using in- or out-of-network providers. *In-network* providers have contracted with the provider for services at lower costs, while *out-of-network* providers have not contracted with the provider. Therefore, every time you decide to use a provider outside the network to obtain better benefits or services, be prepared to pay a co-payment or a deductible.

Types of health care plans

There are variations on a few main themes in health care delivery. The four main types of programs are fee-for-service, independent practice associations, preferred provider organizations, and health maintenance organizations. They vary by who bears the risk of incurring costs and who decides what treatments are necessary.

Fee-for-service (unmanaged care)

In the not-too-distant past, most patients in the U.S. had insurance that simply paid doctors and hospitals for treatment with no strings attached. This type of arrangement is called fee-for-service. You see the doctor of your choice, and he is free to prescribe treatments, drugs, or referrals to specialists without input from the insurance company.

Under a fee-for-service system, the insurer pays the doctor for each visit or service. Doctors spend as much time with each patient as they want, can order as many tests as they wish, and write prescriptions for the drugs they choose. Patients are free to hire and fire doctors, as well as go to any hospital of their choice. Insurers are treated as uninvolved third parties in the financial interactions between health care providers and patients.

Today, most fee-for-service policies include managed care elements such as preauthorization for surgeries, precertification, utilization review, and sometimes a list of approved drugs.

Health maintenance organization (HMO)

Managed care has been around since the 1920s, when doctors first contracted with businesses to provide medical care for their workers for a set fee. In 1973, companies in the United States with 25 or more employees were required to offer a choice between traditional insurance and a health maintenance organization (HMO). Enrollment in managed care has soared in the past two decades—from 6 million subscribers in the mid-1970s to over 70 million in 1997—forever changing the way in which medicine is practiced and patients are treated.

Managed care is a catchall term describing a system that combines coverage of health care costs and delivery of health care for a prepaid premium. Instead of paying claims submitted by independent doctors or hospitals, managed care companies employ or have contracts with doctors and hospitals that set policies for what they can or can't do.

For instance, in order to cut down on self-defined unnecessary procedures and reduce money spent on prescription drugs, HMOs use an authorization process to limit access to specialists. While the process might seem logical to providers, it is illogical to the parent whose child has recently been diagnosed with hydrocephalus or needs a shunt revision, and who is required to jump through hoops in order to receive proper care.

Even if you keep the same doctor you had before joining an HMO, with managed care she may be working under guidelines created by the insurance company that you aren't aware of. Rather than permitting doctors to treat their patients as needed, decisions about your care are established by the HMO based on what it feels is more cost-effective for a larger percentage of the population—not your individual needs. This means that the amount of time your doctor spends with you on an appointment, what tests or treatment alternatives to offer, and which hospital you will be treated in are the call of the HMO—not necessarily your doctor.

> *Learn more about your HMO's policy regarding the use of doctors and facilities outside of the plan. We had one heck of a time trying to get our HMO to let us go outside the plan to see a pediatric neurosurgeon. It took us a few weeks to finally convince the HMO to authorize us taking Brandon outside their network. The way we finally pulled it off was to have the HMO's neurosurgeon write a letter stating that he felt our son needed specialized care that he couldn't provide. And since he was the top neurosurgeon in the plan, his letter must have carried more weight.*

> *When the HMO finally authorized us to go outside their plan, they told us we would have to pay the first $500 for any charges incurred, which we thought was fair, because at least we knew our son was going to see someone who knew what he was doing.*

Preferred provider organization (PPO)

Preferred provider organizations (PPOs) are groups of hospitals and/or physicians who, directly or through a third party, develop contractual agreements with payers to provide a specified set of health care services under defined financial arrangements. PPO services require co-payments for such things as office and emergency room visits as well as some other services.

An exclusive provider organization (EPO) is similar to a PPO in its organization and purpose. The main difference between the two is that EPOs limit subscribers to participating providers for their health care services. Most PPOs offer their customers an EPO option because it aids in controlling the cost of health care. EPOs are usually implemented by employers whose primary concern is providing low-cost health benefits to employees.

Independent practice association (IPA)

An independent practice association (IPA) is a group of independent, private-practice physicians who have banded together in an association that contracts with various HMOs. The doctors agree to accept a set monthly fee per patient (capitation) in exchange for providing all medical care for HMO members. They are not compensated for the actual medical care given.

All of the risk moves from the insurers to the physicians and from a very large pool of people to a much smaller pool of people—those seen by a single practice. For instance, if one patient treated by the group needs a quarter-million dollar kidney transplant, that could consume all of the profits for the year. In extreme cases (an unlucky year for patients) the doctors could go broke by giving their patients the care they need.

These flat-fee systems encourage doctors to take on as many healthy patients as possible because they lose money treating patients with complicated or time-consuming illnesses—such as hydrocephalus. Capitation systems create a stark ethical conflict for doctors: treat patients and lose money. The threat of financial risk (or in extreme cases, insolvency) diminishes their ability to be caring and objective physicians.

Government plans

You may have a government plan if you are in the military or covered by Medicare or Medicaid. Medicare and Medicaid are managed by the Health Care Financing Administration (HCFA), part of U.S. Department of Health and Human Services (DHHS).

TriCare

TriCare, formerly known as CHAMPUS, is the Department of Defense's response to rising health care costs. TriCare was first implemented in March 1995 in the states of Washington and Oregon. The program is designed to expand access to care and control health care costs for patients and the taxpayer. TriCare is available for active duty members, qualified family members, CHAMPUS-eligible retirees and their families, and survivors of all uniformed services. It is currently being implemented by region throughout the U.S., and should be nationwide by the end of 1998.

For additional information about TriCare, contact:

TriCare Management Activity (TMA)
TMA Benefit Services
16401 E. Centretech Parkway
Aurora, Colorado 80011-9043
Phone: (303) 676-3526
Email: *questions@ochampus.mil*
http://www.ochampus.mil/

Medicaid

Medicaid is a health care program for indigent and needy persons, regardless of age. It is financed by general taxation. Every state in the country contributes to the general pool, and the federal government matches those contributions to supplement the program. Medicaid can be used for five basic services:

- Doctor visits.

- Inpatient treatment at a hospital.

- Outpatient treatment at a hospital or authorized medical clinic.

- Laboratory tests and X-rays.

- Medical services provided by nursing homes.

Eligibility for Medicaid varies from state to state. To obtain more information about your state's Medicaid program and information on how to apply for Medicaid, contact your state insurance director. The listing for your state insurance director can be found in the blue pages of your phone book.

Medicare

Medicare is a federally funded, national health insurance program for elderly people in the United States. People who are covered by Medicare are required to pay 20 percent of the bill for all covered medical services. While this might work well for older Americans who are in good health, persons who have serious or chronic health conditions could lose their life savings. For example, if an elderly man on Medicare needed to have his shunt revised and the bill came to $50,000, he would be required to pay $10,000 of that bill. If his shunt were to fail more than once in a year, the cost could be devastating.

Medicare benefits include:

- Inpatient treatment at a hospital for up to 90 days per illness.

- Outpatient services offered by hospitals.

- Inpatient psychiatric care, up to a maximum of 190 days total.

- Extended care services following hospitalization for up to 100 days per illness.

- Home health care services following hospitalization for up to 100 visits per year.

Socialized medicine

Canada, the United Kingdom, Sweden, and Australia have socialized medicine—a system in which every citizen in the population is provided medical care and treatment, and the government picks up the tab. Citizens of countries with socialized medical systems often pay higher income taxes (Canada's highest tax bracket is near 60 percent, compared to 36 percent in the U.S.), have larger amounts of their income deducted, or pay additional sales taxes and sin taxes (taxes on tobacco and alcohol).

The government collects tax dollars and distributes this money to the hospitals, doctors, imaging centers, labs, etc., throughout the country. In some countries, if you earn more than a certain dollar amount annually, you are required to pay a nominal monthly or quarterly premium for the right to receive care under the plan. The government determines how much the doctors will earn, as well as how and when doctors can treat patients.

We experienced Canada's socialized medical system in 1991 when my wife needed to have her shunt revised. At the time (according to her neurosurgeon), neurosurgeons in the province of British Columbia were limited to only eight hours of nonemergency surgery per week. When you compute the time that it takes to perform a shunt placement or revision, including pre- and postop, this regulation restricted neurosurgeons to performing only two to four nonemergency operations per week. With their hands tied by the government, patients in need of surgery were placed on waiting lists by their doctors.

In the case of my wife's first shunt revision that year, the neurosurgeon determined it was a routine shunt revision, and therefore she remained on a waiting list for nearly four months to have her shunt revised. Meantime, her condition continued to worsen, and there was nothing that her neurosurgeon could do. All we could do was sit and wait until the neurosurgeon could get her in, and hope that nothing went terribly wrong.

Sure, when the bill arrived, we didn't have to pay a dime. We paid $0 of a $42,000+ bill that included eight days of intensive care treatment for her following the revision. Or did we?

In the U.S., where insurance pays for costs, millions of Americans go without medical care because they simply cannot afford to pay the premiums or because of a preexisting condition that makes it impossible to obtain coverage. Any system of health care payment and delivery has problems and inequities. The more familiar you are with the system you are working under—and the more assertive you are about your own rights—generally, the better off you will be.

Hospital billing

Bills can be one of the lasting nightmares of hospital stays. Even when you have good insurance and your hospital stay is short, it pays to keep good records, stay alert for billing inaccuracies, and get problems resolved quickly. Even bills for short stays or simple procedures can quickly reach very large amounts.

When treatment is long and complex, the potential for errors escalates and the consequences of not having records or of ignoring problems can be financially devastating. For all families, knowing what expenses are tax-deductible will help you keep the necessary records now and potentially save you money at tax time.

Keeping financial records

Accurate records are a necessary defense against hospital overbilling. Poor organization of bills can mean you will be hounded by collection companies. However, many simple systems exist for keeping financial records.

For most financial records, you will need only an expandable folder. If your treatments for hydrocephalus involve many or lengthy hospital stays, you will probably need a well-organized file cabinet. Financial records are a major headache for many patients or parents, but keep organized records to protect your credit and your ability to support your family's other wants and needs.

- Whenever you open an envelope containing medical billing or insurance information, file the contents immediately. Don't put it on a pile or throw it into a drawer.

- Keep a notebook with a running log of all tax-deductible medical expenses, including the date and type of service, the charges, if the bill has been paid, the date it was paid, and the check number.

- Don't pay a bill unless you have checked over each item listed to make sure that it is correct.

- Set up a file cabinet just for medical expense records. Have hanging files for hospital bills, doctor bills, all other medical bills (such as lab work or imaging), insurance explanations of benefits (EOBs), prescription receipts, tax-deductible receipts (bridge or road tolls, parking, motels, meals, etc.), and any applicable correspondence.

Hospital billing problems

Not everyone experiences billing problems. People who have managed health care plans or receive public assistance may never see their bills. Other people have no problems with billing throughout the treatment. But many people do encounter billing problems. To avoid these problems:

- Keep all records filed in an organized fashion.

- Check every bill from the hospital to make sure there are no charges for treatments not provided, or errors, such as double-billing.

- Check to see if the hospital has financial counselors. If so, make contact early in the hospitalization. Counselors provide services in many areas, including help with understanding the hospital's billing system, billing insurance carriers, explaining benefits, hospital and insurance correspondence, dealing with Medicaid and Medicare, working out a payment plan, designing a ledger system for tracking insurance claims, and resolving disputes.

- Compare each hospital bill to the explanation of benefits (EOB) you receive from your insurance company. Track down discrepancies.

- Call the hospital immediately if you find a billing error. Write down the date, the name of the person you talk to, and the plan of action.

- Call and talk to the billing supervisor if the error is not corrected on your next bill. Explain politely the steps you have already taken and how you would like the problem resolved.

- Write a brief letter to the billing supervisor if the problem is not corrected. Explain the steps you have taken and request immediate action. Keep a copy of each letter you write.

- Ask the hospital billing department and your insurance company, in writing, to audit your account if you are inundated with a constant stream of bills and there are major discrepancies between the hospital charges and your records of the treatment provided. This is a common practice. Insist on a line-by-line explanation for each charge.

- Ask a family member or friend to help if you are too tired or overwhelmed to deal with the bills. He could come every other week, open and file all bills and insurance papers, make phone calls on your behalf, and write all necessary letters. A friend also could enter your records in a computer database or spreadsheet if you do not have access to one.

- Don't let billing problems accumulate. Your account may end up at a collection agency, which can quickly become a huge headache.

Emily had been having problems with recurring numbness to her left side, and the local neurosurgeons couldn't come up with an explanation. They were unwilling to go beyond having an MRI done, so we took our daughter to a major university medical center to be examined by one of the top neurosurgeons in the country. After examining her and performing a shunt tap to test the cerebrospinal fluid for any abnormalities, he sent us on our way.

Three weeks later, we received a bill in the mail from the university for $3,000 for neurosurgery! We were flabbergasted! I called the billing office right away, and asked what the bill was for, and of course they didn't know. I explained to them that they should go back and check the medical records because our daughter did not have an operation, but rather a simple ten-minute procedure.

Another two weeks went by, and still no response, so I phoned them again. This time, they said that they were waiting for the medical records to be sent to billing by the neurosurgical department. When I asked where billing was in relationship to the neurosurgical department, the lady informed me that they were just in the building next door.

Trying not to lose my cool, I explained to her that I didn't want this to go on our credit record or for our insurance company to think that our daughter was operated on when she wasn't. I continued by stating that I had written our insurance company telling them not to pay the claim because I was disputing the charge. This must have struck a chord, because she phoned back the next day saying she had Emily's record, and noted the erroneous charge, and said that she would resubmit the claim for a shunt tap—a $150 outpatient procedure.

Tax-deductible medical expenses

Insurance may not cover many expenses, including gas, car repairs, motels, meals while you're away from home, health insurance deductibles, and prescriptions. Many of these items can be deducted from your federal income tax. To find out what can be legally deducted while you or your child undergoes medical treatment, get IRS publication 502. This booklet is available at many public libraries and at most IRS offices. It can also be ordered by calling 1-800-TAX-FORM (1-800-829-3676) from 8 a.m. to 5 p.m. weekdays, and 9 a.m. to 3 p.m. on Saturdays. IRS publications can also be ordered online from the IRS web site at: *http://www.irs.gov/*.

The Hydrocephalus Association also offers a free information sheet, *Tax Considerations for Parents of Disabled Children*. Contact information to request a copy is listed in Appendix B, *Associations and Organizations*.

Managing bills and paperwork

Overcharges account for a large percentage of all hospital bills. If you come across any errors in your bill, don't be afraid to be assertive. Keeping copies of all the forms you need to submit will give you a record of what is paid and what is outstanding. Maintain a separate file with medical bills and information. Then if there are any future questions regarding unpaid bills/ expenses you know exactly where to obtain that information.

If you suspect an error on your bill, insist that you be sent an itemized list with descriptions of services that have been provided during your hospital stay. Make sure the list has services listed and not just codes. Your hospital records are another great resource; you can compare what's actually been done and what your bill states is due. It's a wise idea to verify the bill before submitting it to your insurance provider.

In hospitals, there are no freebies. Everything they supply from slippers to toothpaste has a price tag—a high price tag! Bring as many of these personal items from home as possible to avoid being charged luxury rates.

Insurance claims and denials

You can obtain maximum benefit from your insurance policy by keeping accurate records and challenging any claims your provider denies:

- Make photocopies of everything you send to your insurance company, including claims, letters, and bills.

- Pay bills by check and keep copies of all canceled checks.

- Keep all correspondence you receive from billing and insurance companies.

- Write down the date, the name of the person contacted, and the details of all telephone conversations related to insurance.

- Keep accurate records of all medical expenses and claims you submit.

Establish a contact person

If you suspect problems or if complications arise, your first step should be to contact your insurance provider. On your initial call, you will be transferred to the first available representative. If, for whatever reason, you don't like the person you are speaking with, ask to be transferred to a different representative. Insurers can sometimes assign you a specific person to review your claims and answer any questions you may have regarding benefits.

When you reach the representative who will be handling your claims, you should write down the representative's name and her extension number. Having someone who is familiar with your case history will save countless hours of having to reexplain your situation each time you call. By developing a cooperative relationship with your insurance representative, you will help to make things run more smoothly and eliminate at least one element of stress.

> I was having trouble trying to communicate my son's needs to the representative on the other end of the phone one day. After having taken Brian from doctor to doctor, and getting a cranky representative on the other end of the line, I was about to lose it. I told her that my son has a very serious condition, which requires specialized care and treatment. She just didn't get it.

My solution was to mail her a nice letter, introducing myself and explaining hydrocephalus to her, in brief. I also included a couple photos of Brian—one of him wearing his soccer uniform, the other of him lying in a hospital bed, shortly after a recent shunt revision. I received a call from her the day she received the letter and photos, and our relationship changed instantly. From that point forward, she's been Brian's advocate on the inside.

If you are insured through your employer, the human resources (HR) representative at work is another person you can turn to when you have questions about your medical coverage. Your HR contact should be familiar with all the details of your health plan. In many cases, your HR representative can act as a liaison between you and the insurance company in the event of any billing discrepancies or denied claims.

Right to appeal denials

You have the right to appeal claims denied by your insurance company. Don't be afraid to ask questions and be persistent:

- Keep original documents in your files and send photocopies to the insurance company with a letter outlining why you think the claim should be covered. Sample appeal letters are provided for your use at the end of this chapter.

- Demand a written reply.

- Talk to your state insurance commissioner (or other office with similar duties) to learn how to file a complaint. Find out what power the state has to help you resolve your dispute.

- Contact your congressional delegation. All senators and members of the House of Representatives have staff members who help constituents with problems.

- Take your claim to small claims court or hire an attorney skilled in insurance matters to sue the insurance company if you've exhausted all other means to resolve the dispute.

Grievances and appeals

Problems fall into two broad categories: grievances and appeals. Grievances are complaints about service, such as a rude doctor or waiting too long for an appointment. Appeals are a procedure used when the plan denies or terminates a service you think you need, or refuses to pay for care you've already received.

To file a grievance with your HMO, take the following steps:

- Talk to the person with whom you had the problem to see if it can be resolved.

- Call the member services department and explain the problem. Make sure to write down the date and time, the phone number, and the first and last names of the person with whom you spoke. Keep a record of what was said and note the person's direct phone line number.

- If the problem is not resolved, write to the plan to ask for an investigation. Different states (as well as each plan) have varying amounts of time they allow for response. To find out your state's regulations, call your state department of insurance.

- Call frequently to ask about the status of the investigation..

Take the following steps to begin the appeal process:

- First, make an appointment with your primary care physician to explain your problem and ask for help. For example, if the problem is refusal to refer you to a specialist, ask her for the reasons (medical and economic) why she refuses to refer you. Tell her clearly why you think the referral is necessary. You may just change her mind.

- Your plan is required to notify you in writing about any denial, reduction, or termination of services. If you have not received it, ask for a written response explaining the medical and financial reasons for refusing the treatment or payment. Demand that the names of all persons involved in the decision, including any "medical advisors" and their qualifications, be included. You should also ask for articles from the medical literature that support the plan's position. If the administration can't or won't provide any, your case is strengthened. In the meantime, locate articles that support your position and attach them to your appeal.

- Take the written denial to your primary care doctor to ask her to write a letter of appeal on your behalf. For instance, if your doctor thinks you need a sophisticated diagnostic test, but the HMO refuses to pay for it, she might be willing to go to bat for you. If she refuses, try to get the plan to send you to another doctor in the network for a second opinion. If they refuse, or if you feel it is important to get an out-of-network view, pay for an independent second opinion yourself.

- Write a letter of appeal yourself and send it to the insurance carrier and your employment benefits manager. Send the letter by certified mail and get a receipt with the signature of the person who accepted the letter. The letter should include a clear and concise definition of the problem, as well as your name, policy number, doctors' statements, lab results, and other pertinent materials. Make sure to state in the letter what action you want the group to take to resolve the problem. Don't delay writing the letter: your right to start an appeal may expire in as few as thirty days. Keep copies of all correspondence for your records.

- The appeal process begins when you write the letter asking for reconsideration of the HMO's decision. The plan generally must complete this reconsideration of their decision within sixty days. Keep calling to find out the status of the appeal. If you need an expedited appeal because your health could be in peril if you wait the sixty days, request it in writing, and enclose supporting documentation from a doctor.

- Consider hiring a medical claims assistance professional. She will organize paperwork, research appeals procedures, and gather medical reports.

- To go outside the HMO for help, send a copy of your written complaint and related documents to the state insurance commissioner as well as your local and state medical societies.

- Send your appeal to your state senators and representatives, and your U.S. senators and representatives. These elected officials have staff members who try to help their constituents. In addition, it helps them as they ponder how to vote on health-care-related bills to know the struggles that members of managed care organizations sometimes face.

- If you are insured through your place of employment, contact the benefits department or union benefits manager to see if they will support your position. If enough problems arise, your company may threaten to find another health care plan, and this threat may help resolve your problem favorably.

- Don't pay a bill that your insurance or Medicaid should pay, even if the claim is taking a long time going thorough the system and you are being hounded by collection agencies. Many public assistance programs, such as Medicaid, have no provision for reimbursing you once you have paid. Keep your providers informed about your efforts to get payment.

A lawyer suggests:

- If you still have the problem, tell the HMO staffers that you will go to the local and national press after a certain date if the problem is not resolved. Sometimes the threat of bad press will help, while other times it hurts.

- Contact Physicians Who Care, an advocacy group of more than 3,500 doctors. Call their complaint hot line (1-800-800-5154) and leave a message about any abuse or ill effects (denial of access to specialists or procedures, reimbursement problems, denials of needed treatments, etc.) resulting from your HMO care. They will contact you by letter within a week. All information is confidential.

- Contact a consumer advocacy group such as the Consumer Federation of America's insurance group at (202) 547-6426. Or the Center for Patient Advocacy at 1-800-846-7444 or online at *http://www.patientadvocacy.org/*. Families USA provides a list of state agencies regulating health care and information on state managed care laws at (202) 628-3030 or *http://www.familiesusa.org/*.

- Contact the local media, including newspapers and radio and television stations. Nearly all forms of media have a writer or reporter who covers consumer complaints to help people in their community resolve their problems.

- Get a lawyer. Lawsuits can take years, and involve endless maneuvering. Most people who go through the process say they underestimated how hard it would be, especially to relive the medical trauma. And then, of course, there is the possibility that you have a legitimate case but will be unable to prove it in court, or state laws may limit your right to collect. Nevertheless, legal help may be your last chance to get the care you need. Contact your local bar association to find an attorney skilled in insurance litigation.

Try to remember that many managed care organizations are used to passive consumers. Proactive, savvy HMO consumers can get excellent and comprehensive health care from an HMO if they choose wisely and have a good relationship with their doctor. Even when you are happy with your care, check the status of your HMO periodically, because they are being bought, sold, and merged at a rapid rate. Make sure that economic forces have not changed the quality of the care provided by your plan.

Sample letters of appeal

The following sample letters are provided for use in appealing denied claims or services by your insurance company. The First Level Appeal letter should be sent out upon notice that a particular service or claim has been denied. The Second Level Appeal letter should be sent either after your initial letter was ignored or if the claim or service was denied a second time.

When sending letters of appeal to your insurance company, it is important that you sign and date each letter and retain a copy for your own files. Make sure that your full name, mailing address, and phone number are at the top of each letter.

These letters are provided courtesy of Cynthia Solomon, Medical Management Resources, Sonoma, California. They were presented at the Hydrocephalus Association's 5th National Conference on Hydrocephalus, March 26-29, 1998.

First Level Appeal

Your Name
Your Address
Your City/State/Province/Zip/Postal Code
Your Phone Number

DATE

Name of Insurance Company
Address
City/State/Province/Zip/Postal Code

Re:
Patient Name:
Date of Birth: Month, Day, Year
Patient ID/Subscriber Number: xxxxxxxxxx

Dear Sir/Madam:

You recently denied a claim for services provided by (name of provider) on (date of services).

I feel denial of this claim was not justified and I am herewith appealing the denial. Please be aware that my child, (name of the patient), has a serious and potentially life-threatening condition and his/her access to care is critical to his/her well-being.

Please review this claim again. The information is correct (or has been corrected) to reflect the appropriate diagnosis and treatment. If you need a medical report, please inform me within 10 days.

I can be reached at the following telephone number(s):

Daytime: (000) 555-1212
Evening: (000) 555-1212

Thank you for your prompt attention to this matter.

Sincerely,

(Your signature goes here)

Second Level Appeal—Request for Hearing

Your Name
Your Address
Your City/State/Province/Zip/Postal Code
Your Phone Number

DATE

Name of Insurance Company
Address
City/State/Province/Zip/Postal Code

Attention: Claims Supervisor

Re:
(Name of Patient)
Date of Birth: Month, Day, Year
Patient ID/Subscriber Number: xxxxxxxxxx

Dear Sir/Madam:

On (date of the first letter), I appealed a denied claim (or service request) for my child. A copy of that claim and appeal letter is enclosed.

I have not heard from you (or the claim remains denied; state reason here). I am herewith requesting a hearing to resolve this matter. I feel that denial and non-payment of this claim has jeopardized my child's access to health care.

If I do not hear from you within 10 days, I am referring this matter to Consumer Assistance, and the State Insurance Commission, and may also seek legal counsel.

In my opinion, you have failed in your obligation to provide acceptable and adequate service. Be assured that I intend to use every available means to get this matter resolved.

Sincerely,

(Your signature here)

cc: Employer Benefits Manager
Physician Hospital Billing Office

Certified Mail

CHAPTER 11

The Well-Informed Patient

A scientist who is also a human being cannot
rest while knowledge which might be used to
reduce suffering rests on the shelf.

—Dr. Albert Sabin
New York Times

WITH A DIAGNOSIS OF HYDROCEPHALUS, many people feel their lives have spun out of control. By becoming a well-informed patient or parent, you can learn to deal with the intricacies of hydrocephalus and how it impacts daily life. There are things that you can learn and do that will enhance your chances for a longer and healthier life, as well as allow you to regain a measure of control.

This chapter first looks at managing the condition medically: knowing your history, having access to records, and passing on your history to doctors. Knowing your history will help you to be alert to medications, tests, or lifestyle choices that might be dangerous and which you should avoid. Since getting good and appropriate medical care depends in part on communication, we also briefly address the doctor-patient relationship.

Next, we look at planning ahead for emergencies: telling people around you what symptoms to look for; ordering a MedicAlert bracelet to warn EMTs and hospital staff of your condition(s); carrying a surgical shunt card in your wallet with views of your latest CT or MRI scan; preparing a Durable Power of Attorney for Health Care.

Now that you are becoming more informed about hydrocephalus, you might want to look up medical reports and journal articles that apply to your particular condition. We give a quick look at finding medical texts, including two recommended online databases, and how to order the full text of articles whose abstracts look interesting.

We close the chapter with a look at some of the medical legislation in the United States, including the Americans with Disabilities Act, the Biomaterials Access Assurance Act, the Family and Medical Leave Act, and Social Security. By the end of this chapter, you should be well on your way to being a well-informed patient—capable of making knowledge-based decisions about the care you or your child receives.

Managing your medical condition

Managing your medical condition means many things. You need to know all of your medical history—the types of surgeries you've had and when, what medications you're on, and what reactions you've had to them. There's a lot to know, and in many ways, keeping track of your medical history is just as much work as going through all of the exams, tests, and operations. Additionally, you need to be able to make wise, informed lifestyle choices and manage the relationships you have with your doctors to ensure you receive the best care possible.

Knowing your medical history

A thorough knowledge of your medical history is essential for assertive patients. You will need this knowledge to educate all of your doctors on the particulars of your medical past, as well as to ensure that your current care is state-of-the-art.

If possible, try to obtain copies of all your medical records. When you see a new doctor or specialist, bring your copies with you. The new doctor can make copies for herself and familiarize herself with your medical history. Having this information available is especially helpful if you relocate. Allow doctors to copy your records, but make sure that you have them all back when you leave.

> We keep copies of all of Evan's medical records, and have numbered each page with a sticker in the lower right corner. This way, we know before we go to the doctors how many pages we are taking with us as a way of ensuring that we get all of them back if they need to make any copies.

Additionally, ask your doctors to send copies of any correspondence or reports to your home address so you can keep your own records up to date.

Obtaining past records

Medical records are the property of the hospital or the doctor, not yours. However, most states have laws that permit you the right to review, copy, and request amendments to your medical records. One way you can learn more about your state law is to contact your state legislator's office and ask them to provide the medical record access law for your state.

> *When we take Lee to see any of her specialists, we let them know that we want to receive copies of all correspondence and of entries made to her medical record. This way, we are aware of what's going on and what's being discussed between the various doctors. Knowing what's going on behind the scenes is very important—and often enlightening.*

Provisions that your state law might contain are:

- You will need to submit a written request to review all or part of your medical records.

- You have the right to review your medical records at a hospital or doctor's office.

- The review may be supervised to ensure the contents of the records are kept intact. Keep in mind that the staff person who supervises your review of the records should not be considered qualified to answer questions about the contents of your records.

- If you have a question regarding an entry in your medical records, you have the right to ask the doctor about it when he is available.

- During the review, you can usually indicate which copies of the records you would like to receive. The law also might specify that your doctor doesn't have to provide you with copies of your records on the spot. It might specify a timeframe (for example, 30 days) in which your doctor can provide you with the copies you've requested.

- A fee schedule for copies might also be specified in the law, including a search fee to locate your chart, and a maximum fee for each page copied.

- Patients who either cannot, do not want, or are unable to conduct a personal review can usually specify what copies they want (i.e., surgical, pathology, and imaging reports; discharge summaries, etc.) or request the complete medical record.

Don't be too surprised if you encounter varied responses from your doctors when you request to read or receive a copy your chart.

> When I asked my neurosurgeon for copies of my records and any correspondence he had about me, he looked amused and said, "Now why would you want to read through all that?" After I explained to him that my husband and I wanted to piece together my medical history so we could learn more about my condition, his attitude changed and he said he'd help out any way he could.

If you run into problems obtaining copies of your records, it sometimes helps to phone or write the medical records administrator of the hospital or medical group and ask for help. In addition, copies of medical records are usually provided directly to a new health care provider without fee upon receipt of a written authorization. If you are having trouble getting access to your records, you might authorize another doctor or even your dentist to receive the records and turn them over to you for your review.

Organizing records

Once you have copies of your medical records, take the time to read through them and organize them in chronological order. Place the records and reports in a file folder with the most recent material on top. That way, if you need to refer to a recent test or exam, it is right on top. This also makes it easy to refer back to when going over medical bills and insurance claims.

> One thing that we have done is to compile a summary of my wife's medical history, as it pertains to her hydrocephalus. The hardest part for us was going back into the 1970s to obtain copies of her medical records, some of which were destroyed. However, we were able to piece together the original cause of her hydrocephalus (an astrocytoma), and have compiled a two-page summary sheet, which is organized from the past to the present.

Recommended information to include in a medical summary:

- **Dates.** These include admission and discharge dates from the hospital, tests, and when imaging studies were done.

- **Description.** A brief description of what happened on a particular date; whether it was an operation, imaging study, or change in medications.

- **Attending physician.** Include the name, address, and phone number of the attending physician for that particular event (if known).

- **Place of service.** Where the operation or imaging study was performed.

- **Diagnosis/treatment.** A brief description of the diagnosis and/or treatment.

- **Medications.** List all the medications you are taking, as well as any to which you are allergic.

By compiling this information and keeping it all in one place, you will be able to provide this summary to new doctors and specialists at the first appointment. This summary helps them by giving a quick overview of your medical history. If physicians need to find out additional information, they can always refer to the copies of the medical records you have provided.

Lifestyle choices

Living with hydrocephalus, for some, requires minor lifestyle changes. You should check with your neurosurgeon about particular circumstances for your case.

> *Growing up with hydrocephalus, I led a very active life. I was in school, I rode with the Westernaires, a high-speed, mounted drill riding organization, and I was in the school play.*

Some neurosurgeons recommend that their patients:

- Avoid impact to the head. Some neurosurgeons recommend that their patients avoid contact sports altogether, such as American football or rugby. If you play soccer, you will want to avoid "heading" the ball. And you'll want to wear protective headgear for biking, in-line skating, and other sports.

- Fly only on airplanes with pressurized cabins. Changes in outside pressure could affect ICP. Commercial flights have pressurized cabins, and loss of air pressure is rare. Flying in private, unpressurized planes should be avoided. Avoid sudden or prolonged increases in gravitational forces or flying that includes going upside down, such as during stunt flying or testing aircraft performance.

- Avoid all scuba diving. People with hydrocephalus are extremely sensitive to changes in ICP. As scuba divers descend, pressure on the body increases. Swimming closer to the surface (e.g., snorkeling or swimming underwater) poses no problems.

• Avoid other health-compromising behavior such as smoking, drinking alcohol to excess, taking drugs, or engaging in risky behavior.

I lived life like the normal college student, sleeping little, partying with friends, not eating the healthiest of meals, and drinking alcohol. The headaches/hangovers I had as a result of drinking alcohol definitely exceeded my friends', especially for the amount of alcohol I consumed—I did not drink that much.

What I think should be the biggest concern for an individual with a shunt partying with his/her college buddies is not the direct effect that the alcohol has on the CSF and the brain, but rather, the actions that an alcohol-impaired person may take. That person's judgment is impaired, and his decision-making process is not at its best. This should always be a part of a shunted individual's decision-making process.

As at other levels of schooling, it is important that an individual's college classmates and teachers are aware of the condition just in case of an emergency. In my situation, my shunt malfunctioned in college and it was my roommates who brought me to the hospital, where I met my parents and neurosurgeon. I wouldn't want to think of the potential outcome if my roommates did not know of my hydrocephalus and shunt. It is because of this kind of situation that I am a strong supporter of wearing a MedicAlert necklace or bracelet.

Pregnancy and hydrocephalus

Modern treatment for hydrocephalus has been around only since John Holter invented the flow-control valve in 1957. As such, many women who have received shunts since the 1960s are part of the first generation of childbearing age. How hydrocephalus and shunts are affected during pregnancy and labor has been a relatively unknown factor, untracked by most neurosurgeons.

To help track the effects of pregnancy on women with hydrocephalus, Nancy Bradley has created the Maternal Hydrocephalus Study. Nancy is a mother of two and has been shunted for hydrocephalus since birth. The study, which began in May 1994, collected data from 37 women from the United States,

Canada, and the United Kingdom, who had a total of 77 pregnancies. The results of her study were published in the September 1998 issue of the journal *Neurosurgery.*

For additional information on the Maternal Hydrocephalus Study, or to participate in the continuing study, contact:

Nancy Bradley
8403 Boyne Street
Downey, CA 90242
Phone: (562) 869-3689
Email: *hydrowoman@aol.com*

The doctor-patient relationship

Times have changed since the first code of the American Medical Association was written in 1847, which included these words:

> *There is a class of patients much dreaded by physicians, namely, those who insist upon being taken into a medical consultation with regard to the treatment. Such patients desire not only to know what medicines are prescribed, but to discuss the reasons therefor; they are not content without exercising their own judgment concerning therapeutic indications and the means of fulfilling them.*

Knowledgeable patients no longer blindly follow the advice of their physicians, and with good reason. With the explosion of medical knowledge in the last few decades, one doctor cannot know it all. In addition, doctors are trained to treat disease, not to balance the beneficial with the detrimental consequences of treatment for individuals. However, if you think of the proposed therapy in terms of your philosophy of life, family situation, and job, and discuss the therapy with your doctor in that light, your treatment can be tailored more personally for you.

The process of working with your doctor to find an optimal treatment plan tailored to all your needs can be easy or difficult, depending on what you find out in your research and the personalities and communication skills you and your doctor possess. The following story from a mother whose child has hydrocephalus illustrates the conflicts that sometimes arise over sharing medical information and decision-making:

> *We always seemed embroiled in one conflict after another with our daughter's neurosurgeon. Caley had just been through her fifth shunt*

revision in less than three months, and we were furious. We wanted to know what was causing the problems that required her shunt to be revised. We wanted to know if there was a different type of shunt that could be used. We wanted to know if there was a different place the shunt could be located. And when we asked the question, "Is there a more quali-fied and skilled neurosurgeon out there to treat Caley?" the neurosurgeon became enraged—like we personally attacked his self-esteem!

All we want is the best care for our daughter, but he seems to be too caught up in his ego to even listen to us. Just because we aren't colleagues of his shouldn't mean that we should be blocked out of the treatment and decision-making process for our daughter.

Some strategies for improving understanding prior to making joint deci-sions are:

- You and your physician should compare definitions of the problem, goals of treatment, and preferred methods of treatment.

- Ask the doctor why she thinks the recommended treatment is best and if there are any guidelines for treating your illness or condition.

- Explain as clearly as you can your life circumstances that make one treatment more appropriate than another. If, for instance, you have three preschool children at home, you will not want to take an antiseizure medication that would cause you to sleep most of the day.

- Repeat back instructions and explanations to make sure you under-stand. One way to do this is to say, "Let me see if I fully understand. You think the problem is _____, caused by _____. You want me to take ___ medication and call you back in a week if things improve, and sooner if they get worse."

- If you find yourself getting overwhelmed by information during an appointment, say so and ask to come back another time to complete your discussion.

- Bring a list of all of your prescription and over-the-counter medications with you to each appointment. Your doctor can be tired or hurried, and she may forget one or more of your medications or conditions. When-ever your doctor writes a prescription for a new medication, take out your list and go over it together to make sure that all of the medications are compatible. At this time, remind the doctor of any chronic health conditions, such as diabetes, congestive heart failure, or asthma.

Ask questions

The only stupid question is one that goes unasked. This is particularly true when you're dealing with a medical condition that can be as potentially life-threatening as hydrocephalus.

Because of the resources that are available, many patients today are more educated than in the past. Some patients demand to know what exactly is being prescribed and why. This can make many physicians uncomfortable. Just remember, the more you know about your medical history and the medications you're on, the better you will be able to form a partnership with your doctor to get excellent health care.

Patients should be afforded an opportunity to ask questions if they have them. If you ask questions every time you see your doctor, it helps to keep the lines of communication open and shows the doctor that you have an interest in the care you or your child receives. It helps to build a solid doctor-patient relationship that's based on trust. Even if the only thing you can think of is, "Are there any new treatments or procedures available for treating my condition?"—ask it. In addition to gathering information, asking questions has been shown actually to improve a patient's response to treatment.

> I always ask questions when I go to see my neurosurgeon. There are times when I might have a weird pain in my head or abdomen, and I'm not sure whether it's associated with my VP shunt or not. I make a list of all the questions I want to ask, then bring that along with me. He's pretty good about answering them, too.

If you are not used to asking your doctor questions, it can be intimidating to start. Don't let doctors intimidate you. If you have a question about your condition, a test, or a procedure, you have every right to ask for a clarification from your doctor. To survive and thrive, it is important that you know as much as possible about your condition. Think about it this way: for most doctors, medicine is a passion and consumes virtually all of their time. Just like anyone with a passion, they tend to enjoy talking about it. So keep asking questions—it's one of many ways to learn what you need to heal.

Change how you talk to your doctor

Communication is a two-way street. Many patients find that when they consciously change the way they interact with their doctor, the relationship shifts. One mother of a child with a serious illness was irritated when the doctor said at every visit, "I'm surprised to see him doing so well." After several variations of this gloomy comment, she finally responded, "Really, we rejoice in each day, and expect many more." The mother continued to talk in a positive manner and saw a gradual shift in her doctor's outlook.

> *I talk to my neurosurgeon the same way I'd like him to talk to me. I try not to be confrontational, which can be hard sometimes when I don't seem to get the answers I'm looking for. But I try to remember that he's busy, just like me, and it won't do my child any good if I get in his face.*

Show appreciation

Doctors, like patients, are grateful for encouragement, expressions of appreciation, or a pat on the back. Thank-you notes for kind deeds or excellent work are treasured by doctors because they don't often get such tangible expressions of thanks. Patients who show appreciation for their doctors and nurses help smooth over the rough spots that are inevitable in relationships and bring some much-needed pleasure into the sometimes grim work of medical caregivers. Praise shows that you appreciate the difficulty of their jobs. Feedback also gives doctors vital information on how their actions help or hurt their patients. Rewarding good deeds is one of the most effective methods to alter behavior.

> *This might sound strange to some, but I sent my wife's neurosurgeon a thank-you card after her last checkup. I always go to the doctor with my wife, mainly so there's someone else there to help interpret things that are said. I thought he handled all of her questions and concerns in a very professional and kind manner, and I appreciated that.*

Not only are expressions of thanks appreciated, but they help establish a more balanced relationship. You are relating in an active, human way rather than being a passive recipient of an exam and medical advice. It also creates a "goodwill bank." When you make many deposits, an occasional withdrawal will not be as noticeable.

A positive relationship between patient and doctor thrives on clear and frequent communication. Good communication can improve the quality of care you or your child receives. Poor communication can leave doctors, parents, and children feeling angry and resentful. Doctors should explain things clearly and listen well, and parents should feel comfortable asking questions and expressing concerns before they become grievances.

Preparing for emergencies

Think about all of the times that you or your child are alone during the day or with people who may not know about your condition. If your shunt were to malfunction, or if your child were to have a seizure when he was with friends, would they know what to do? This section contains tips on how to help others help you in case of an emergency.

Family and friends

Make sure as many people as possible around you know about your hydrocephalus. If you're uncomfortable discussing your condition, inform those closest to you and most likely to be present should an emergency arise. It's not important to tell others all the details about every operation or revision, but do give them enough information so they are aware of possible shunt complications.

> Since our son plays with most of the local kids, we invited all of the parents over to our house to let them know about Max's hydrocephalus. We told them to bring their kids so they could all play together outside, while inside we told the parents about Max's condition and educated them on what to look for in case of a shunt problem. Afterward, we had a question-and-answer session to help calm some of the concerns that some of the parents had.

By keeping everyone around you up to date on how you or your child is doing, you enable them to help in case of an emergency. It also helps to build a valuable support system around you.

MedicAlert®

MedicAlert offers bracelets and necklaces that you can wear to inform emergency medical services personnel and others about your medical condition in case of an emergency. Founded by a physician whose daughter nearly died from an allergic reaction, MedicAlert is a nonprofit membership organization. It has been endorsed by leading medical and health organizations nationwide. There are nearly 2.3 million individuals who are members of the MedicAlert network, and more than 80,000 people have credited MedicAlert with saving their lives.

The initial membership fee for MedicAlert is a minimum of $35 and can go as high as $115, depending on the style and size of the bracelet or necklace you order. After that, the annual renewal fee is only $15. Your fee provides one-year membership, including:

- Setting up and maintaining your computerized medical file with personal ID number.

- Membership card to carry in your wallet or purse.

- Custom engraved emblem with chain (you have a choice of the type of metal and size).

- 24-hour Emergency Response Center (ERC), which is staffed around the clock to receive calls from people with information from your bracelet in case of an emergency.

- Unlimited free record updates.

- Member publications.

MedicAlert is more than just a bracelet or necklace. When you become a MedicAlert member, vital information about you is maintained in a central database to help provide EMS personnel information that could save your life in an emergency. Information that is kept on file includes:

- Your name, date of birth, address, and phone number.

- Emergency contacts, including names and phone numbers.

- Your doctor's name, address, and phone number. You can list up to two doctors in your record; the recommended option would be to list your primary care physician and your neurosurgeon.

- Information about your health coverage, including the name of the plan, policy number, subscriber number, and a phone number to contact for approval of emergency procedures.

- A list of medications and the dosages you are taking.

You can update the information at any time by calling MedicAlert's toll-free number. Your $15 annual renewal fee helps pay for maintaining your record in the MedicAlert database.

The following information is engraved on one side of the MedicAlert bracelet:

- The member identification number.

- Phone number for MedicAlert's ERC, with directions to call collect.

- Essential emergency medical information about your condition. The amount of information that can be engraved depends on the size of the bracelet. The small bracelet holds up to 60 spaces, while the large bracelet holds up to 90 spaces (not including the emergency phone number or your member identification number). The engraving on the Medic-Alert bracelets is guaranteed for five years. The engraving on the reverse of a MedicAlert bracelet might read:

HYDROCEPHALUS
VP SHUNT
ASTHMA
DIABETES INSIPIDUS
123456789

The series of numbers on the last line is your identification number.

An example of how MedicAlert works follows. Your son is in an accident while playing with friends and he is knocked unconscious, and a bystander calls 911. When EMS personnel arrive, one thing they will look for while examining him is any sign of emergency medical identification. When the MedicAlert bracelet is found, the EMT or paramedic will call the dispatcher and give her the identification number found on the bracelet. She, in turn, will call MedicAlert's Emergency Response Center, which can then relay information back to the EMS personnel that may be vital to your child's survival. Additionally, the EMS dispatcher will be given the emergency phone numbers you have provided, and will contact you and your child's doctors.

The fees you pay for MedicAlert can be deducted from your taxes as a medical expense. Applications for MedicAlert can be found at most pharmacies and drug stores. For additional information, or to order a MedicAlert bracelet or necklace, contact:

MedicAlert
2323 Colorado Avenue
Turlock, CA 95382
Phone: (800) 432-5378
Fax: (209) 669-2450
http://www.medicalert/org/index.html

Wallet-sized CTs and MRIs

Shunt malfunctions can happen anytime, anywhere. Another way to protect yourself and inform medical personnel about your condition is to carry around copies of your latest CT or MRI with you. The only problem is that the films are big and bulky. One company, BelMed, has come up with a solution to this problem by creating the surgical shunt card.

This wallet-sized card is customized with six views of your CT or MRI scan on one side and critical information about your medical history on the reverse. The images on the card enable medical personnel to know what your ventricles should look like when your shunt is functioning properly.

When you apply for a surgical shunt card, your neurosurgeon selects six images from your latest CT or MRI scan and sends them with an order form. Information included on the opposite side of the scans includes:

- Patient name.

- Type of scan (CT or MRI) and the date it was taken.

- Type of shunt placement (e.g., ventriculoperitoneal shunt).

- Shunt manufacturer and pressure setting of the valve (e.g., PS Medical, medium-pressure).

- Name of the patient's neurosurgeon, address, phone number, and the hospital at which he practices.

The card is heavily laminated and is about the size of a credit card, so it fits in your wallet. The surgical shunt card costs $25 for the first card and $10 for each additional card. Once produced, the cards will be mailed to your home address, and the films will be returned to your neurosurgeon. For additional information about the surgical shunt card or to request an order form, contact:

BelMed, Inc.
6255 Barfield Road, #191
P.O. Box 888321
Atlanta, GA 30356-0321
Phone: (404) 851-1965
Fax: (404) 851-1800; or (800) 727-6137

Durable Power of Attorney

If you are unconscious, comatose, or cannot speak for yourself, do you know who will make medical decisions on your behalf? If you don't have a

Durable Power of Attorney for Health Care (DPAHC) in place, the decisions about your medical care will be made by the medical professionals, and not by someone who knows what your wishes are.

What is a Durable Power of Attorney for Health Care?

A Durable Power of Attorney for Health Care is a legal document that must be signed by a competent adult. It allows you to transfer medical decision-making authority from yourself to a person you designate (known as an agent) to make those decisions for you in the event that you become incapacitated.

The person you select to be the agent of your DPAHC should be someone you know and trust, and whom you feel is capable of making decisions based on your wishes. You can also specify more than one agent, just in case the primary agent is incapacitated or unable to execute the DPAHC. This person must be 18 years of age or older.

The DPAHC guarantees that your health care choices will be carried out according to your wishes, values, and beliefs. Once signed and witnessed by either a lawyer or a notary public (a person authorized by the state to notarize legal documents such as wills and powers of attorney), the DPAHC can be executed only if you are unable to make the decisions yourself.

How is the DPAHC executed?

The DPAHC must be presented to the attending physician by your agent to serve as legal proof of her decision-making authority. A copy of the DPAHC will be placed in your medical records and will remain there until you are capable of making your own decisions, or if the DPAHC is revoked. The DPAHC can be revoked only by you, regardless of your mental state, and can be done so orally or in writing to your agent and your health care provider.

Before signing a DPAHC, you should understand that the person you choose to be your agent in the DPAHC will have control over the health care you receive while incapacitated. This means that she can dictate the type of treatment, service, or procedure to maintain, diagnose, or treat your physical or mental condition. Things she cannot consent to include:

- Admitting you for inpatient mental health services.
- Convulsive treatment.

- Psychosurgery.

- Abortion.

The DPAHC is a legal document, requiring your doctor to comply with the instructions or requests of your agent. If he disagrees with the terms or fails to comply with your DPAHC, he must transfer your care to another physician.

Sample Durable Power of Attorney for Health Care

On the following pages is a sample Durable Power of Attorney for Health Care, which is reprinted with permission from the web site of the Texas Medical Association (TMA, *http://www.texmed.org/*).

Researching medical texts

A plethora of scientific data and information is available at low or no cost to those who take the time to find it. But that's the key—*you* have to find it. Nobody is going to walk up to you with a silver platter heaped with the latest journal articles. And nobody is going to give you the answers to unasked questions.

Public libraries

When people start learning more about hydrocephalus, the first place many turn is to their local public library. Most libraries are connected to powerful computer databases that store information about all of the books available within their network (usually within the same county or city) and access to medical journals to which they subscribe. Medical journals that most libraries subscribe to include:

- *Journal of the American Medical Association (JAMA)*.

- *New England Journal of Medicine (NEJM)*.

- *The Lancet.*

By doing a simple search on the library's database, you can access medical textbooks and journals, as well as consumer publications (such as *Time, Newsweek,* and *People* magazines), that carry human interest stories on medical conditions and ratings of health care organizations.

Durable Power of Attorney for Health Care Form

Designation of Health Care Agent

I: (insert your name) _____

appoint: Name: _____

Address: _____

_____

Phone: _____

as my agent to make any and all health care decisions for me, except to the extent I state otherwise in this document. This Durable Power of Attorney for Health Care takes effect if I become unable to make my own health care decisions and this fact is certified in writing by my physician.

LIMITATIONS ON THE DECISION MAKING AUTHORITY OF MY AGENT ARE AS FOLLOWS:

_____

_____

_____

Designation of Alternate Agent

(You are not required to designate an alternate agent but you may do so. An alternate agent may make the same health care decisions as the designated agent if the designated agent is unable or unwilling to act as your agent. If the agent designated is your spouse, the designation is automatically revoked by law if your marriage is dissolved.)

If the person designated as my agent is unable or unwilling to make health care decisions for me, I designate the following persons to serve as my agent to make health care decisions for me as authorized by this document, who serve in the following order:

A. First Alternate Agent   B. Second Alternate Agent

Name: _____   Name: _____

Address: _____   Address: _____

_____   _____

Phone: _____   Phone: _____

The original of this document is kept at_____

The following individuals or institutions have signed copies:

Name: _____   Name: _____

Address: _____   Address: _____

_____   _____

Duration

I understand that this power of attorney exists indefinitely from the date I execute this document unless I establish a shorter time or revoke the power of attorney. If I am unable to make health care decisions for myself when this power of attorney expires, the authority I have granted my agent continues to exist until the time I become able to make health care decisions for myself.

(IF APPLICABLE) This power of attorney ends on the following date: _____

Prior Designations Revoked

I revoke any prior Durable Power of Attorney for Health Care.

Acknowledgment of Disclosure Statement

I have been provided with a disclosure statement explaining the effect of this document. I have read and understand that information contained in the disclosure statement.

(YOU MUST DATE AND SIGN THIS POWER OF ATTORNEY)

I sign my name to this Durable Power of Attorney for Health Care on _____ day

of _____ 19_____ at _____

(City and State)

_____
(Signature)

_____
(Print Name)

Statement of Witness

I declare under penalty of perjury that the principal has identified himself or herself to me, that the principal signed or acknowledged this Durable Power of Attorney in my presence, that I believe the principal to be of sound mind, that the principal has affirmed that the principal is aware of the nature of the document and is signing it voluntarily and free from duress, that the principal requested that I serve as witness to the principal's execution of this document, that I am not the person appointed as agent by this document, and that I am not a provider of health or residential care, an employee of a provider of health or residential care, the operator of a community care facility, or an employee of an operator of a health care facility.

I declare that I am not related to the principal by blood, marriage, or adoption and that to the best of my knowledge I am not entitled to any part of the estate of the principal on the death of the principal under a will or by operation of law.

Witness Signature: _____   Witness Signature: _____

Print Name: _____   Print Name: _____

Address: _____   Address: _____

_____   _____

Date: _____   Date: _____

If you are not familiar with how to operate the computer system, don't worry. The computer screen has keyboard commands listed along the bottom of the screen and clear instructions on what to do. Or, if you're not the do-it-yourself type, you can ask for assistance from the reference librarian.

Many of the books you will find about neurosurgery and neurologic conditions will be located in the library's reference section. Books and publications in the reference section are for in-house use only, meaning you can't take them outside the library.

> At first, we looked upon having to stay in the library to read books in the reference section as yet another obstacle to obtaining the information we needed. But once we realized the value of the information we were finding, we found ourselves spending hours in the library, combing over the medical texts.

If you don't have precious hours to spend in your public library, you can always find what you are looking for and make copies for personal use. Most libraries have photocopy machines that charge from 10 to 25 cents per page. Considering the time you might save, it's a relatively small price to pay— plus you will be able to read the articles at your leisure, and not just when the library is open.

The downside of trying to access information through your public library is that the library may not have access to the medical journals and texts you need. If you find yourself in this situation, don't give up. There are other places you can turn in your community to find the information you're looking for, including medical libraries.

Medical libraries

When it comes to looking for specific medical information, there is no better place to look than a medical library. The only problem is that medical libraries aren't listed in the telephone directory in the same way public libraries are—you have to find them.

Finding one in your area, however, could be as simple as calling the hospitals in your area to find out if they have a medical library that is open to the public. Another place to look for a medical library would be at a university medical center, if there is one in your area. If you can't find a medical library in your area, you could ask your family doctor and neurosurgeon if they know of one that is open to the public.

Hospital-based medical libraries serve many functions. Primarily, most medical libraries are located at hospitals as a quick reference area for the doctors and residents who practice at the hospital. They also serve the people in the community by allowing them access to hard-to-find medical texts and journals. For instance, while your public library may not subscribe to the *Journal of Neurosurgery, Neurosurgery,* or *Pediatric Neurosurgery,* chances are that a hospital- or university-based medical library will. For a listing of medical journals of interest to patients with hydrocephalus, see Appendix C, *Medical Libraries and Journals.*

The heart of any medical library is the textbooks, particularly if the hospital or university medical center library is located in a teaching hospital. Libraries play a crucial role in providing up-to-date information for both students and their instructors. Additionally, they have valuable archive material in case you are interested in how certain techniques and operations have evolved over the years.

Online resources

Today you can research medical journals online, on your personal computer. Entering something as simple as the word "hydrocephalus" in one of the Internet's search engines can bring you thousands of possible links to turn to. Some of these links, however, may not be all that valuable. When you are researching medical information online, there are two sites in particular that you should turn your attention to: PubMed and Internet Grateful Med.

PubMed

PubMed (*http://www.ncbi.nlm.nih.gov/PubMed/*) is a web site run by the National Libraries of Medicine (NLM). Here you will have access to over 9 million journal articles, dating as far back as 1966. When you conduct a search on PubMed, the results you see will be a list of citations (database entries which list the title of the article, author, and publication information). You can also opt to view an abstract report, which will show you the published abstract (summary) of the journal article.

In a sample session, if you go to PubMed and search for articles that contain the word *hydrocephalus*, your search will return almost 14,000 citations and abstracts. In order to get closer to finding the information you are looking for, you'll need to be more specific with your search criteria.

For example, if you want to find articles on subdural hematomas as they relate to hydrocephalus, enter the following into the search window and press return:

hydrocephalus,subdural hematoma

This search will result in more than 300 citations and abstracts. You can narrow the search further by including a specific journal:

J Neurosurg,hydrocephalus,subdural hematoma

This search query looks for the articles on hydrocephalus and subdural hematomas only in the *Journal of Neurosurgery* (*J Neurosurg* is the MEDLINE abbreviation for the title of the journal). You'll get about 20 articles to choose from. This is a great way to find articles from journals to which your medical library subscribes.

Internet Grateful Med

The Internet Grateful Med (IGM; *http://igm.nlm.nih.gov/*) is a powerful search engine built by the National Library of Medicine. The site allows users to perform MEDLINE searches to access approximately 9 million articles in its database. Although PubMed and IGM have access to the same MEDLINE records, IGM enables you to search 11 other databases as well.

In a sample session, after getting to IGM's home page, you will see a line of text that says something like, *Internet Grateful Med V2.3.2,* with a button next to it that says "Proceed." If you click on that button, you will be taken to IGM's search interface. The search interface is more complex than the one found on PubMed. Here you can enter up to three query items using options of subject, author name, and/or title word. The next part of the search interface allows you to apply limits to the query terms you've requested. Limits you can specify include:

- **Language.** This allows you to specify the language the article is published in, including English, French, German, Italian, Japanese, Russian, Spanish, all non-English, or all of the above.

- **Study groups.** This option relates to medical research subjects. The options here are human, animal, or all of the above.

- **Age groups.** Allows you to select the age range of those in the studies. The options include: infant/newborn (0-1 month), infant (1 to 23 months), child/preschool (2 to 5 years), child (6 to 12 years), adolescence (13 to 18 years), all child (0 to 18 years), adult (19 to 44 years), middle age (45 to 64 years), aged (65 years and over), aged 80 (80 years and over), all adult (19 years and over).

- **Publication types.** The type of article in the publication. Options include clinical trial, editorial, letter, meta-analysis, practice guideline, randomized control trial, and review.

- **Gender.** Choose from male, female, or both.

- **Journal type.** Choose from all medical journal types, or select dental or nursing journals specifically.

- **Year range.** Allows you to specify the beginning and ending year range for the article types in your search. An alternative to selecting a range of years is a checkbox that allows you to specify one specific year for your search.

Let's use the example from the previous PubMed search, and expand on it a bit. Start by entering "hydrocephalus" and "subdural hematoma" in the fields for Query Terms, and select the following for the limits:

Languages: All languages.
Study groups: Human subjects only.
Age groups: All child (0 to 18 years).
Publication types: All.
Gender: All.
Journals: All.
Year range: From 1990 to 1998.

This search resulted in 13 journal articles that met all of the criteria. The title of each article is a link that takes you to the MEDLINE record for that particular article, including the abstract.

By using a combination of PubMed and the Internet Grateful Med, you should be able to find just about any article you're looking for. All you need is a connection to the Internet—at home, work, or your public library—and you're on your way. Appendix E, *Internet Resources,* lists online resources that you can research.

Loansome Doc™

Although PubMed and Internet Grateful Med are great for searching specific journals and topics, and for reading the abstracts of the articles you've

found, you're still not given access to the full text of the article. Both search services provide abstracts, but you have to locate the journal article yourself to read the full text. What can you do if both the public and medical library don't have a subscription to the journal you're looking for? The answer is another feature of the NLM, called Loansome Doc.

Loansome Doc is a way for PubMed and Internet Grateful Med users to order articles by accessing a network of over 4,500 medical libraries throughout the United States. But in order to use Loansome Doc, you must first have access to a registered medical library. Medical libraries that are registered to use Loansome Doc are given a library identification number (LIBID), which is used by the medical librarian when requesting materials. This means that in order for you to request a journal article from Loansome Doc, you will need to request it through the librarian at the medical library to which you have access.

Loansome Doc is not a free service. Articles requested through Loansome Doc are subject to processing and handling fees, so check with the librarian about the costs before requesting 20 or 30 journal articles.

For more information about libraries that participate in Loansome Doc, call 1-800-338-7657, Monday through Friday, 8:30 a.m. to 5:00 p.m. in all time zones. For a complete list of regional medical libraries, see Appendix C, *Medical Libraries and Journals*.

Know your legal rights

It's important to know your rights as a patient. Legally, you or your child cannot be treated without your consent. If your neurosurgeon proposes a procedure that you do not feel comfortable with, keep asking questions until you feel fully informed. You have the right to refuse the procedure if you do not think it's necessary. However, if the hospital feels that you are wrongfully withholding permission for treatment of your child, it can take you to court.

There are also governmental regulations you should know about that might apply to your situation.

Family and Medical Leave Act of 1993

The Family and Medical Leave Act (FMLA) was signed into law on February 5, 1993, as a means of granting family members up to 12 weeks of unpaid

medical leave from their jobs without fear of losing their jobs and source of income. The purpose of this Act is to balance the demands of the workplace with the needs of families, to promote the stability and economic security of families, and to promote national interests in preserving family integrity. The Act entitles employees to take reasonable leave for medical reasons, for the birth or adoption of a child, and for the care of a child, spouse, or parent who has a serious health condition.

To be eligible for a medical leave of absence under the FMLA, the law requires that:

- You have worked for your employer for at least 12 months.
- You have worked at least 1,250 hours for your employer during the 12-month period.
- Your employer must have at least 50 employees within 75 miles of the company.

FMLA outlines provisions for paid and unpaid medical leave, including reduced work hours. Under the law, family members are eligible for up to 12 weeks of job-protected medical leave from their employer as long as they meet the eligibility requirements stated above. You are not required to take all 12 weeks at the same time. You can opt to take the leave intermittently, or use time from the 12 weeks to reduce the amount of hours you work in a day.

Also, during the time you are on medical leave under the FMLA, your employer is required to maintain your medical coverage unless you fail to return to work.

For additional information about the Family and Medical Leave Act of 1993, contact your employer's human resources representative or these online resources:

- Family and Medical Leave Act of 1993 (full text):

    ftp://ftp.loc/gov/pub/thomas/c103/h1.enr.txt

- Seyfarth, Shaw, Fairweather & Geraldson, "Clinton Signs Family Leave Bill":

    http://www.seyfarth.com/insights/FAMLVBIL.HTM

Biomaterials Access Assurance Act of 1997

At the time of this writing, no other bill before the U.S. Congress could potentially benefit patients with hydrocephalus more than the Biomaterials Access Assurance Bill.

In February 1997, the Biomaterials Access Assurance Act (HR 872 and S 364) was introduced to the 105th Congress in both the U.S. House of Representatives and the Senate. The intent of this bill is to establish laws governing product liability actions against suppliers of raw materials and bulk components used in the manufacture of medical devices and implants.

As noted in this Act, under the Federal Food, Drug, and Cosmetic Act (21 U.S.C. 301 et seq.), manufacturers of medical devices are required to demonstrate that the medical devices are safe and effective, that they are properly designed, and that they have adequate warnings or instructions.

Since suppliers of raw materials do not actually design, manufacture, or test medical devices, the Biomaterials Access Assurance Act of 1997 would protect raw materials manufacturers from liability in any lawsuit brought against the product manufacturer. The Act would protect suppliers of raw materials used to make medical devices that are to be implanted in a human being. In recent years, people who have been suing silicone breast manufacturers have also filed suit against the smaller companies who supplied materials to make the implants. Since many of these companies are small and have nothing to do with how the implants are manufactured, many have gone out of business as a result of multimillion dollar settlements brought against them.

Under this Act, an implant is defined as:

- A medical device that is intended by the manufacturer of the device to:
  - Be placed into a surgically or naturally formed or existing cavity of the body for a period of at least 30 days; or
  - Remain in contact with bodily fluids or internal human tissue through a surgically produced opening for a period of less than 30 days.
- Suture materials used in implant procedures.

How does HR 872 and S 364 affect hydrocephalus patients? Nearly all shunt valves and catheters are made from silicone and are implanted in the body. If the Biomaterials Access Assurance Act does not pass, many smaller companies that supply raw materials to manufacture the silicone implants could be held liable for damages if someone were to sue the shunt manufacturer. And since many of the raw material suppliers are small operations, they could potentially go out of business if a multimillion dollar lawsuit or judgment were brought against them. The result would be fewer companies who are willing to provide raw materials and components for use as surgical implants.

The way that U.S. lawsuits are currently structured is for a suit to be brought against all parties who potentially have any liability. Otherwise, other defendants in the suit can point to an absent party as the party at fault, and the suit could be held up and/or lost. Unfortunately, suing multiple defendants and trying to get the most money possible in compensatory damages can discourage suppliers from providing raw materials, even though they have nothing to do with the way the device was manufactured, tested, or sold to the patient.

HR 872 and S 364 in no way prevents a patient from recovering damages against the manufacturers of faulty or defective medical devices, nor does it excuse a biomaterials supplier from liability if the supplier is also the manufacturer or seller of the implant.

Social Security

The Social Security Administration (SSA) provides Social Security Disability Insurance (SSDI). You must demonstrate having a disability in order to be eligible, and the amount you can collect depends on the amount you have paid through tax deductions from your work life to date. If you are under 18, the determination is based on your parents' account(s). If you qualify, you collect monthly checks that are not taxable.

In 1972, the Supplemental Security Income Program (SSI), an amendment to the Social Security Act, was introduced. SSI guaranteed a minimum income to elderly, blind, and disabled individuals who could not sustain gainful employment. SSI and SSDI recipients became eligible for Medicare, a federal health insurance program, and Medicaid, a program administered by the states, which covers medical expenses.

The SSA has designed the programs to encourage people with disabilities to work. According to the Government Accounting Office, 42 percent of people with disabilities would like to work, and 33 percent of Social Security beneficiaries have the ability to work.

You are allowed a trial work period of nine months—which do not have to be consecutive—plus an additional three months, during which you can still collect your benefits no matter how much you earn. But when the time is up, the benefits end. If you work a month here and a month there, you might be surprised to find you have used up your trial period, so be careful how you use that time.

There is an "extended period of eligibility" (EPE)—36 months—during which you can collect a benefit in a month when you make less than $500, or go back on regular benefits if you must stop working.

Medicare and Medicaid benefits are another part of this formula. You must be on SSI or SSDI for 24 months before you can qualify. You can maintain your Medicare benefits during the EPE, and in some cases can continue Medicare on your own beyond that time. You might pay some premiums yourself, which will be deducted from your check if you still receive benefits.

Social Security offers some vocational rehabilitation (VR) services that contribute to education, counseling, equipment, or job placement. The SSA is experimenting with a program to allow you to choose approved outside providers of VR paid by SSA.

You are allowed to deduct expenses, including access modifications, some attendant care (getting dressed for work, for example), transportation, or even the cost of a canine helper. Money you have to spend to be able to work can be subtracted from the calculation of your monthly income.

If you are able to get and maintain a well-paying job with health coverage, then the 12-month period is a blessing. It allows you to make all the money you want and still collect your tax-free disability income. You could do this on a contract or part-time basis while still covered on Medicare, to encourage an employer to give you a try and then hire you full time with benefits once your benefits lapse. It could also give you time to start a business, because 40 hours of work per month also counts as a trial work month.

If you earn $200 or more per month, SSA considers that to be a trial work month. If you continue to earn at this level for nine months, you will lose your benefits. People with low income potential have problems retaining benefits. At the end of an EPE, you need to be at a level of $500 of gross income per month to be considered as doing "substantial gainful activity." This is when you will be considered ineligible for that monthly check. Certainly this is not enough to live on. Unless you can make a lot more than $200 per month—or $500 after an EPE—getting a job is probably not a very attractive option to staying on disability.

Part-time work is often the only option for people with limited stamina, frequent medical procedures, or the occasional need for time off to tend to demands of their disability. Part-time jobs, however, usually do not offer medical coverage and are not a reliable long-term source of income. Yet they are a way to stay active, participate in the community, and take pride in earning at least part of one's own income.

Getting approved for SSA benefits can be difficult. There are plenty of stories of people who have had to struggle with a complicated bureaucracy, dealing with staff who do not provide full or accurate information. In the mid-1990s, as part of a federal government cutback, Social Security staff was reduced, overloading the system further.

It can be just as hard to get Social Security to stop the money as it is to receive it in the first place. When you complete a trial work period, the Social Security Administration is likely to keep sending you checks. No matter how efficiently you fill out their forms reporting your income, they often keep sending you money for months to come. And once they finally get to your case, they'll come calling to get that money back.

Americans with Disabilities Act (ADA)

The Americans with Disabilities Act is a civil rights act.

It guarantees, for instance, that you cannot be discriminated against for a job based on your disability. It says that employers must provide "reasonable accommodation" for you to do a job you are otherwise equally qualified to perform. If you can show an employer how you can do the job using a certain adaptive device, he cannot refuse you the job in favor of an otherwise lesser candidate.

Of course, the ADA does not automatically stop such events from taking place. But it does mean you have recourse. In such situations, you can take legal action because your civil rights have been violated.

Some people with hydrocephalus use wheelchairs for mobility. Section 504 of the ADA provides federal funds to ensure that people with disabilities have access to all public services. As of January 1992, activities ranging from school board meetings to city picnics need to accommodate people with disabilities.

You are entitled to access to public and commercial areas, where you are protected from discrimination "in the full equal enjoyment of the goods, services, facilities, privileges, advantages, or accommodations of any place of public accommodation." Banks, shopping centers, transportation terminals, and theaters need to provide a clear path to restrooms, drinking fountains, telephones, and elevators.

The ADA also addresses public and private transportation, and requires telecommunications options for people with hearing disabilities.

Pediatric Neurosurgeons

THIS LIST OF PEDIATRIC NEUROSURGEONS has been provided by Dr. Marion L. Walker, Chairman of the American Board of Pediatric Neurological Surgeons (ABPNS). Updates to this list can be found on the ABPNS web site at *http://www.abpns.org/*, and may also be obtained from the Hydrocephalus Association as a printed booklet. The information provided here is the most current as of time of publication. Neurosurgeons are listed alphabetically by last name, under their state or province. For more information about the ABPNS and its certification requirements, see Chapter 3, *Selecting a Neurosurgeon*.

United States

Alabama

Timothy Mapstone, M.D.
Children's Hospital of Alabama
1600 Seventh Avenue S., #ACC400
Birmingham, AL 35233
Phone: (205) 939-9653

W. Jerry Oakes, M.D.
Professor of Neurosurgery
Chief, Pediatric Neurosurgery
Children's Hospital of Alabama
1600 Seventh Avenue S., #ACC400
Birmingham, AL 35233
Phone: (205) 939-9653

Arizona

Kim H. Manwaring, M.D.
Director, Pediatric Neurosurgery
Faculty, Phoenix Children's Hospital
Phoenix Children's Hospital
909 E. Brill Street
Phoenix, AZ 85006
Phone: (602) 239-4880

S. David Moss, M.D.
Phoenix Children's Hospital
909 E. Brill Street
Phoenix, AZ 85006
Phone: (602) 239-4880

Harold L. Rekate, M.D.
Chief, Pediatric Neurosurgery
Clinical Professor, University of Arizona
Barrow Neurological Institute
2910 N. Third Avenue
Phoenix, AZ 85013
Phone: (602) 406-3632

Arkansas

Frederick A. Boop, M.D.
Arkansas Children's Hospital
800 Marshall Street
Little Rock, AR 72202
Phone: (501) 320-1448

Charles Teo, M.D.
Vice Chief, Division of Pediatric Neurosurgery
Arkansas Children's Hospital
Division of Pediatric Neurosurgery
800 Marshall Street
Little Rock, AR 72202
Phone: (501) 320-1448

California

Leslie D. Cahan, M.D.
Associate Professor
Division of Neurological Surgery
University of Southern California, Fourth Floor—Neurosurgery
1505 N. Edemont Street
Los Angeles, CA 90027
Phone: (213) 667-4704

Michael S.B. Edwards, M.D.
Edwards and Ciricillo Medical Corporation
Pediatric Neurosurgery and Neuro-Oncology
2800 L Street, Suite 340
Sacramento, CA 95816
Phone: (916) 454-6850; or (800) 250-3208

Clarence S. Greene, Jr., M.D.
University of California at Irvine Medical Center
Department of Neurological Surgery
101 The City Drive, Bldg. 3
Suite 313, Rte. 81
Orange, CA 92668
Phone: (714) 456-6301

Hector E. James, M.D.
Clinical Professor, Neurosurgery/Pediatrics
University of California at San Diego
7930 Frost Street, #304
San Diego, CA 92123
Phone: (619) 560-4791

J. Gordon McComb, M.D.
Head, Division of Neurosurgery
Children's Hospital, Los Angeles
1300 N. Vermont Avenue, Suite 906
Los Angeles, CA 90027
Phone: (213) 663-8128

Michael G. Muhonen, M.D.
Children's Hospital Orange County
455 S. Main
Orange, CA 92668
Phone: (714) 289-4151

Dachling Pang, M.D.
Chief, Pediatric Neurosurgery
University of California at Davis
2516 Stockton Boulevard, #254
Sacramento, CA 95817
Phone: (916) 734-0362

Warwick J. Peacock, M.D.
Chief, Pediatric Neurosurgery
University of California at San Francisco
533 Parnassus Street, Room 126
San Francisco, CA 94143
Phone: (415) 476-1081

Colorado

Michael H. Handler, M.D.
1010 E. 19th Street, Suite 605
Denver, CO 80218
Phone: (303) 861-6015

Michael D. Partington, M.D.
Assistant Professor, Neurosurgery and Pediatrics
University of Colorado School of Medicine
1056 E. 19th Avenue, B467
Denver, CO 80218
Phone: (303) 764-8228

Ken R. Winston, M.D.
Director of Pediatric Neurosurgery
Professor, University of Colorado
1950 Ogden, B467
Denver, CO 80218
Phone: (303) 861-3995

Connecticut

Charles C. Duncan, M.D.
Yale University School of Medicine
Chief, Pediatric Neurosurgery
P.O. Box 208039
New Haven, CT 06520
Phone: (203) 785-2809

Florida

J. Parker Mickle, M.D.
Shands Children's Hospital at the University of Florida
Department of Neurology
P.O. Box 100265
1600 S.W. Archer Road
Gainesville, FL 32610-0265
Phone: (352) 392-4331

Glenn Morrison, M.D.
Director, Division of Neurological Surgery
Miami Children's Hospital
3200 S.W. 60 Court, #301
Miami, FL 33155
Phone: (305) 662-8386

Jogi V. Pattisapu, M.D.
22 W. Lake Beauty Drive, #204
Orlando, FL 32806
Phone: (407) 649-7686

John Ragheb, M.D.
1501 N.W. Ninth Avenue
Miami, FL 33136
Phone: (305) 243-6946

Georgia

Ann Marie Flannery, M.D.
Associate Professor, Medical College of Georgia
Assistant Dean, Graduate Medical Education
1120 15th Street, BIW 348B
Augusta, GA 30912-4010
Phone: (706) 721-3071

Roger Hudgins, M.D.
Pediatric Neurosurgery Associates, P.C.
Children's Medical Professional Bldg.
5455 Meridan Mark Road, #540
Atlanta, GA 30342
Phone: (404) 255-6509

Mary M. Johnson, M.D.
Scottish Rite Children's Hospital
4514 Chamblee Dunwoody Road, #347
Atlanta, GA 30338-6202
Phone: (404) 233-4109

Mark S. O'Brien, M.D.
Professor of Neurosurgery
Emory University
1900 Century Boulevard, Suite 4
Atlanta, GA 30345
Phone: (404) 321-9234

Illinois

Francisco Gutierrez, M.D.
707 N. Fairbanks Court
Chicago, IL 60611
Phone: (312) 951-9092

Yoon Hahn, M.D.
Director of Pediatric Neurosurgery
Hope Children's Hospital
4440 W. 95th Street, #477S
Oak Lawn, IL 60453
Phone: (708) 346-1013

David G. McLone, M.D., Ph.D.
Head, Pediatric Neurosurgery
Professor of Surgery, Northwestern University
Children's Memorial Hospital
2300 Children's Plaza, Box 28
Chicago, IL 60614
Phone: (312) 880-4373

Tadanori Tomita, M.D.
Director of Brain Tumor Center
Children's Memorial Hospital
2300 Children's Plaza
Chicago, IL 60614
Phone: (312) 880-4373

Indiana

Joel C. Boaz, M.D.
James W. Riley Hospital for Children
1 Children's Square, Suite 2510
Indianapolis, IN 46202
Phone: (317) 274-8852

Thomas G. Luerssen, M.D.
Director, Pediatric Neurosurgery
Associate Professor, Indiana University School of Medicine
James W. Riley Hospital for Children
One Children's Square
Indianapolis, IN 46202
Phone: (317) 274-8852

Michael S. Turner, M.D.
Clinical Assistant Professor, Neurosurgery
1801 N. Senate Boulevard, #535
Indianapolis, IN 46202-1228
Phone: (317) 926-5411

Iowa

Arnold H. Menezes, M.D.
Professor, Vice Chairman, Neurosurgery
University of Iowa
University of Iowa Hospital and Clinics
200 Hawkins Drive, Room 1841, JPP
Iowa City, IA 52242
Phone: (319) 356-2768

Kentucky

Benjamin C. Warf, M.D.
University of Kentucky Medical Center
Division of Neurosurgery
800 Rose Street, Room MS 105A
Lexington, KY 40536-0084
Phone: (606) 323-8986

Louisiana

Joseph M. Nadell, M.D.
Professor of Neurosurgery and Pediatrics
Tulane University
200 Henry Clay Avenue
New Orleans, LA 70118
Phone: (504) 896-9568

Maryland

Benjamin S. Carson, M.D.
Johns Hopkins University Hospital
811 Harvey
600 N. Wolfe Street
Baltimore, MD 21287-8811
Phone: (410) 955-7888

Walker L. Robinson, M.D.
Associate Professor, Head of Pediatric Neurosurgery
Acting Chairman, Division of Neurological Surgery
22 S. Green Street
Baltimore, MD 21201
Phone: (301) 328-6034

Massachusetts

Peter M. Black, M.D.
Franc D. Ingraham Professor of Neurosurgery
Harvard Medical School
Children's Hospital
300 Longwood Avenue
Boston, MA 02115
Phone: (617) 355-6008

Paul H. Chapman, M.D.
Massachusetts General Hospital
32 Fruit Street
Boston, MA 02114-2698
Phone: (617) 726-3887

Liliana C. Goumnerova, M.D.
Instructor of Surgery, Harvard Medical School
Children's Hospital
300 Longwood Avenue, Bader 3
Boston, MA 02115-5724
Phone: (617) 355-6364

Joseph R. Madsen, M.D.
Assistant Professor of Surgery
Harvard Medical School
Children's Hospital
300 Longwood Avenue, Room 312
Boston, MA 02115-5724
Phone: (617) 735-6005

R. Michael Scott, M.D.
Director, Pediatric Neurosurgery
Professor of Surgery, Harvard Medical School
Children's Hospital
300 Longwood Avenue, Bader 3
Boston. MA 02115
Phone: (617) 355-6011

Michigan

Patricia A. Aronin, M.D.
Associate Professor, Neurosurgery
Wayne State University
Department of Neurosurgery, 6E, UHC
4201 St. Antoine Street
Detroit, MI 48201
Phone: (313) 745-4099

Alexa I. Canady, M.D.
Chief, Neurosurgery, Children's Hospital
Vice Chair, Neurosurgery
Wayne State University
3901 Beaubien
Detroit, MI 48201
Phone: (313) 833-4490

Paul M. Kanev, M.D.
Chief of Neurosurgery
Henry Ford Medical Center
2799 W. Grand Boulevard
Detroit, MI 48202-2608
Phone: (313) 876-3528

Karin M. Muraszko, M.D.
Director, Pediatric Brain Tumor Clinic
University of Michigan
2128 Taubman Center
1500 E. Medical Center Drive
Ann Arbor, MI 48109
Phone: (313) 936-5062

Minnesota

Mahmoud G. Nagib, M.D.
Instructor of Neurosurgery
University of Minnesota
305 Piper Building
800 E. 28th Street
Minneapolis, MN 55407-3799
Phone: (612) 871-7278

Corey Raffel, M.D.
Mayo Clinic
Department of Neurosurgery
200 First Street, S.W.
Rochester, MN 55905-0001
Phone: (507) 284-2611

Mississippi

Andrew Parent, M.D.
University of Mississippi Medical Center
2500 N. State Street
Jackson, MS 39216-4505
Phone: (601) 984-5702

Missouri

David F. Jimenez, M.D.
Director, Pediatric Neurosurgery
University of Missouri Health Science Center
One Hospital Drive, Room N521
Columbia, MO 65212
Phone: (573) 882-4908

Bruce A. Kaufman, M.D.
Assistant Professor
Washington University School of Medicine
St. Louis Children's Hospital
1 Children's Place, #1S46
St. Louis, MO 63110
Phone: (314) 454-2812

Tae Sung Park, M.D.
St. Louis Children's Hospital
Department of Neurosurgery
1 Children's Place
St. Louis, MO 63110
Phone: (314) 454-2810

Thomas Pittman, M.D.
Associate Professor of Surgery
St. Louis University Medical Center
1465 S. Grand
St. Louis, MO 63110-1003
Phone: (314) 577-5306

Nebraska

Leslie C. Hellbusch, M.D.
Chief, Pediatric Neurosurgery
Clinical Associate Professor
University of Nebraska Medical Center
111 N. 84th Street
Omaha, NE 68114
Phone: (402) 398-9243

New Jersey

Peter W. Carmel, M.D.
Professor, Neurological Surgery
Division Chief, Neurological Surgery
University of Medicine and Dentistry of New Jersey (U.M.D.N.J.)
U.M.D.N.J. University Hospital
DDC-7300
90 Bergen Street
Newark, NJ 07103-2499
Phone: (201) 972-2323

New Mexico

Bruce B. Storrs, M.D.
Chief, Pediatric Neurosurgery
Professor of Surgery and Pediatrics
Children's Hospital of New Mexico
2211 Lomas Boulevard N.E.
Albuquerque, NM 87131
Phone: (505) 272-3401

New York

Rick Abbott, III, M.D.
Assistant Professor
Beth Israel Medical Center
170 East End Avenue
New York, NY 10128
Phone: (212) 870-9600

Mark S. Dias, M.D.
Chief of Neurosurgery
Children's Hospital of Buffalo
219 Bryant Street
Buffalo, NY 14222
Phone: (716) 878-7386

Michael R. Egnor, M.D.
Chief, Pediatric Neurosurgery
Assistant Professor
State University of New York (S.U.N.Y.)—Stony Brook
Stony Brook, NY 11794
Phone: (516) 444-1210

Fred J. Epstein, M.D.
Chairman of Neurosurgery
Director of Institute of Neurology/Neurosurgery
Beth Israel Medical Center
170 East End Avenue
New York, NY 10128
Phone: (212) 870-9600

Neil Arthur Feldstein, M.D.
Neurological Institute
710 W. 168th Street
New York, NY 10032-2603
Phone: (212) 305-1396

Arno H. Fried, M.D.
Chief of Neurosurgery
Westchester Medical Center
Munger Pavilion, #329
Valhalla, NY 10595
Phone: (914) 285-8392

James T. Goodrich, M.D., Ph.D.
Director, Division of Pediatric Neurosurgery
Associate Professor of Neurosurgery
Montefiore Medical Center
111 E. 210th Street
Bronx, NY 10467
Phone: (718) 920-4196

John I. Miller, M.D.
Director, Division of Pediatric Neurosurgery
S.U.N.Y. Health Sciences Center, Brooklyn
450 Clarkson Avenue
Box 1189
Brooklyn, NY 11203-2098
Phone: (718) 270-3920
Also:
St. John's Queens Hospital
Department of Neurosurgery
95-25 Queens Boulevard, 2nd Floor
Rego Park, NY 11374
Phone: (718) 459-7700

Steven J. Schneider, M.D.
410 Lakeville Road, #204
New Hyde Park, NY 10042
Phone: (516) 354-3401

John B. Waldman, M.D.
Associate Professor of Surgery and Pediatrics
Albany Medical College
Division of Neurosurgery, A-61-NE
Albany, NY 12180
Phone: (518) 262-5088

Jeffrey H. Wisoff, M.D.
Director, Division of Pediatric Neurosurgery
Associate Professor, New York University Medical Center
550 First Avenue
New York, NY 10016
Phone: (212) 263-6419

North Carolina

Herbert C. Fuchs, M.D.
Assistant Professor
Duke University Medical Center
Box 3272
Durham, NC 27710
Phone: (919) 681-4850

C. Scott McLanahan, M.D.
Charlotte Neurosurgical Associates
1010 Edgehill Road N.
Charlotte, NC 28207
Phone: (704) 376-1605

Ohio

Henry M. Bartkowski, M.D.
Clinical Assistant Professor
Ohio State University
Neurosurgical Associates
931 Chatham Lane
Columbus, OH 43221
Phone: (614) 457-4880

Thomas S. Berger, M.D.
Professor of Clinical Neurosurgery
Director, Division of Pediatric Neurosurgery
University of Cincinnati
506 Oak Street
Cincinnati, OH 45219
Phone: (513) 569-5255

Alan R. Cohen, M.D.
Chief, Pediatric Neurosurgery
Rainbow Babies and Children's Hospital
11100 Euclid Avenue
Cleveland, OH 44106
Phone: (216) 844-5741

Kerry R. Crone, M.D.
Associate Professor
Children's Hospital
3333 Burnet Avenue
Cincinnati, OH 45229
Phone: (513) 559-4726

Edward J. Kosnik, M.D.
Chief, Neurosurgery, Children's Hospital
Professor of Neurosurgery, Ohio State University
931 Chatham Lane
Columbus, OH 43221
Phone: (614) 457-4880

Robert L. McLaurin, M.D.
Professor, Neurological Surgery
University Hospital, University of Cincinnati
900 4th and Vine Tower
Cincinnati, OH 45202
Phone: (513) 381-9291

Oregon

Martin Johnson, M.D.
Director, Pediatric Neurosurgery
Emanuel Children's Hospital
2800 N. Vancouver, #106
Portland, OR 97227
Phone: (503) 287-2646

Joseph H. Piatt, Jr., M.D.
Assistant Professor, Neurosurgery and Pediatrics
Oregon Health Sciences University
3181 S.W. Sam Jackson Park Road, L472
Portland, OR 97201
Phone: (503) 494-8070

Pennsylvania

P. David Adelson, M.D.
Assistant Professor
Department of Pediatric Neurological Surgery
Children's Hospital of Pittsburgh
3705 Fifth Avenue
Pittsburgh, PA 15213-2583
Phone: (412) 692-6347

A. Leland Albright, M.D.
Chief, Pediatric Neurosurgery
Professor of Neurosurgery, University of Pittsburgh
Children's Hospital of Pittsburgh
3705 Fifth Avenue
Pittsburgh, PA 15213-2583
Phone: (412) 692-8142

Karin S. Bierbrauer, M.D.
Assistant Professor, Neurosurgery
Temple University
St. Christopher's Hospital
Pediatric Neurosurgery
Erie Avenue at Front Street
Philadelphia, PA 19134
Phone: (215) 427-5196

Ann-Christine Duhaime, M.D.
Associate Neurosurgeon
Assistant Professor of Neurosurgery
University of Pennsylvania
Children's Hospital of Philadelphia
34th Street and Civic Center Boulevard
Philadelphia, PA 19104
Phone: (215) 590-2780

Dennis L. Johnson, M.D.
Director of Pediatric Neurosurgery
Associate Professor, Penn State University
Hershey Medical Center
P.O. Box 850
Hershey, PA 17033
Phone: (717) 531-8807

Gary Magram, M.D.
Chief Pediatric Neurosurgeon
St. Christopher's Hospital for Children
Erie Avenue at Front Street
Philadelphia, PA 19134
Phone: (215) 427-5196

Ian F. Pollack, M.D.
Children's Hospital of Pittsburgh
3705 Fifth Avenue
Pittsburgh, PA 15213-2583
Phone: (412) 692-5881

Donald H. Reigel, M.D.
Director, Pediatric Neurosurgery
Allegheny General Hospital
320 E. North Avenue, 7th Floor
Pittsburgh, PA 15212
Phone: (412) 359-6200

Leslie N. Sutton, M.D.
Chairman, Division of Neurosurgery
Children's Hospital of Philadelphia
34th Street and Civic Center Boulevard
Philadelphia, PA 19104-4399
Phone: (215) 590-2780

Luis Schut, M.D.
Chief, Neurosurgery
Professor, Neurosurgery
University of Pennsylvania
Children's Hospital of Philadelphia
34th Street and Civic Center Boulevard
Philadelphia, PA 19104-4399
Phone: (215) 590-2780

South Carolina

Lenwood P. Smith, Jr., M.D.
Palmetto-Richmond Memorial Hospital
3 Medical Park, Suite 310
Columbia, SC 29203
Phone: (803) 256-7112

Tennessee

Michael S. Mulbauer, M.D.
University of Tennessee Medical School
Semmes-Murphy Clinic
930 Madison Avenue, #600
Memphis, TN 38103
Phone: (901) 522-7761

R. Alexander Sanford, M.D.
Chief, Pediatric Neurosurgery
LeBonheur Hospital
University of Tennessee Medical School
Semmes-Murphy Clinic
930 Madison Avenue, #600
Memphis, TN 38103
Phone: (901) 522-7762

Noel Tulipan, M.D.
Associate Professor of Neurosurgery
Vanderbilt University Hospital
RM T-4224, MCN
Nashville, TN 37232-2380
Phone: (615) 322-6875

Texas

Derek A. Bruce, M.D.
Clinical Associate Professor
University of Texas-Southwestern Medical School
1935 Motor Street
Dallas, TX 75235
Phone: (214) 640-6660

William R. Cheek, M.D.
Texas Children's Hospital
Clinical Care Center, #950
6621 Fannin, MC 3-3435
Houston, TX 77030
Phone: (713) 798-1750

Robert C. Dauser, M.D.
Assistant Professor
Baylor College of Medicine
6621 Fannin, MC 3-3435
Houston, TX 77030
Phone: (713) 770-3950

Sarah J. Gaskill, M.D.
4499 Medical Drive, Suite 397
San Antonio, TX 78229
Phone: (210) 615-1218

John P. Laurent, M.D.
Assistant Professor, Neurosurgery
Baylor College of Medicine
Clinical Care Center, MC3-3435
6621 Fannin, #0-202
Houston, TX 77030
Phone: (713) 770-3950

Arthur E. Marlin, M.D.
Clinical Professor, Pediatrics
University of Texas Health Science Center
4499 Medical Drive, #397
San Antonio, TX 78229
Phone: (210) 615-1218

Jack E. McCallum, M.D.
800 Seventh Avenue
Fort Worth, TX 76104
Phone: (817) 336-1300

Kenneth N. Shapiro, M.D.
Clinical Associate Professor, Neurosurgery
University of Texas-Southwestern Medical School
1935 Motor Street
Dallas, TX 75235
Phone: (214) 640-6660

Frederick H. Sklar, M.D.
Clinical Associate Professor, Neurosurgery
University of Texas-Southwestern Medical School
1935 Motor Street
Dallas, TX 75235
Phone: (214) 640-6660

John W. Walsh, M.D.
6411 Fannin, Box 61
Houston, TX 77030
Phone: (713) 793-6445

Ronald J. Wilson, M.D.
Chief, Neurosurgery
Brackenridge Hospital
1313 Red River, #120
Austin, TX 78701
Phone: (512) 474-5152

Utah

Lyn M. Carey, M.D.
Assistant Professor, Neurosurgery and Pediatrics
Primary Children's Medical Center
100 North Medical Drive
Salt Lake City, UT 84113
Phone: (801) 588-3400

Marion L. Walker, M.D.
Professor and Head, Pediatric Neurosurgery
University of Utah
Children's Medical Center
100 North Medical Drive, Suite 2400
Salt Lake City, UT 84113
Phone: (801) 588-3400

Virginia

John D. Ward, M.D.
Professor, Neurosurgery
Chief, Pediatric Neurosurgery
Medical College of Virginia
MCV Station, Box 980631
Richmond, VA 23298
Phone: (804) 828-9165

Washington

Richard G. Ellenbogen, M.D.
Associate Professor
Department of Neurological Surgery
Children's Hospital and Regional Medical Center, E-606
Box 359300
Seattle, WA 98195
Phone: (206) 526-2544

Theodore S. Roberts, M.D.
Chief, Pediatric Neurosurgery
Professor, Neurosurgery
University of Washington
Children's Hospital and Medical Center
4800 Sand Point Way, N.E. (Box 5371)
Seattle, WA 98105-0371
Phone: (206) 526-2544

Washington, D.C.

Philip H. Cogen, M.D., Ph.D.
Chairman, Department of Neurosurgery
Children's National Medical Center
111 Michigan Avenue, N.W.
Washington, DC 20010
Phone: (202) 884-3020

David J. Donahue, M.D.
Children's National Medical Center
Department of Neurological Surgery
111 Michigan Avenue, N.W.
Suite W4-100
Washington, DC 20010-2970
Phone: (202) 884-3020

Steven J. Schiff, M.D., Ph.D.
Children's National Medical Center
111 Michigan Avenue, N.W.
Washington, DC 20010
Phone: (202) 884-3020

Canada

Alberta

Keith E. Aronyk, M.D.
Neurosurgery Associates
2D-102 MacKenzie Centre
8440 112th Street
Edmonton, AB Canada
T6G 2B7
Phone: (403) 492-6870

British Columbia

D. Douglas Cochrane, M.D.
Associate Professor, Head of Pediatric Surgery
University of British Columbia
British Columbia Children's Hospial
Department of Neurosurgery
4480 Oak Street
Vancouver, BC Canada
V6H 3V4
Phone: (604) 875-2094

John R.W. Kestle, M.D.
British Columbia Children's Hospital
Department of Neurosurgery
4480 Oak Street
Vancouver, BC Canada
V6H 3V4
Phone: (604) 875-2094

Paul Steinbok, M.D.
Associate Professor, University of British Columbia
British Columbia Children's Hospital
4480 Oak Street, Room A325
Vancouver, BC Canada
V6H 3V4
Phone: (604) 875-2094

Ontario

James M. Drake, M.D.
Hospital for Sick Children
1504D-555 University Avenue
Toronto, ON Canada
M5G 1X8
Phone: (416) 813-6125

Harold J. Hoffman, M.D.
Professor of Surgery, University of Toronto
Hospital for Sick Children
1504-555 University Avenue
Toronto, ON Canada
M5G 1X8
Phone: (416) 813-6426

Robert D. Hollenberg, M.D.
McMaster University Medical Center
Department of Surgery, #4U4
Hamilton, ON Canada
L8N 3Z5
Phone: (905) 521-2100, ext. 5235

Robin P. Humphreys, M.D., FRCSC, FACS
Professor of Surgery and Anatomy
University of Toronto
1504-555 University Avenue
Toronto, ON Canada
M5G 1X8
Phone: (416) 813-6427

James T. Rutka, M.D.
Hospital for Sick Children
1504-555 University Avenue
Toronto, ON Canada
M5G 1X8
Phone: (416) 813-6425

Enrique C.G. Ventureyra, M.D.
Division of Neurosurgery
Children's Hospital of Eastern Ontario
401 Smythe
Ottawa, ON Canada
K1H 8L1
Phone: (613) 737-2316

Quebec

Jean-Pierre Farmer, M.D.
Division of Neurosurgery
Montreal Children's Hospital
2300 Tuper Street
Montreal, QC Canada
H3H 1P3
Phone: (514) 934-4400

Jose L. Montes, M.D.
Montreal Children's Hospital
2300 Tuper Street, Room C-811
Montreal, QC Canada
H3H 1P3
Phone: (514) 934-4400, ext. 5224

Associations and Organizations

Hydrocephalus information and support

Hydrocephalus Association
Emily S. Fudge, Executive Director
Jennifer Henerlau, Assistant Director
Pip Marks, Outreach Coordinator
870 Market Street, Suite 955
San Francisco, CA 94102
Phone: (415) 732-7040
Fax: (415) 732-7044
Email: *hydroassoc@aol.com*
Web: *http://neurosurgery.mgh.harvard.edu/ha/*

The Hydrocephalus Association is a nonprofit organization, founded in 1983, that provides support, education, and advocacy to individuals, families, and professionals. Its goal is to provide comprehensive services to empower individuals and families to seek out the best medical care, programs, and resources that will meet their needs now and in the future.

Hydrocephalus Association of North Texas (HANT)
Jana Dransfield
P.O. Box 670552
Dallas, TX 75637-0552
Phone: (214) 528-2877
Fax: (214) 528-8097

Hydrocephalus Family Support Group of Central Florida
Pediatric Neurosurgery
Kay Taylor, R.N.
22 Lake Beauty Drive, Suite 204
Orlando, FL 32806-2040
Phone: (407) 649-7686
Fax: (407) 649-7692
Email: *mrssm1000@aol.com*

Hydrocephalus Foundation, Inc. (HyFI)
Greg Tocco, Executive Director and Founder
910 Rear Broadway
Saugus, MA 01906
Phone: (617) 942-1161
Web: *http://neurosurgery.mgh.harvard.edu/HyFI/*

The Hydrocephalus Foundation was established to help assist patients and their families during the transition from their diagnosis to a resumption of their normal lifestyles. The primary focus of the Hydrocephalus Foundation is to contribute emotional support to patients of hydrocephalus and their families. The foundation will promote and encourage research that assists in the comprehensive treatment of people with hydrocephalus and the training of competent professionals.

Hydrocephalus Research Foundation
Ann Marie Liakos, Executive Director
1670 Green Oak Circle
Lawrenceville, GA 30243
Phone: (770) 995-9570
Email: *Ann_Liakos@atlmug.org*

Hydrocephalus Support Group, Inc. (HSG)
Debby Buffa, Founder/Chairman
P.O. Box 4236
Chesterfield, MO 63006-4236
Phone: (314) 532-8228
Fax: (314) 995-4108
Email: *hydro@inlink.com*

The Hydrocephalus Support Group, Inc. (HSG) is a nonprofit organization providing education and support to individuals with hydrocephalus and their families. HSG has periodic meetings for anyone interested, a quarterly newsletter, parent referrals, and a library with more than 300 articles and tapes on hydrocephalus. HSG sponsors a one-day conference on hydrocephalus every year.

National Hydrocephalus Foundation (NHF)
Debbi Fields, Executive Director
12413 Centralia
Lakewood, CA 90715-1623
Phone: (562) 402-3523
Email: *hydrobrat@earthlink.net*

The National Hydrocephalus Foundation (NHF) was incorporated in 1980 as a voluntary, nonprofit, 501(c)3, public service organization. The objectives of NHF are:

- To assemble and disseminate information pertaining to hydrocephalus, its treatments, and outcomes.

- To establish and facilitate a communication network among affected families and individuals.

- To help others gain a deeper understanding of those areas affected by hydrocephalus, such as education, insurance, tax and estate planning, employment and family.

- To increase public awareness and knowledge of hydrocephalus.

- To promote and support research on the causes, treatment, and prevention of hydrocephalus.

In addition to providing the public with informational pamphlets, the NHF maintains a reference library and videos on hydrocephalus, promotes and helps support groups, and offers parent-to-parent and adult-to-adult referrals. NHF also issues a quarterly newsletter, *Life-Line*. The Foundation is supported by donations and membership fees.

Pregnancy and Maternal Hydrocephalus Database
Nancy Bradley, Coordinator
8403 Boyne Street
Downey, CA 90242
Phone: (562) 869-3689
Email: *HydroWoman@aol.com*

Seeking Techniques Advancing Research in Shunts (STARS)
Parent Support Group
Hydrocephalus/Shunt Research Fund Raising
Rosemary Ricelli
Steve Scheidt
1289 N. Glenhurst
Birmingham, MI 48009
Phone: (248) 644-STAR
Fax: (248) 647-5711

Related disorders

National Organization of Rare Disorders (NORD)
P.O. Box 8923
New Fairfield, CT 06812
Phone: (203) 746-6518; or (800) 999-6673
Web: *http://www.rarediseases.org*

Arnold-Chiari Malformation

World Arnold-Chiari Malformation Association
31 Newtown Woods Road
Newtown Square, PA 19073
Phone: (610) 353-4737
Email: *internautbhm@worldnet.att.net*
Web: *http://www.pressenter.com/~wacma/*

Attention deficit disorder

Children and Adults with Attention Deficit Disorders (CHADD)
499 N.W. 70th Avenue, Suite 101
Plantation, FL 33317
Phone: (800) 233-4050
Fax: (954) 587-4599
Email: *national@chadd.org*
Web: *http://www.chadd.org/*

Children and Adults with Attention Deficit Disorders (CHADD) is a nonprofit organization that was started by parents of children with attention deficit disorder (ADD) and professionals who work with such children. The objectives of CHADD include maintaining support groups for parents, providing a forum for continuing education, being an information resource, and ensuring that the best educational experiences are available to children and adults with ADD. CHADD sponsors a national conference on ADD and also publishes *Attention! Magazine,* the premiere magazine written for people with ADD/ADHD and those who work with them. CHADD's web site provides a listing of local chapters in the United States.

National Attention Deficit Disorder Association (ADDA)
9930 Johnnycake Ridge Road, Suite 3E
Mentor, OH 44060
Phone: (440) 350-9595; or (800) 487-2282
Fax: (440) 350-0223
Email: *NatlADDA@aol.com*
Web: *http://www.add.org/*

ADDA's mission is to help people with ADD lead happier, more successful lives through education, research, and public advocacy. Whether you have ADD yourself or someone special in your life does, or if you treat, counsel, or teach those who do, ADDA is an organization for you. ADDA is especially focused on the needs of ADDults and young adults with ADD. Parents of children with ADD are also welcome.

ADDA's mission is not only to educate, teach, and lobby for rights, but to cultivate and rally the varied talents from within the ADD community. ADDA supports training, conferences, and research into ADD's causes and treatment. Through a growing Support Group Network, ADDA is working to help people discover how to cope with the challenges of ADD while celebrating and leveraging its many positive aspects.

Brain tumor/head injury

Brain Injury Association USA
105 North Alfred Street
Alexandria, VA 22314
Phone: 703-236-6000
Fax: 703-236-6001
Email: *FamilyHelpline@biausa.org*
Web: *http://www.biausa.org/*

Brain Tumor Foundation of Canada
650 Waterloo Street, Suite 100
London, ON Canada
N6B 2R4
Phone: 519-642-7755
Fax: 519-642-7192
Email: *BTFC@gtn.net*
Web: *http://www.btfc.org/*

The Brain Tumor Society (TBTS)
Elain R. Cohen, Executive Director
84 Seattle Street
Boston, MA 02134-1245
Phone: (800) 770-8287; or (617) 783-0340
Fax: (617) 783-9712
Email: *info@tbts.org*
Web: *http://www.tbts.org/*

National Brain Tumor Foundation (NBTF)
785 Market Street, Suite 1600
San Francisco, CA 94103
Phone: (415) 284-0208; or (800) 934-CURE
Fax: (415) 284-0209
Email: *nbtf@braintumor.org*
Web: *http://www.braintumor.org/*

National Head Injury Foundation (NHIF)
1776 Massachusetts Avenue, N.W.
Suite 100
Washington, DC 20036
Phone: (800) 444-6443; or (202) 296-6443
Fax: (202) 296-8850

Diabetes insipidus

Nephrogenic Diabetes Insipidus Foundation (NDIF)
Main Street
P.O. Box 1390
Eastsound, WA 98245
Phone: 888-376-6343
Fax: 888-376-3842
Email: *info@ndif.org*
Web: *http://www.ndif.org/*

Epilepsy

The Cleveland Clinic Foundation
Departments of Neurology and Neurological Surgery
9500 Euclid Avenue
Cleveland, Ohio 44195-5125
Phone: (216) 444-5559; or (800) 223-2273, ext. 45559
Fax: (216) 444-0266
TTY: (216) 444-0261
Web: *http://www.neus.ccf.org/*

The Cleveland Clinic Foundation's Epilepsy Center, formed in 1978, is a national and international pacesetter in the treatment of epilepsy in both children and adults. The center provides a comfortable, caring environment where the staff members do everything possible to bring seizures under control.

The Epilepsy Foundation
4351 Garden City Drive
Landover, MD 20785-2267
Phone: (301) 459-3700; or (800) EFA-1000
Fax: (301) 577-2684
Web: *http://www.efa.org/*

The Epilepsy Foundation, founded in 1968, is a network of more than 60 affiliated organizations offering services in 125 communities across the United States. National programs include a toll-free public information and referral service, research, professional education, public and family education, legal and legislative advocacy, and employment assistance. Local affiliate services may include outreach to schools and the community, support groups, camping, information and referral, employment services, respite care, and help with living arrangements for families. The Epilepsy Foundation also publishes a quarterly newsletter, *In Touch,* which provides tips and stories by people who have seizures and epilepsy.

Spina bifida

Spina Bifida Association of America
590 MacArthur Blvd. N.W., Suite 250
Washington, DC 20007-4226
Phone: (202) 944-3285; or (800) 621-3141
Fax: (202) 944-3295
Email: *ir@sbaa.org*
Web: *http://www.sbaa.org/*

Spina Bifida and Hydrocephalus Association of Canada (SBHAC)
220-388 Donald Street
Winnipeg, MB Canada
R3B 2J4
Phone: (204) 957-1784; or (800) 565-9488
Fax: (204) 957-1794
Email: *spinab@mts.net*
Web: *http://www.sbhac.ca/*

Disability and neurological organizations

The National Information Center for Children and Youth with Disabilities (NICHCY)
P.O. Box 1492
Washington, DC 20013
Phone: (202) 884-8200 (V/ TTY); or (800) 695-0285 (V/ TTY)
Fax: (202) 884-8441
Email: *nichcy@aed.org*
Web: *http://www.nichcy.org/*

NICHCY is the national information and referral center that provides information on disabilities and disability-related issues for families, educators, and other professionals. Its special focus is children and youth (birth to age 22).

National Institute for Neurological Disorders and Stroke (NINDS)
Office of Scientific and Health Reports
P.O. Box 5801
Bethesda, MD 20824
Phone: (800) 352-9424; or (301) 496-5751
Web: *http://www.ninds.nih.gov/*

The NINDS is an agency of the U.S. federal government and a component of the National Institutes of Health (NIH) and the U.S. Public Health Service. NINDS is the lead agency for the congressionally designated *Decade of the Brain* and the leading supporter of biomedical research on disorders of the brain and nervous system.

The National Parent Network on Disabilities (NPND)
Patty McGill Smith, Executive Director
1200 G Street N.W., Suite 800
Washington, DC 20005
Phone: (202) 434-8686 (V/TDD)
Fax: (202) 638-7299
Email: *npnd@cs.com*
Web: *http://www.npnd.org/*

NPND was established to provide a presence and national voice for parents of children, youth, and adults with special needs. NPND shares information and resources in order to promote and support the power of parents to influence and affect policy issues concerning the needs of people with disabilities and their families.

TASH (formerly the Association for People with Severe Handicaps)
29 Susquehanna Avenue, Suite 210
. Baltimore, MD 21204
Phone: (410) 828-8274
Fax: (410) 828-6706
TDD: (410) 828-1306
Email: *info@tash.org*
Web: *http://www.tash.org/*

TASH is a nonprofit, international, advocacy association of people with disabilities, their family members, other advocates, and people who work in the disability field. There are 38 chapters and members from 34 different countries and territories. Since its inception in 1974, TASH has gained international acclaim for its uncompromising stand against separatism, stigmatization, abuse, and neglect. TASH actively promotes the full inclusion and participation of persons with disabilities in all aspects of life. TASH believes that no one with a disability should be forced to live, work, or learn in a segregated setting, that all individuals deserve the right to direct their own lives. TASH's mission is to eliminate physical and social obstacles that prevent equity, diversity, and quality of life.

TASH is a civil rights organization for, and of, people with mental retardation, autism, cerebral palsy, physical disabilities, and other conditions that make full integration a challenge. TASH is a member-based organization. Members of TASH receive a monthly newsletter, the *Journal of the Association of Persons with Severe Handicaps,* and also receive a reduced registration fee for attending the annual conference.

Medical and professional associations

American Academy of Neurology (AAN)
1080 Montreal Avenue
St. Paul, MN 55116-2325
Phone: (612) 695-1940
Fax: (612) 695-2791
Web: *http://www.neurology.org/*

The American Academy of Neurology publishes the monthly journal *Neurology* and provides fact sheets and brochures on various neurological disorders, including brain tumors, epilepsy, headache, and head injuries. Its brochure, *Epilepsy: What You Should Know,* includes useful information for patients who have epilepsy. It also has a section on its web site called *Neurology News,* which provides people with the latest information on neurologic disorders.

American Association of Neurological Surgeons (AANS)
22 South Washington Street
Park Ridge, IL 60068-4287
Phone: (847) 692-9500
Fax: (847) 692-2589
Email: *info@aans.org*
Web: *http://www.neurosurgery.org/* or *http://www.aans.org/*

American Board of Clinical Neuropsychology
Department of Psychiatry
The University of Michigan Hospitals
1500 East Medical Center Drive
Ann Arbor, Michigan 48109-0704
Phone: (734) 936-8269
Fax: (734) 936-9761
Web: *http://www.med.umich.edu/abcn/*

The American Board of Clinical Neuropsychology (ABCN) is the affiliated specialty board of the American Board of Professional Psychology (ABPP), which is responsible for the examination for the diploma in Clinical Neuropsychology.

American Board of Professional Neuropsychology (ABPN)
Michael J. Raymond, Ph.D.
Director, Neuropsychological/Cognitive Services
Allied Services
John Heinz Institute of Rehabilitation Medicine
150 Mundy Street
P.O. Box 2096
Wilkes-Barre Township, PA 18702
Phone: (717) 826-3800
Fax: (717) 826-3898
Web: *http://www.people.memphis.edu/~clong/abpn-hp.htm*

The American Board of Professional Neuropsychology (ABPN) was created by a group of clinical neuropsychologists in response to the growing need to formally assess competency in the practice of clinical neuropsychology. The ABPN maintains a directory of neuropsychologists who have received the ABPN's diploma.

American Board of Medical Specialties (ABMS)
1007 Church Street, Suite 404
Evanston, Illinois 60201-5913
Phone: (847) 491-9091
Fax: (847) 328-3596
Web: *http://www.abms.org/*

American Board of Neurological Surgery (ABNS)
6550 Fannin Street
Suite 2139
Houston, TX 77030-2701
Phone: (713) 790-6015
Fax: (713) 794-0207
Web: *http://www.abns.org/*

American Board of Pediatric Neurological Surgery (ABPNS)
930 Madison Avenue
Suite 600
Memphis, TN 38103
Web: *http://www.abpns.org/*

American Society of Pediatric Neurosurgeons (ASPN)
Web: *http://www.aspn.org/*

International Neuropsychological Society
700 Ackerman Road, Suite 550
Columbus, Ohio 43202-1559
Phone: (614) 263-4200
Fax: (614) 263-4366
Email: *osu_ins@postbox.acs.ohio-state.edu*
Web: *http://www.med.ohio-state.edu/ins/index.html*

The International Neuropsychological Society is dedicated to promoting research, service, and education in neuropsychology and to enhancing communication among the scientific disciplines that contribute to the understanding of brain-behavior relationships. The society has more than 3,500 members worldwide.

Insurance

Agency for Health Care Policy and Research (AHCPR)
Publications Clearinghouse
Office Center, Suite 500
2101 East Jefferson Street
Rockville, MD 20852
Phone: (410) 381-3150; or (800) 358-9295
TDD: (888) 586-6340 (hearing impaired only)
Email: *info@ahcpr.gov*
Web: *http://www.ahcpr.gov/*

American Association of Health Plans (AAHP)
1129 20th Street, N.W., Suite 600
Washington, DC 20036-3421
Phone: (202) 778-3200
Fax: (202) 331-7487
Web: *http://www.aahp.org/*

Joint Commission on Accreditation of Healthcare Organizations (JCAHO)
One Renaissance Blvd.
Oakbrook Terrace, IL 60181
Phone: (630) 792-5889
Fax: (630) 792-5005
Web: *http://www.jcaho.org/*

The National Committee for Quality Assurance (NCQA)
2000 L. Street N.W.
Suite #500
Washington, DC 20036
Phone: (202) 955-3500
To order publications, phone: (800) 839-6487
For information about conferences, phone: (202) 955-5697
Fax: (202) 955-3599
Web: *http://www.ncqa.org/*

International organizations

Arbeitsgemeinschaft Spina bifida und Hydrocephalus e.V. (ASbH e.V.)
Bundesverband
Münsterstr.13
D-44145 Dortmund
Germany
Phone: (0231) 86 10 50-0
Fax: (0231) 86 10 50-50
Email: *asbh@asbh.de*
Web: *http://www.asbh.de/*

Association for Spina Bifida and Hydrocephalus (ASBAH)
Teresa Cole, Vice President
42 Park Road
Peterborough, United Kingdom
PE1 2UQ
Phone: 01733 555988
Fax: 01733 555985
Email: *postmaster@asbah.demon.co.uk*
Web: *http://www.asbah.demon.co.uk/*

ASBAH, the Association for Spina Bifida and Hydrocephalus, was formed in 1966 and serves England, Wales, and Northern Ireland. Through a network of professional advisers backed up by specialists in mobility, continence management, education, and medical matters, ASBAH provides advice and practical support to people with these disabilities, their families, and their care providers. ASBAH aims to improve services for people with spina bifida and/or hydrocephalus, to work with them to extend their choices, and maximize opportunities for independence and achievement.

International Federation for Hydrocephalus and Spina Bifida
13D Chemin du Levant
F-01210 Ferney-Voltaire
France
Phone: +33 (0) 450 40 01 02
Fax: +33 (0) 450 40 01 19
Email: *ifhsb@msn.com*
Web: *http://www.asbah.demon.co.uk/ifhsb.html*

The International Federation for Hydrocephalus and Spina Bifida (if) is the worldwide umbrella organization for these two disabilities and has a contact network on every continent. Its members are national organizations for spina bifida and hydrocephalus in more than 30 countries. These national organizations support people with spina bifida and hydrocephalus in their daily lives.

Irish Association for Spina Bifida and Hydrocephalus
Claire Gill, Hon Secretary, Irish ASBAH
Old Nangor Road
Clondalkin, Dublin 22
Phone: Dublin 003531 4572326

New Zealand Spina Bifida Trust
P.O. Box 19281
Avondale, Auckland
New Zealand

Scottish Spina Bifida Association
National Office
190 Queensferry Road
Edinburgh, Scotland
EH4 2BW
Phone: (0131) 332 0743
Fax: (0131) 343 3651
Email: *101677.765@compuserve.com*
Web: *http://ourworld.compuserve.com/homepages/ssbahq/*

Spina Bifida Group of New South Wales
P.O. Box 4055
Parramatta, NSW 2124
Australia

The Spina Bifida Association of Western Australia (Inc.)
37 Hampden Road
Nedlands, Western Australia 6009
Australia
Phone: (08) 9389 8311; or +61 8 9389 8311 (international)
Fax: (08) 9389 8331; or +61 8 9389 8331 (international)
Email: *sbawa@swannet.com.au*
Web: *http://www.swannet.com.au/sbawa/*

Medical Libraries and Journals

Regional medical libraries (RML)

For more information about specific network programs in your region, call the regional medical library in your area at its direct number (see the list below) or call the toll-free phone number for all regional medical libraries: 1-800-338-7657.

For general network information contact:

National Network of Libraries of Medicine
National Library of Medicine
8600 Rockville Pike, Building 38, Room B1-E03
Bethesda, MD 20894
Phone: (301) 496-4777
Fax: (301) 480-1467
Email: *nnlm-info@nlm.nih.gov*
http://www.nnlm.nlm.nih.gov

New England Region

Connecticut, Maine, Massachusetts, New Hampshire, Rhode Island, and Vermont:

University of Connecticut Health Center
Lyman Maynard Stowe Library
263 Farmington Avenue
Farmington, CT 06030-5370
Phone: (860) 679-4500
Fax: (860) 679-1305
http://www.nnlm.nlm.nih.gov/ner

Middle Atlantic Region

Delaware, New Jersey, New York, and Pennsylvania:

The New York Academy of Medicine
1216 Fifth Avenue
New York, NY 10029
Phone: (212) 822-7396
Fax: (212) 534-7042
http://www.nnlm.nlm.nih.gov/mar

Southeastern/Atlantic Region

Alabama, Florida, Georgia, Maryland, Mississippi, North Carolina, South
Carolina, Tennessee, Virginia, West Virginia, the District of Columbia, Puerto
Rico, and the U.S. Virgin Islands:

University of Maryland at Baltimore
Health Sciences Library
601 W. Lombard Street
Baltimore, MD 21201-1583
Phone: (410) 706-2855
Fax: (410) 706-0099
http://www.nnlm.nlm.nih.gov/sar

Greater Midwest Region

Iowa, Illinois, Indiana, Kentucky, Michigan, Minnesota, North Dakota, South
Dakota, Ohio, and Wisconsin:

The University of Illinois at Chicago
Library of the Health Sciences (M/C 763)
1750 W. Polk Street
Chicago, IL 60612-7223
Phone: (312) 996-2464
Fax: (312) 996-2226
http://www.nnlm.nlm.nih.gov/gmr

Midcontinental Region

Colorado, Kansas, Missouri, Nebraska, Utah, and Wyoming:

University of Nebraska Medical Center
Leon S. McGoogan Library of Medicine
Regional Medical Library
986706 Nebraska Medical Center
Omaha, NE 68198-6706
Phone: (402) 559-4326
Fax: (402) 559-5482
http://www.nnlm.nlm.nih.gov/mr

South Central Region

Arkansas, Louisiana, New Mexico, Oklahoma, and Texas:

Houston Academy of Medicine-Texas Medical Center Library
1133 M.D. Anderson Boulevard
Houston, TX 77030-2809
Phone: (713) 799-7880
Fax: (713) 790-7030
Email: *nnlmscr@library.tmc.edu*
http://www.nnlm.nlm.nih.gov/scr

Pacific Northwest Region

Alaska, Idaho, Montana, Oregon, Washington:

Health Sciences Libraries and Information Center
Box 357155
University of Washington
Seattle, WA 98195-7155
Phone: (206) 543-8262
Fax: (206) 543-2469
Email: *nnlm@u.washington.edu*
http://www.nnlm.nlm.nih.gov/pnr

Pacific Southwest Region

Arizona, California, Hawaii, Nevada, and U.S. territories in the Pacific Basin:

University of California, Los Angeles
Louise M. Darling Biomedical Library
12-077 Center for the Health Sciences
Box 951798
Los Angeles, CA 90095-1798
Phone: (310) 825-1200
Fax: (310) 825-5389
http://www.nnlm.nlm.nih.gov/psr

Medical journals

The following is a list of medical journals that publish articles on or related to hydrocephalus and health care. We have included the full name of the journal, as well as its MEDLINE abbreviation to aid you in conducting searches on PubMed. Web addresses are provided for those journals that have web sites.

MEDLINE: Journals that Offer Full Text
http://www.ncbi.nlm.nih.gov/PubMed/fulltext.html

ACTA Neurologica Latinoamericana
MEDLINE: *Acta Neurol Latinoam*
http://www.anla.com/

Advances and Technical Standards in Neurosurgery
MEDLINE: *Adv Tech Stand Neurosurg*

Advances in Neurology
MEDLINE: *Adv Neurol*

American Journal of Diseases of Children
MEDLINE: *Am J Dis Child*

Annals of Neurology
MEDLINE: *Ann Neurol*

Archives of Disease in Childhood
MEDLINE: *Arch Dis Child*

Archives of Disease in Childhood: Fetal and Neonatal Edition
MEDLINE: *Arch Dis Child Fetal Neonatal Ed*

Archives of Neurology
MEDLINE: *Arch Neurol*
http://www.ama-assn.org/public/journals/neur/neurhome.htm

Archives of Pediatric and Adolescent Medicine
MEDLINE: *Arch Pediatr Adolesc Med*
http://www.ama-assn.org/public/journals/ajdc/ajdchome.htm

Behavioral Neuropsychiatry
MEDLINE: *Behav Neuropsychiatry*

British Journal of Neurosurgery
MEDLINE: *Br J Neurosurg*

British Medical Journal
MEDLINE: *Br Med J*
http://www.bmj.com/

Canadian Hospital
MEDLINE: *Can Hosp*

Canadian Journal of Neurological Sciences
MEDLINE: *Can J Neurol Sci*

The Harvard Brain
No MEDLINE record
http://hcs.harvard.edu/~husn/BRAIN/

International Journal of Developmental Neuroscience
MEDLINE: *Int J Dev Neurosci*

Irish Medical Journal
MEDLINE: *Ir Med J*
http://www.imj.ie/

Journal of the American Medical Association (JAMA)
MEDLINE: *JAMA*

Journal of Child Neurology
MEDLINE: *J Child Neurol*

Journal of the International Neuropsychological Society
MEDLINE: *J Int Neuropsychol Soc*

Journal of Learning Disabilities
MEDLINE: *J Learn Disabil*

Journal of Neuroendocrinology
MEDLINE: *J Neuroendocrinol*

Journal of Neurology, Neurosurgery, & Psychiatry
MEDLINE: *J Neurol Neurosurg Psychiatry*
http://www.bmjpg.com/data/jnnp.htm

Journal of Neuro-ophthalmology
MEDLINE: *J Neuroophthalmol*

Journal of Neurosurgery
MEDLINE: *J Neurosurg*

Journal of Neurosurgical Nursing
MEDLINE: *J Neurosurg Nurs*

Journal of Pediatric Ophthalmology
MEDLINE: *J Pediatr Ophthalmol*

The Lancet
MEDLINE: *Lancet*
http://www.thelancet.com/

Medical Journal of Australia
MEDLINE: *Med J Aust*
http://www.mja.com.au/

Minimally Invasive Neurosurgery
MEDLINE: *Minim Invasive Neurosurg*
http://www.thieme.com/cgi-win/thieme.exe/onGIMLKAGHLILJ/display/765

Neurocirugía—Journal of the Spanish Neurosurgery Society
MEDLINE: *Neurocirugia*
http://www.mundivia.es/empresas/neurocirugia/

Neurosurgery
MEDLINE: *Neurosurgery*
http://www.wwilkins.com/neurosurgery/

New England Journal of Medicine
MEDLINE: *N Engl J Med*
http://www.nejm.org/

Pediatric Neurology
MEDLINE: *Pediatr Neurol*

Pediatric Neurosurgery
MEDLINE: *Pediatr Neurosurg*

Pediatrics
MEDLINE: *Pediatrics*
http://www.pediatrics.org/

Perspectives in Neurological Surgery
No MEDLINE record
http://www.thieme.com/cgi-win/thieme.exe/onGIMLKAGHLILJ/display/768

Research in Developmental Disabilities
MEDLINE: *Res Dev Disabil*

Suggested Reading

Hydrocephalus

About Normal Pressure Hydrocephalus: A Book for Adults and Their Families.
Hydrocephalus Association. To receive a copy, contact the Hydrocephalus
Association (see listing under "Hydrocephalus information and support" in
Appendix B, *Associations and Organizations*).

Eye Problems Associated with Hydrocephalus (Information Sheet). Adapted from
a presentation made by Marijean Miller, M.D., Children's National Medical Center, at the 5th National Conference on Hydrocephalus for Families
and Professionals, and an article by I. M. Rabinowic, M.A., R.R.C.S., D.O.,
for the Spina Bifida Association. Provided courtesy of the Hydrocephalus
Association, © 1998. This fact sheet can be obtained from the Hydrocephalus Association at no cost (see Appendix B for contact information).

The Shunt Book. J. M. Drake and C. Sainte-Rose. Blackwell Science, 1995.

For children and teens

The Human Brain Coloring Book. M. C. Diamond, A. B. Scheibel, and L. M.
Elson. HarperPerennial, 1985.

Just Like Any Other Beagle. Cordis Corporation. 1992. Copies of this coloring
book are available from Cordis Corp., P.O. Box 025700, Miami, FL 33102-
5700. Phone: (800) 327-7714, or (305) 824-6040. Fax: (305) 824-2050.

*Keeping a Head in School: A Student's Book about Learning Abilities and Learning
Disorders.* Mel Levine. 1994.

Shelly, the Hyperactive Turtle. Deborah Moss. 1989.

Healthcare

*The HMO Health Care Companion: A Consumer's Guide to Managed Care Net-
works.* Alan G. Raymond. HarperPerennial, 1994.

The HMO Survival Guide. Sue Berkman. Villard Books/Random House, Inc., 1997.

Hospital Smarts: The Insider's Survival Guide to Your Hospital, Your Doctor, the Nursing Staff—and Your Bill!. Theodore Tyberg and Kenneth Rothaus. Hearst Books, 1995.

The Intelligent Patient's Guide to the Doctor-Patient Relationship. Barbara M. Korsch, M.D., and Caroline Harding. Oxford University Press, 1997.

Managed Care Beware: Five Steps You Need to Know to Survive HMOs and Get the Care You Deserve. Harvey M. Shapiro, M.D. Dove Audio, Inc., 1997.

Medical-Surgical Care Planning, 2nd Edition. Nancy M. Holloway, RN, MSN. Springhouse Corporation, 1993.

Medical Records: Getting Yours. Public Citizen, 1995.

Medicare Made Simple: A Consumer's Guide to the Medicare Program. Denise Knaus. Health Information Press, 1996.

Mind Body Medicine: How to Use Your Mind for Better Health. Daniel Goleman and Joel Gurin, eds. Fairfield, OH: Consumer Reports Books, 1993. 9180 LeSaint Drive, Fairfield, OH 45014.

Mosby's Diagnostic and Laboratory Test Reference, 3rd Edition. Kathleen D. Pagana, Ph.D., R.N., and Timothy J. Pagana, M.D., F.A.C.S. Mosby-Year Book, Inc., 1997.

Naked to the Bone: Medical Imaging in the Twentieth Century. Bettyann H. Kevles. Rutgers University Press, 1997.

The PDR Pocket Guide to Prescription Drugs, Revised and Updated. Medical Economics Company, Inc., 1997. Printed by Pocket Books, a division of Simon & Schuster, Inc.

Take Charge of Your Hospital Stay: A "Start Smart" Guide for Patients and Care Partners. Karen Keating McCann. Plenum Press, 1994.

Take this Book to the Hospital with You. Charles Inlander. St. Martin's Mass Market Paper, 1997.

Working with Your Doctor: Getting the Healthcare You Deserve. Nancy Keene. O'Reilly & Associates, Inc., 1998.

Your Child in the Hospital: A Practical Guide for Parents, Second Edition. Nancy Keene and Rachel Prentice. O'Reilly & Associates, 1999.

Support

Armfuls of Time: The Psychological Experience of the Child with a Life-Threatening Illness. Barbara M. Sourkes, Ph.D. Pittsburgh: University of Pittsburgh Press, 1995.

Directory of Hydrocephalus Support Groups. Hydrocephalus Association, 1998. This directory is a listing of all known hydrocephalus support groups including address, telephone number, contact person(s), and a description of services and resources provided. To receive a copy, contact the Hydrocephalus Association (see listing in Appendix B).

Making Therapy Work: Your Guide to Choosing, Using, and Ending Therapy. Fredda Bruckner et al. New York: Harper & Row, 1988. Excellent book full of practical advice on how to find the right therapist and get the most out of your sessions, and when to end therapy.

Organizing and Maintaining Support Groups for Parents of Children with Chronic Illness and Handicapping Conditions. Minna Newman Nathanson. Association for the Care of Children's Health. 19 Mantua Road, Mount Royal, NJ 08061; phone: (609) 224-1742; fax: (609) 423-3420; email: *amkent@smarthub.com*; Web: *http://www.aach.org/.*

Starting/Running Support Groups, 3rd Edition. Buz Overbeck and Joanie Overbeck. TLC Group, 1992.

Vistas of Challenge: Profiles of Inspiring People and Their Courage. Seryl Sander. New York: Mesorah Publications, 1996. (800) MESORAH, or (721) 921-2000.

When You Worry About The Child You Love: Emotional and Learning Problems in Children. Edward Hallowell. Fireside, 1997.

Education

Education of the Handicapped Act Amendments of 1990 (EHA). Public Law 101-476 (S. 1824). This law is a series of amendments, including changing the name from EHA to the Individuals with Disabilities Education Act (IDEA). The text of this law can be obtained from the Library of Congress, or online: *http://thomas.loc.gov/home/thomas2.html.*

Educational Care: A System for Understanding and Helping Children with Learning Problems at Home and in School. Mel Levine. Educators Publishing Service, 1994.

Individuals with Disabilities Education Act Amendments of 1997. Public Law 105-17 (H.R. 5). Better known as IDEA 97, this law amends P.L. 101-476 with stronger provisions for guaranteeing access to specialized education for children with disabilities. The text of this law can be obtained from the Library of Congress, or on the Web at: *http://thomas.loc.gov/home/thomas2.html.*

Negotiating the Special Education Maze: A Guide for Parents and Teachers, 3rd Edition. Winifred Anderson, Stephen Chitwood, and Deidre Hayden. Woodbine House, 1997.

Smart Kids with School Problems: Things to Know and Ways to Help. Priscilla Vail and Patricia Vail. New American Library Trade, 1989.

The Special Education Sourcebook: A Teacher's Guide to Programs, Materials, and Information Resources. Michael S. Rosenberg and Irene Edmond-Rosenberg. Woodbine House, 1994.

"What Does IDEA '97 Say About Evaluations, Eligibility, IEPs and Placements." Rud Turnbull, Kate Rainbold, and Amy Buchele-Ash. *TASH Newsletter.* December 1997/January 1998.

Learning disabilities

ADD and Adolescence: Strategies for Success from CHADD. CHADD. Paperback, 134 pp. Can be ordered only from CHADD's distributor, Caset, by calling (800) 545-5583, or from the ADD Warehouse Catalog at (800) 233-9273.

ADD and the College Student: A Guide for High School and College Students with Attention Deficit Disorder. Patricia O. Quinn. Magination, 1994.

Driven to Distraction: Recognizing and Coping with Attention Deficit Disorder from Childhood through Adulthood. Edward M. Hallowell and John J. Ratey. Simon & Schuster, 1995. Two cassette tapes.

Learning About Learning Disabilities, 2nd Edition. Bernice Y. L. Wong. Academic Press, 1998.

Maybe You Know My Kid: A Parent's Guide To Identifying, Understanding, and Helping Your Child With Attention Deficit Hyperactivity Disorder. Mary Fowler. Birch Lane Press, 1999.

Nonverbal Learning Disabilities: The Syndrome and the Model. Byron P. Rourke. Guilford Press, 1989.

Nonverbal Learning Disorder Syndrome Information Sheet. Emily Fudge. Adapted from a paper by Rochelle Harris, David H. Bennett, Brian Belden, Lynne Covitz, and Vicki Little, of the Section of Developmental Medicine and Psychology, Children's Mercy Hospital, Kansas City, MO.

Out of the Fog: Treatment Options and Coping Strategies for Adult Attention Deficit Disorder. Kevin R. Murphy and Suzanne LeVert. Hyperion, 1995.

Women With Attention Deficit Disorder: Embracing Disorganization at Home and in the Workplace. Sari Solden. Underwood Books, 1995.

Internet Resources

THE FOLLOWING LIST OF WEB SITE ADDRESSES is intended to provide you with additional resources to locate information about hydrocephalus and related topics. Many of the organizations in Appendix B, *Associations and Organizations*, have web sites as well. Links to the web resources in this book are available online at:

http://www.patientcenters.com/hydrocephalus/

Hydrocephalus

Beth Israel Medical Center—Hydrocephalus
http://www.bimc.edu/inn/hydro/hyd_ind.html

Hydrocephalus Brochure
(Available from the American Association of Neurological Surgeons)
http://www.aans.org/pubpages/patres/hydrobroch.html

Hydrocephalus Facts & Links
http://members.nova.org/~twinkee/HydroLinks.htm

Hydrocephalus Index, Bowman Gray/Wake Forest
http://www.bgsm.edu/bgsm/surg-sci/ns/hyceph.html

Hydrocephalus Project at the Cleveland Clinic Foundation
http://www.neus.ccf.org:80/Hydroceph/

Hydrocephalus, Syrinx, Myelomeningocele Resource Guide
http://neurosurgery.mgh.harvard.edu/hyd-rsrc.htm

Spina Bifida, Syrinx, Hydrocephalus Home Page at Massachusetts General Hospital/Harvard Medical School
http://neurosurgery.mgh.harvard.edu/pedi-hp.htm

The University of Adelaide, Paediatric Neurosurgery Department—Hydrocephalus
http://www.health.adelaide.edu.au/paed-neuro/hydro.html

Personal home pages

Chris Riccio's Home Page
http://members.aol.com/CARiccio/

Nancy Bradley's Maternal Hydrocephalus Page
http://members.aol.com/HydroWoman/index.html

Chat rooms and listservs

HYCEPH-L (The Hydrocephalus Listserv)
http://www.geocities.com/HotSprings/Villa/2020/

Hydrohaven Chat Room
http://www.geocities.com/Heartland/6950/HydroHav.html

Massachusetts General Hospital Neurology—Neurology Web-Forum
http://neuro-www.mgh.harvard.edu/forum/

Disabilities and special education

Americans with Disabilities Act Document Center
http://janweb.icdi.wvu.edu/kinder/

Council for Exceptional Children (CEC)
http://www.cec.sped.org/

National Institute on Disability and Rehabilitative Research (NIDRR)
http://www.ed.gov/offices/OSERS/NIDRR/

National Library Service for the Blind and Physically Handicapped
http://lcweb.loc.gov/nls/nls.html

Office of Special Education and Rehabilitative Services (OSERS)
http://www.ed.gov/offices/OSERS/

OSERS: Office of Special Education Programs (OSEP)
http://www.ed.gov/offices/OSERS/OSEP/

OSERS: IDEA '97 Home Page
http://www.ed.gov/offices/OSERS/IDEA/

Rare Genetic Diseases in Children: Disability Resources Directory
http://mcrcr2.med.nyu.edu/murphp01/disable.htm

U.S. Department of Justice ADA Home Page
http://www.usdoj.gov/crt/ada/adahom1.htm

U.S. Department of Justice: Americans with Disabilities Act (ADA)
http://www.usdoj.gov/crt/ada/pubs/ada.txt

Neurosurgery

AANS Glossary of Neurosurgical Terms
http://www.aans.org/pubpages/whatis/glossary.html

The Cleveland Clinic Foundation, Department of Neurological Surgery
http://www.neus.ccf.org/

MGH Neurology—Neurology Web-Forum
http://neuro-www.mgh.harvard.edu/forum/

Neurosurgery://On-Call
(American Association of Neurological Surgeons)
http://www.aans.org/

Neurosurgery at Massachusetts General Hospital/Harvard Medical Center
http://neurosurgery.mgh.harvard.edu/

Neurosurgery Links
http://www.wwilkins.com/neurosurgery/0148-396Xlinks.html

Pediatric Neurosurgery—Hydrocephalus
http://cpmcnet.columbia.edu/dept/nsg/PNS/Hydrocephalus.html

Third Ventriculostomy
http://www.neuro.hscsyr.edu/teachfile/3V/3Vtop.html

The University of North Carolina-Chapel Hill, Division of Neurosurgery
http://sunsite.unc.edu/Neuro/Neuro.html

Imaging (CT, MRI, and radiology)

Joint Program in Nuclear Medicine
http://www.med.harvard.edu/JPNM/

Nuclear Medicine at Children's Hospital, Boston
http://nucmedweb.tch.harvard.edu/

Shields Health Care Group
http://www.shields.com/

What Is Computed Tomography?
(Advanced Research and Applications Corporation—ARACOR)
http://www.aracor.com/faqs/whatisCT.html

The Whole Brain Atlas
http://www.med.harvard.edu:80/AANLIB/home.html

Shunt manufacturers

Elekta
http://www.elekta.com/

Medtronic: PS Medical
http://www.medtronic.com/neuro/psmedical/

Radionics: Hydrocephalus Shunt Products
http://www.radionics.com/products/hydrocephalus_shunt/

Neuropsychology

Neuropsychology Central
http://www.premier.net/~cogito/neuropsy.html

Pediatric Neuropsychology in Medial Settings
http://netpsych.com/health/neuropsych.htm

Hospitals and medical centers

Beth Israel Hospital—Institute for Neurology and Neurosurgery
http://www.bethisraelny.org/inn/

Children's Hospital Boston
http://www.childrenshospital.org/

Children's Hospital of Pittsburgh
http://www.chp.edu/

The Children's Hospital of Philadelphia
http://www.chop.edu/

The Hospital for Sick Children
http://www.sickkids.on.ca/

HospitalWeb
http://neuro-www.mgh.harvard.edu/hospitalweb.shtml

Montreal Neurological Institute and Hospital
http://www.mcgill.ca/mni/

Shands for Kids
http://www.shandskids.com/

Health care information

Centers for Disease Control and Prevention (CDC): Prevention of Neural Tube Defects (NTDs)
http://www.cdc.gov/nceh/programs/infants/brthdfct/prevent/ntd_prev.htm

Dr. Koop's Community
(by Dr. C. Everett Koop, former U.S. Surgeon General)
http://www.drkoop.com/

MedicineNet
http://www.medicinenet.com/

Mediconsult.com
http://www.mediconsult.com/

National Health Information Resource Center (NHIRC)
http://www.nhirc.org/

OnHealth!
http://www.onhealth.com/

Public Citizen: Health Research Group
http://www.citizen.org/hrg/

ThriveOnline
http://www.thriveonline.com/

Government and health care law

Centers for Disease Control and Prevention (CDC)
http://www.cdc.gov/

Federation of State Medical Boards (FSMB)
http://www.usmle.org/boards.htm

Health Industry Manufacturers Association (HIMA)
http://www.himanet.com/

Health Policy Sites at George Washington University
http://www.gwu.edu/~ihpp/Hpolicy.html

Legislation: Bills, Amendments, and Laws
http://lcweb.loc.gov/global/legislative/bill.html

National Institutes of Health (NIH)
http://www.nih.gov/

Selected Internet Resources in Health Law and Policy
http://lawlib.slu.edu/centers/hlthlaw/hlthlnk.htm

State Insurance Commissioners
http://www.surrogacy.com/insurance/insurcom.html

THOMAS—U.S. Congress on the Internet
http://thomas.loc.gov/

Search sites

GALEN II—The UCSF Digital Library
http://www.library.ucsf.edu/

Internet Grateful Med
http://igm.nlm.nih.gov/

PubMed
http://www.ncbi.nlm.nih.gov/PubMed/

U.S. National Library of Medicine (NLM)
http://www.nlm.nih.gov/

WelchWeb: Welch Medical Library, Johns Hopkins University
http://www.welch.jhu.edu/

Glossary

Abducens nerve
Also known as the sixth cranial nerve, the abducens nerve is responsible for controlling the lateral rectus muscle of each eye, which turns the eye outward, away from the nose.

Acquired hydrocephalus
Hydrocephalus that is caused later in life; noncongenital.

Alzheimer's disease
A neurological form of dementia that is commonly confused with normal pressure hydrocephalus (NPH) in elderly patients. Some of the signs of Alzheimer's disease are shared by those of NPH, including urinary incontinence, disturbances of gait, and dementia.

Amblyopia
Dimness of vision in an eye without changes in the eye structures. (Also called lazy eye or wandering eye.)

Anaphylactic shock
A serious allergic reaction, causing swelling, constriction of the bronchioles in the lungs, heart failure, circulatory collapse, and sometimes death.

Anencephaly
A congenital birth defect where the bones at the back of the skull and the cerebral hemispheres are absent.

Anesthesia
A medical technique that reduces or eliminates consciousness, pain, and voluntary movements by administering medications that create a sleep-like state.

Anesthesiologist
A physician who studies and administers anesthesia.

Angled gantry
A technique used during computed tomography (CT) scans to reduce the amount of radiation the patient receives during the scan.

Antimicrobial agent
  An antibacterial chemical that is applied to a new brand of shunt catheters to help reduce the risk of infection.

Aqueduct of Sylvius
  A small passageway that connects the third and fourth ventricles of the brain. Also known as the cerebral aqueduct.

Aqueductal stenosis
  A blockage of the aqueduct of Sylvius that causes a form of non-communicating hydrocephalus.

Arachnoid granulations
  Protrusions of the arachnoid membrane of the brain. Arachnoid granulations, or villi, are similar to a one-way valve, allowing CSF to drain from the subarachnoid space into the superior sagittal sinus, where the fluid is reabsorbed into the bloodstream.

Arachnoid villi
  See *Arachnoid granulations*.

Arrhythmia
  An abnormal heart rate or rhythm.

Ataxia
  Unsteady gait or shaky movements.

Atrial introducer
  A device used during the placement of the distal catheter of a ventriculoatrial shunt for introducing the distal catheter into a blood vessel located in the patient's neck (either the right common facial vein or the internal jugular vein).

Babinski reflex
  A test performed to check the plantar reflex. Babinski reflexes are checked by drawing a blunt object, such as the handle of an instrument, along the outer edge of the sole of the foot from the heel to the little toe.

Barium sulfate
  A contrast material used to enhance the imagery of X-rays, CTs, and MRIs.

Basilar artery
  A large artery located at the base of the brain below the third ventricle.

Benign extra-axial fluid of infancy
  See *Benign subdural hygroma*.

Benign subdural hygroma

An accumulation of CSF in the subdural space that usually presents itself at birth or within the first few months after birth. An indication of a benign subdural hygroma is an increase in head circumference. Imagery will reveal there is no intracranial mass and normal-sized or slightly enlarged ventricles. This fluid accumulation will, over time, be reabsorbed by the brain. Benign subdural hygromas may also be referred to as *benign extra-axial fluid of infancy* and *external hydrocephalus.*

Betadine

A solution, made up of iodine and alcohol, used to help cleanse and sterilize an area prior to surgery.

Brain stem

The structure that connects the brain with the spinal cord. The brain stem is comprised of three sections: the pons, medulla, and the midbrain.

Bulb reservoir

A small dome on most shunt valves. As CSF flows into the valve from the ventricles of the brain via the proximal catheter, CSF will accumulate inside the bulb. If depressed, CSF should flow through the valve and out of the distal catheter. The bulb reservoir is used by medical professionals to test the condition of the shunt system.

Burr hole

A small hole that is drilled through the skull during a shunt placement procedure or to drain a subdural hematoma. The burr hole, or twist-drill hole, allows the neurosurgeon access to the brain.

Carotid artery

Either of two large arteries in the neck that supply the brain and other areas of the head and neck with oxygenated blood.

Catheter

A small, flexible tube made of silicone material that can be inserted into narrow openings to drain or administer fluids. There are two catheters as part of a shunt system: the proximal and distal catheters. The proximal catheter is inserted into the ventricles of the brain and connected to the shunt valve. The distal catheter is connected to the opposite end of the shunt valve, with the distal end of the catheter being placed in an area where CSF can be reabsorbed by the body (e.g., the peritoneal cavity). Also see *Distal catheter* and *Proximal catheter.*

Cerebellum

Area of the brain located below the occipital lobes and behind the brain stem, primarily responsible for coordinating movements and muscle

tone, and for controlling the body's sense of balance. It is made up of two distinct hemispheres.

Cerebral aqueduct
See *Aqueduct of Sylvius.*

Cerebral hemisphere
Two cerebral hemispheres—the left and right—make up the brain.

Cerebrospinal fluid (CSF)
A clear, colorless fluid produced mainly by the choroid plexus of the lateral ventricles. CSF is made up mostly of water with a few trace proteins and nutrients that are needed for the nourishment and normal function of the brain. CSF circulates around the brain and spinal cord, protecting them from injury and trauma.

Chiari Malformation (CM)
A rare, congenital anomaly in which two parts of the brain, the brain stem and cerebellum, are longer than normal and protrude down into the spinal cord.

Choroid plexus
A network of tiny blood vessels located in the ventricles of the brain. The choroid plexus is responsible for the production of CSF.

Cistern
Fluid-filled cavity. CSF naturally accumulates in three cisterns of the brain: the prepontine, interpeduncular, and the cisterna magna (or large cistern).

Communicating hydrocephalus
A type of hydrocephalus where CSF is allowed to flow freely through the ventricular system of the brain. However, hydrocephalus is caused because the fluid cannot be reabsorbed properly.

Computed tomography (CT)
A scan for examining the soft tissues and internal structures of the body using low doses of ionizing radiation to do the imaging and computer technology to interpret and produce the images. A head CT scans the head in thin slices. (Also known as computed axial tomography—CAT.)

Congenital hydrocephalus
Hydrocephalus that is caused by a congenital, or birth-related, malformation or defect within the brain that causes an obstruction in the flow and drainage of CSF.

Corpus callosum
A broad band of fibers that allows one side of the brain to communicate with the other.

Craniosynostosis
A congenital anomaly characterized by the premature closure of one or more of the cranial sutures before the brain has fully grown.

Cyst
Benign sacs or closed cavities that are filled with fluid. While cysts may occur anywhere in the body, cysts in the brain are normally filled with CSF.

Dandy-Walker syndrome
A congenital brain malformation that involves the fourth ventricle and the cerebellum. It is defined as an enlargement of the fourth ventricle, and is accompanied by the absence of the cerebellar vermis (the narrow, middle area between the hemispheres of the brain) and cysts in the posterior fossa. The combination of these malformations is what causes hydrocephalus in patients with Dandy-Walker syndrome.

Distal catheter
Catheter connected to the shunt valve and placed in an area of the body where CSF can drain and be reabsorbed.

Diuretic
Any medication that is used to increase the output of urine.

Downward gaze
The ability to look down. A loss of downward gaze, or sunsetting of the eyes, is often a sign of increased intracranial pressure.

Dura
The outermost layer of the meninges.

Electrocardiogram
An electrocardiogram (ECG or EKG) produces a graphic record of heart rhythms.

Endoscope
A small camera used during surgery that allows the surgeon to observe internal structures of the body on a television monitor.

Endoscopic surgery
Surgery aided by the use of an endoscope.

Epinephrine
A type of adrenaline that stimulates heart and breathing rates. Injected into patients who have an allergic reaction to medication (see *Anaphylactic shock*).

Esotropia
Crossed eyes.

External hydrocephalus
See *Benign subdural hygroma.*

External ventricular drainage (EVD)
Drainage system often used when the ventricles of the brain have been compromised by infection. The entire shunt system (i.e., the valve and proximal and distal catheters) is replaced by a single proximal catheter that is connected to a bag to collect CSF as it drains from the ventricles. An EVD also permits the doctors to administer antibiotics directly into the ventricles through the catheter.

Falx cerebri
The fold of the meninges that extends downward between the left and right hemispheres of the brain.

Femoral artery
A large artery that supplies oxygenated blood to the legs and lower extremities.

Fluoroscope
An instrument that consists of a fluorescent screen and is coated with chemicals. Neurosurgeons use fluoroscopes for mass chest X-ray examination after placing a shunt. Images can be viewed without the pictures being developed.

Fogarty catheter
A catheter with a tiny balloon on one end. Used in third ventriculostomy procedures to help enlarge holes that are punctured in the floor of the third ventricle. The neurosurgeon will insert the balloon end of the Fogarty catheter through the hole, inflate it slightly, and then pull the balloon back through the hole to help enlarge it.

Follicle stimulating hormone (FSH)
A hormone produced by the anterior region of the pituitary gland, FSH is responsible for stimulating the ripening of the follicles in the ovaries, and the formation of sperm in the testes.

Fontanel
An opening between the sutures of the skull in infants and young children. If hydrocephalus is present, the fontanel may be enlarged or tense.

Foramen
Narrow passages that permit CSF to flow from one ventricle to another. The ventricular foramina (plural of foramen) consist of the foramen of Monro, which connects the lateral ventricles with the third ventricle, and the foramina of Luschke and Magendie (see below) of the fourth ventricle, which allow CSF to exit the ventricular system.

Foramen of Monro
Small passageway that connects the lateral ventricles with the third ventricle.

Foramina of Luschke and Magendie
Outlets of the fourth ventricle that permit CSF to flow from the ventricular system to the brain.

Frontal lobe
A division located at the front part of each cerebral hemisphere that extends back to the middle of the brain. The frontal lobe makes up approximately one third of each hemisphere of the brain.

Gait
The term used to refer to the way a person walks. When someone is said to have an *unsteady gait,* they may have difficulty walking or maintaining their balance while standing.

Gait disturbance
A reduction or loss of motor skills.

Gamma camera
A special imaging device used to take photographs of parts of the body that have been injected with a contrast-enhancing imaging agent.

Gonadotrophin (GnRH)
Hormone produced by the hypothalamus, responsible for releasing other sex hormones (i.e., FSH, LH, and SHBG) into the bloodstream, causing the production of ova and sperm.

Hemiparesis
Paralysis to one side of the body, caused by damage to the opposite side of the brain.

Hydranencephaly
A rare condition where the brain's cerebral hemispheres are absent at birth, and are replaced by sacs filled with CSF.

Hydrothorax
A condition caused by excessive fluid in the pleural space that surrounds the lungs.

Hyperglycemia
The term used when there is too much sugar in the bloodstream.

Hypoglycemia
The term used when there is not enough sugar in the bloodstream.

Hypothalamus
Part of the brain responsible for regulating body temperature, thirst, emotions, sleep, hunger, eating, water balance, and sexual behavior.

Inelastic
Something that does not stretch.

Internal jugular vein
A vein in the neck that returns blood from the head to the right atrium of the heart. The internal jugular vein is one of the possible locations of the distal catheter for placement of a ventriculoatrial shunt.

Intracranial
Within the cranium; within the skull.

Intracranial pressure (ICP)
The pressure of CSF within the brain.

Intraventricular hemorrhage (IVH)
A bleed within the ventricular system.

Laparoscopic surgery
Abdominal surgery performed with the aid of a laparoscope. As it pertains to hydrocephalus shunt surgery, laparoscopic surgery may be performed on the peritoneal cavity for one of three reasons: to retrieve a disconnected or stray distal catheter; to reinsert the distal catheter if it is pulled out of the peritoneum; to remove and reinsert the distal catheter during shunt lengthening procedures.

Lobe
One of four distinct sections of each cerebral hemisphere: the frontal, temporal, parietal, and occipital lobes.

Lumbar puncture
Procedure performed to measure intracranial pressure, to remove CSF for pathological testing, or to test the shunt system for a possible proximal obstruction. (Also known as a spinal tap.)

Luteinizing hormone (LH)
Hormone produced by the anterior region of the pituitary gland, responsible for producing ovulation, progesterone, and corpus luteum formation, which prepares the uterus for implantation. LH is also responsible for androgen synthesis by the testes, which stimulates development of the male sex organs.

Macrocrania
An enlarged cranium, mainly seen in infants and small children as a result of increased intracranial pressure.

Magnetic resonance imaging (MRI)
A computerized body-imaging process that uses radio waves and powerful magnets to provide three-dimensional images of the body.

Manometer

A graduated scale that is connected to the hub of the needle used to perform a lumbar puncture. The manometer is used to read intracranial pressure as well as to retrieve a sample of CSF for testing.

Medulla

Part of the brain stem, responsible for controlling breathing and heart rate. (Also referred to as medulla oblongata.)

Meninges

Protective layering that surrounds the brain and spinal cord. The three layers that make up the meninges are the dura, arachnoid, and pia.

Meningitis

A life-threatening infection—either viral or bacterial—that causes swelling and inflammation of the meninges. Hydrocephalus develops when scarring of the meninges restricts the flow of CSF in the subarachnoid space, or when it passes through the aqueducts of the ventricular system.

Meningocele

A type of spina bifida where the spinal cord develops normally but the meninges protrude from an opening on the spine.

Motor cortex

Part of the brain responsible for controlling voluntary movements of the muscles and limbs of the body.

Myelomenigocele

The severest form of spina bifida, in which the spinal cord and its protective covering (the meninges) protrude from an opening in the spine.

Neurologist

A doctor who specializes in the study of the structure and function of the body's nervous system. This includes the brain, spinal cord, and peripheral nerves.

Neuro-ophthalmologist

An ophthalmologist who has a subspecialty in neurology and specializes in treating visual problems that are caused by neurological conditions such as hydrocephalus.

Neuropsychologist

A psychologist who specializes in determining where the brain is damaged through a battery of tests and by monitoring the physical and emotional reactions of the patient to the tests.

Neurosurgeon

A doctor who is specially trained and board-certified to operate on the brain and nervous structures of the body.

Non-communicating hydrocephalus
   Hydrocephalus caused when there is a complete obstruction in the flow of CSF within the ventricular system, including the outlets of the fourth ventricle—the foramina of Luschke and Magendie. (Also known as obstructive hydrocephalus.)

Normal-pressure hydrocephalus (NPH)
   Hydrocephalus where the ventricles of the brain are enlarged, yet there is little or no increase in the production of CSF. NPH can be divided into two classifications: those where the cause of the hydrocephalus is known, as in aqueductal stenosis; and *ideopathic,* where the cause of NPH is not yet known.

Nuclear radiologist
   A radiologist who is trained in nuclear medicine.

Nystagmus
   Jerky or unsteady eye movements.

Obstructive hydrocephalus
   See *Non-communicating hydrocephalus.*

Occipital lobe
   The rear of each cerebral hemisphere, responsible for interpreting sight.

Occiput
   In reference to the back of the head or the area near the occipital lobe of the brain.

Oculomotor nerve
   Also known as the third cranial nerve. The oculomotor nerve is responsible for controlling four of the six main muscles of the eye as well as those of the upper eyelid. The fibers of the oculomotor nerve help control eye movements and reactions of the pupils to light.

Optic nerve
   Also known as the second cranial nerve. The optic nerve is responsible for transmitting visual images from the eyes to the occipital lobe. The optic nerves are made up of approximately one million tiny fibers that receive information from the rod and cone cells of the retina.

Papilledema
   Swelling of the optic nerve caused as a result of increased ICP. The increase of ICP causes swelling of the meninges, which constricts the optic nerve at the back of the eye.

Parietal lobe
   One of the four lobes of the brain, the parietal lobe is located above the temporal lobe and between the frontal and occipital lobes. Located

within the parietal lobe is the primary sensory area, which is responsible for receiving sensations from nerves in the body.

Pediatrician

A doctor who specializes in and is board-certified to treat the medical needs of infants and children.

Periostium

The protective layering that surrounds all bones. The periostium lies between bones and muscle tissue.

Peritoneal cavity

The space of the abdomen, below the diaphragm, where the intestines are located. In a ventriculoperitoneal shunt placement, the tip of the distal catheter is placed into the peritoneal cavity. This allows CSF to flow from the ventricles of the brain through the shunt valve, and to be reabsorbed by blood vessels which line the peritoneal cavity.

Peritoneal pseudocysts

One of the rare side effects of having a VP shunt. Pseudocysts are cysts made up of CSF and other debris that can form in the peritoneal cavity near the distal catheter. Although rare, pseudocysts can block the tip of the distal catheter, either reducing the flow of CSF through the shunt system or completely obstructing the distal end.

Pia mater

The innermost layer of the meninges, which hugs the surface of the brain and spinal cord and is filled with blood vessels that supply the nerve tissue below.

Pleural space

The area surrounding the lungs.

Polydypsia

Constant thirst.

Polyuria

Frequent urination.

Pons

The part of the brain stem responsible for relaying information between the two hemispheres of the brain.

Porencephaly

A condition in which communication between the lateral ventricle and the surface of the brain is abnormal.

Primary care physician (PCP)

Your primary, or family, doctor.

Proximal catheter
A catheter placed in the ventricles of the brain. (Also known as the ventricular catheter.)

Pulse oximeter
A device used to measure the amount of oxygen in the bloodstream.

Radioisotope
A radioactive isotope used widely in medicine to enhance CT and MRI imaging studies of shunt systems and the bloodstream.

Radioisotope cisternography
A procedure that is often performed on the patient when NPH is suspected. It monitors the flow of CSF within the subarachnoid spaces, the ventricles, and the basal cisterns.

Radionuclide shuntogram
A test that is performed to determine if the shunt system has been compromised by infection, obstruction, or degradation of the shunt catheters.

Radiopaque material
A material that often contains iodine, used as contrast media in radiography.

Schizencephaly
A rare developmental disorder characterized by abnormal slits or clefts in the brain's cerebral hemispheres.

Sex hormone binding globulin (SHBG)
A hormone produced by the ovaries and testes, responsible for sexual development and stimulating reproductive functions.

Sheath
A layer of connective tissue that encases nerves, arteries, tendons, and muscles.

Silicone
A synthetic plastic polymer material that is rigid yet flexible enough to allow it to bend without kinking.

Slit ventricle syndrome
A syndrome commonly associated with shunt dependency. Ventricles are determined to be slit-like based on their appearance in imaging series, which reveal very narrow or almost nonexistent ventricles.

Spina bifida
A neural tube defect characterized by incomplete development of the brain, spinal cord, and/or their protective coverings.

Staphylococci aureus
Bacteria that can cause shunt infections.

Stenosis
A blockage, as in *Aqueductal stenosis*.

Strabismus
Eye misalignment.

Subarachnoid
The area between the pia and arachnoid mater known as the subarachnoid space, where CSF flows over the surface of the brain and spinal cord.

Subarachnoid cyst
A sac filled with CSF and lined with matter from the arachnoid membrane.

Subdural hematoma
An accumulation of blood (hematoma) between the dura mater and the arachnoid layers of the meninges. This area is known as the subdural space.

Sunsetting of the eyes
Eyes are deviated downward with the eyelids retracted.

Superior sagittal sinus
A large vein that runs sagittally near between the two cerebral hemispheres near the top of the brain. The superior sagittal sinus, in conjunction with the arachnoid granulations (or villi), plays a key role in the circulatory flow of CSF.

Superior vena cava
The superior vena cava, or "large vein," is located in the neck near the carotid artery, and is responsible for returning blood flow from the brain, upper body, and arms to the right atrium of the heart. In most ventriculoatrial (VA) shunt placements, this is where the distal catheter will be placed.

Supine
When you are lying flat on your back.

Sutures
(1) Stitches used to close an incision; (2) the area of the skull formed when the bones of the skull are joined together.

Temporal lobe
Lobe located at the side of the brain within the temple of the cranium.

Tentorium
The fold of the meninges that covers the upper surface of the cerebellum and supports the occipital lobes.

Thalamus

The relay station for all sensory pathways of the brain. With the exception of the sense of smell, all sensory input enters the thalamus before being transmitted to the primary sensory cortex in the parietal lobe.

Third ventriculostomy

A procedure where small holes are punctured through the floor of the third ventricle to permit the flow of CSF from the third to the fourth ventricle of the brain.

Trachea

The windpipe. Part of the air passage between the larynx and the bronchi that carries air to the lungs.

Trocar

A sharp, pointed surgical instrument used in combination with a cannula to draw fluids from the peritoneal cavity.

Trochlear nerve

Also known as the fourth cranial nerve. The trochlear nerve is responsible for rotating the eyeball while at the same time turning it downward and from side to side.

Tumor

An abnormal growth of tissue that grows independently of the normal rate. This tissue may be benign or malignant.

Ultrasonography

The use of high-frequency sound waves to outline the structures within the cranium.

Upward gaze

The ability to look upward.

Ureter

A long narrow duct that conducts urine from the kidneys to the bladder.

Vasopressin

Also known as the antidiuretic hormone, or ADH, the hormone that regulates fluid reabsorption in the kidneys.

Vein of Galen malformation

A rare vascular disorder that occurs mostly in infants and young children. It occurs when the Vein of Galen balloons and creates an aneurysimal sac.

Ventricles

The four chambers of the brain, which are connected to each other by way of narrow passages called foramen. (See *Foramen.*)

Ventricular catheter
See *Proximal catheter.*

Ventricular foramina
See *Foramen.*

Ventriculocholecystic
Type of shunt system where the tip of the distal catheter is placed in the gall bladder.

Ventriculofemoral
Type of shunt system where the distal catheter is inserted into one of the femoral veins of the leg (near the groin). The distal catheter is then run up through the venous system so that the tip of the catheter resides within the right atrium of the heart (similar to a ventriculoatrial shunt placement).

Ventriculopleural
Type of shunt system where the tip of the distal catheter is located in the pleural space that surrounds the lungs.

Ventriculoureter
Type of shunt system where the tip of the distal catheter is located in the ureter, which leads from the bladder.

Bibliography

American Association of Nurse Anesthetists (AANA). Patient resources and information regarding anesthesia. *http://www.aana.com/documents/preop.htm.* Copyright © 1998, AANA.

Bayston, R., and E. Lambert. "Duration of Protective Activity of Cerebrospinal Fluid Shunt Catheters Impregnated with Antimicrobial Agents to Prevent Bacterial Catheter-related Infection." *Journal of Neurosurgery* 87, no. 8 (August 1997): 247-251.

Benzel, E. C., M. Mirfakhraee, and T. A. Hadden. "Evaluation of CSF Shunt Function: Value of Functional Examination with Contrast Material." *American Journal of Neuroradiology.* 12, no. 1 (1991): 143-147.

Black, P. McL., R. Hakim, and N. O. Bailey. "The Use of the Codman-Medos Programmable Hakim Valve in the Management of Patients with Hydrocephalus: Illustrative Cases." *Neurosurgery* 34, no. 6 (June 1994): 1110.

Black, P. McL., and R. G. Ojemann. *Youmans Neurological Surgery: A Comprehensive Reference Guide to the Diagnosis and Management of Neurosurgical Problems, Second Edition.* W.B. Saunders Company, 1990. Chapter 41, "Hydrocephalus in Adults," 1277-1298.

Chapman, P.H., E.R. Cosman, and M.A. Arnold. "The Relationship Between Ventricular Fluid Pressure and Body Position in Normal Subjects and Subjects with Shunts: a Telemetric Study." *Neurosurgery* 26, no. 2 (February 1990): 181-189.

Chapman, P. H. *Youmans Neurological Surgery, Second Edition.* W. B. Saunders Company, 1990. Chapter 40, "Hydrocephalus in Childhood," 1236-1276.

Clyde, B. L., and A. L. Albright. "Evidence for a Patent Fibrous Tract in Fractured, Outgrown, or Disconnected Ventriculoperitoneal Shunts," *Pediatric Neurosurgery* 23, no. 1 (1995): 20-25.

Diagnostic and Statistical Manual of Mental Disorders, Fourth Edition. Washington, DC: American Psychiatric Association, 1994.

Ersahin, Y., S. Mutluer, and G. Tekeli. "Abdominal Cerebrospinal Fluid Pseudocysts." *Child's Nervous System* 12, no. 12 (1996): 755-758.

Fenichel, Gerald M. *Clinical Pediatric Neurology: A Signs and Symptoms Approach.* W.B. Saunders Company, 1997. Chapter 18, "Disorders of Cranial Volume and Shape," 365-373.

Fouyas, I. P., et al. "Use of Intracranial Pressure Monitoring in the Management of Childhood Hydrocephalus and Shunt-related Problems." *Neurosurgery* 38, no. 4 (1996): 726-732.

Fudge, Emily. *Nonverbal Learning Disorder Syndrome Information Sheet.* Adapted from a paper by Rochelle Harris, David H. Bennett, Brian Belden, Lynne Covitz, and Vicki Little, of the Section of Developmental Medicine and Psychology, Children's Mercy Hospital, Kansas City, Missouri.

Goodman, R. R., "Magnetic Resonance Imaging-Directed Stereotactic Endoscopic Third Ventriculostomy." *(technical note). Neurosurgery* 32, no. 6 (June 1993): 1043.

Haerer, Armin F. *DeJong's The Neurologic Examination, Fifth Edition.* J.B. Lippincott Company, 1992. Chapter 59, "Related Examinations and Procedures," 789-791.

Hamilton, M. G., J. B. Frizzell, and B. I. Tranmer. "Chronic Subdural Hematoma: the Role for Craniotomy Reevaluated." *Neurosurgery* 33, no. 1 (1993): 67-72.

Hallowell, Edward M., and John J. Ratey. *Driven to Distraction: Recognizing and Coping with Attention Deficit Disorder from Childhood Through Adulthood.* Simon & Schuster, 1995.

Hudgins, R. J., and W. R. Boydston. "Hydrocephalus, Part 3: Shunt Complications." *Pediatric Neurosurgery News* 2, no. 1 (1998).

Jaeger, K. M., and T. N. Layton. *New Shunt System for Treatment of Hydrocephalus: in Vitro Testing.* Consensus Conference on Complex Hydrocephalus and Hydrocephalus Complications, Assisi, Italy, April 1997.

James, Hector E. "Hydrocephalus in Infancy and Childhood." *American Family Physician* 45, no. 2 (February 1992): 733-742.

Jimenez, D. F., R. Keating, and J. T. Goodrich. "Silicone Allergy in Ventriculoperitoneal Shunts." *Child's Nervous System* 10, no. 1 (1994): 59-63.

Karp, G. L. *Life on Wheels.* O'Reilly & Associates, 1999. Chapter 9, "Spinal Cord Research."

Ketoff, J. A., R. L. Klein, and K. F. Maukkassa. "Ventricular Cholecystic Shunts in Children." *Journal of Pediatric Neurosurgery* 32, no. 2 (February 1997): 181-183.

Kevles, Bettyann H. *Naked to the Bone: Medical Imaging in the Twentieth Century.* Rutgers University Press, 1997.

Klauschie, J., and S. R. Rose. "Incidence of Short Stature in Children with Hydrocephalus." *Journal of Pediatric Endocrinology and Metabolism* 9, no. 2 (March 1996): 181-187.

Löppönen, T., et al. "Accelerated Pubertal Development in Patients with Shunted Hydrocephalus." *Archives of Diseases in Children* 74, no. 6 (June 1996): 490-496.

Lund-Johansen, M., F. Svendsen, and K. Wester. "Shunt Failures and Complications in Adults as Related to Shunt Type, Diagnosis, and the Experience of the Surgeon." *Neurosurgery* 35, no. 5 (1994): 839.

Lundar, T., and P. Nakstad. "Torkildsen's Operation—50 Years Later." *Tidsskrift for den Norske Laegeforen* 110, no. 5 (February 1990): 584-586. (Article in Norwegian.)

McComb, J. G. *Neurosurgical Emergencies, Vol. II, Acute Shunt Malfunction.* American Association of Neurological Surgeons, 1994. Chapter 21, 327-334.

McComb, J. G. *Surgery of the Third Ventricle, 2nd Ed.* Williams & Wilkins, 1998. Chapter 27, "Methods of Cerebrospinal Fluid Diversion."

Newton, P. "A New Self-adjusting Flow-regulating Device for Shunting of CSF." *Child's Nervous System* 26, no. 10 (October 1996): 619-625.

Philips, M. F., et al. "Ventriculofemoroatrial Shunt: a Viable Alternative for the Treatment of Hydrocephalus" (technical note). *Journal of Neurosurgery* 86, no. 6 (June 1997): 1063-1066.

Piatt, J. H., Jr., and C. V. Carlson. "Hydrocephalus and Epilepsy: an Actuarial Analysis." *Neurosurgery* 39, no. 4 (October 1996): 722-728.

Prockop, Leon D. *Merritt's Textbook of Neurology, Ninth Edition.* Williams & Wilkins, 1995. Section V, "Disorders of Cerebrospinal and Brain Fluids."

Proos, L. A., et al. "Increased Perinatal Intracranial Pressure and Prediction of Early Puberty in Girls with Myelomeningocele." *Archive of Diseases in Childhood* 75, no. 1 (July 1996): 42-45.

Public Law 101-476 (S. 1824), *Education of the Handicapped Act Amendments of 1990 (EHA).* This law is a series of amendments, including changing the name from EHA to the Individuals with Disabilities Education Act (IDEA). The text of this law can be obtained from the Library of Congress, or on the Web: *http://thomas.loc.gov/home/thomas2.html.*

Public Law 105-17 (H.R. 5), *Individuals with Disabilities Education Act Amendments of 1997.* Better known as IDEA '97, this law amends P.L. 101-476 with stronger provisions for guaranteeing access to specialized education for children with disabilities. The text of this law can be obtained from the Library of Congress, or on the Web: *http://thomas.loc.gov/home/thomas2.html.*

Reinprecht, A., T. Czech, and W. Dietrich. "Clinical Experience with a New Pressure-adjustable Shunt Valve." *Acta Neurochirurgica* 134, no. 3-4 (1995): 119-124.

Stamos, J. K., B. A. Kaufman, and R. Yogev. "Ventriculoperitoneal Shunt Infections with Gram-negative Bacteria." *Neurosurgery* 33, no. 5 (1993): 858-862.

Tanaka, J., et al. "Laparoscopic Retrieval of Disconnected Ventriculoperitoneal Shunt Catheters: Report of Two Cases." *Surgical Laparoscopy and Endoscopy* 5, no. 4 (1995): 263-266.

Vernet, O., et al. "Radionuclide Shuntogram: Adjunct to Manage Hydrocephalic Patients." *Journal of Nuclear Medicine* 37, no. 3 (1996): 406-410.

Walker, M. L., et al. *Neurosurgery Clinics of North America, Vol. 4* (A. Butler and D. McLone, eds.). Philadelphia: W.B. Saunders, 1993. "Diagnosis and Treatment of the Slit Ventricle Syndrome," 707-714.

Walker, M. L., and J. Petronio. *Pediatric Neurosurgery: Surgery of the Developing Nervous System, 3rd Edition* (W. Cheek, ed.). Philadelphia: W.B. Saunders, 1994. "Ventriculoscopy," 572-581.

Watson, D. A. *The Delta™ Valve: A physiologic shunt system*. The Consensus Conference on Pediatric Neurosurgery, Assisi, Italy, April 1992.

Wiswell, Thomas E., et al. "Major Congenital Neurologic Malformations: A 17-Year Study." *American Journal of Diseases of Children* 144, no. 1 (January 1990): 61-67.

Index

A

abducens nerve, 153
abnormal head growth, 21-23
acquired hydrocephalus, 10-13
admissions, hospital, 114-116
adult onset hydrocephalus, 37-39
Alzheimer's disease, 33
AMA Directory of Physicians in the United States, 64-65
American Association of Neurological Surgeons (AANS), 67
American Association for Marriage and Family Therapy, The (AAMFT), 188
American Board of Pediatric Neurological Surgery (ABPNS), 62
American Medical Association (AMA), 67
Americans with Disabilities Act (ADA), 272-273
anesthesia, 94-96
    questionnaire, 95-96
    questions to ask before, 96
antiseizure medication, 160-165
    common side effects of, 160-161
    Depakene; Depakote (Valproic acid), 162
    Diamox (Acetazolamide), 162
    Dilantin (Phenytoin sodium), 163
    Klonopin (Clonazepam), 163
    Lamictal (Lamotrigine), 163
    Mysoline (Primidone), 163-164
    Neurontin (Gabapentin), 164

    Phenobarbital (Luminal, Solfoton), 164
    questions to ask about, 160
    Tegretol (Carbamazepine; Atretol, Epitol, Tegretol-XR), 164-165
    Valium (Diazepam), 165
    Zarontin (Ethosuximide), 166
aqueduct of Sylvius, 2
aqueductal stenosis, 2
arachnoid, 5
Arnold-Chiari malformation (ACM), 17
Association for Spina Bifida and Hydrocephalus (ASBAH), 184
attention deficit disorder (ADD), 201-204
    characteristics of, 201-203
    intervention for, 203-204
attention deficit hyperactivity disorder (ADHD), 201-204
    characteristics of, 201-203
    intervention for, 203-204

B

bacterial meningitis, 11-12
benign extra-axial fluid of infancy, 32
Beverly Referential Valve, 90-91
Biomaterials Access Assurance Act of 1997, 269-270
brain
    cerebellum, 9
    cerebral hemispheres, 6-7
    meninges, 4-6

Desmopressin (DDAVP), 170-171
diabetes insipidus, 169-171
    symptoms, tests for, 169-170
    treatment for, 170-171
diagnosis
    adult onset hydrocephalus,
        example, 37-39
    child, informing of, 52-53
    childhood onset hydrocephalus,
        example, 35-37
    congenital hydrocephalus,
        example, 34-35
    CT scans, 28-32
    MRI scans, 28-32
    neurological exam, 25-28
    radioisotope cisternography, 27-
        28
    second opinions for, 33
    ultrasonography (ultrasound), 28
    See also misdiagnoses; responses
        to diagnosis
Diamond™ valve, 92
Diamox (Acetazolamide), 162
differential pressure valves, 79
Dilantin (Phenytoin sodium), 163
disconnected catheters, 141-142
distal catheter, 77
    obstructions, 134-135
doctor-patient relationship, 251-255
    joint decision making and, 252
Durable Power of Attorney for Health
    Care, 258-260
dura mater, 5

E

Elekta Instruments, Inc., 91
emergencies
    Durable Power of Attorney for
        Health Care, 258-260
    family, friends and, 255
    MedicAlert, 255-257
    neurosurgeons and, 56
    wallet-sized CTs, MRIs, 258

employee assistance programs (EAPs),
    190
endoscopic third ventriculostomy,
    100-101
eye, visual problems, 23-24, 152-156
    eye misalignments, 155
    how brain sees, 152-153
    impaired vision, 156
    ophthalmologists, 154-155
    perceptual defects, 156
    sunsetting, 24, 155
    symptoms of, 153-154

F

falx cerebri, 5-6
Family and Medical Leave Act of
    1993, 267-268
fee-for-service (unmanaged care)
    insurance, 228
first aid, seizures and, 166-168
foramen, 7
foramen of Monro, 2
free appropriate public education
    (FAPE), 212
frontal lobes, 6

G

gait disturbance, 23
German measles, 10
government insurance plans
    Medicaid, 231
    Medicare, 231-232
    socialized medicine and, 232-233
    Social Security Disability
        Insurance (SSDI), 270-
        272
    TriCare (CHAMPUS), 230-231

H

Hakim™ Precision Valve System, 87
headaches, 23
head trauma, 13

NeuroCare Group, Heyer-Shulte®
    shunts, 89-91
neuroendoscopic third
    ventriculostomy, 100-
    101
neurological exam, 25-28
    adults, 27
    children, 26-27
    full-term infants, 25
    premature infants, 25
Neurontin (Gabapentin), 164
neuro-opthalmologists, 154
neuropsychological testing, 147-152
    benefits of, 149-150
    described, 151
    paying for, 148-149
    results of, 151-152
    selecting neuropsychologist, 150-
    151
neurosurgeons, 54
    communication skills and, 70
    emergency treatments, 56
    finding new (relocating), 74-75
    interviewing, 68-69
    newly diagnosed patients, 55-56
    personalities of, 70-72
    relationship with, 69-70, 72-73
    selecting new, 56-57
    shunt revisions and, 143-144
    See also referrals
neurosurgeons, selecting
    commercial resources for, 63
    national practitioner data bank,
    67-68
    Official ABMS Directory of Board
        Certified Medical
        Specialists, The, 65-66
    online resources, 66-67
    print resources, 63-66
    16,638 Questionable Doctors, 66
    See also referrals
neurosurgery. See surgery
Newton SaFR™, 92

NMT Neurosciences (U.S.), Inc.,
    Cordis® shunt
    products, 91-92
non-communicating hydrocephalus,
    13-14
nonsurgical treatments, 101
nonverbal learning disorder (NVLD),
    204-210
    causes of, 204-205
    characteristics of, 205-207
    helping with, 207-210
normal-pressure hydrocephalus
    (NPH), 14, 37
Novus™ shunt valve system, 89-90
nuclear cisternography, 27-28

O

obstructions, 133-135
    distal catheter, 134-135
    proximal catheter , 133-134
obstructive hydrocephalus, 13-14
occipital lobe, 7
oculomotor nerve, 153
Official ABMS Directory of Board
    Certified Medical
    Specialists, The, 65-66
Omnishunt® system, 91-92
online resources. See internet
    resources
ophthalmologists, 154-155
    neuro-opthalmologists, 154
    pediatric, 154
optic nerve, 152-153
Orbis-Sigma® system, 91
Otitic hydrocephalus, 13

P

parents, support for, 178-180, 182-
    183
parietal lobes, 6
Parinaud's syndrome, 24
pediatric ophthalmologists, 154
perceptual defects, 156

peritoneal pseudocysts, 142-143
Phenobarbital (Luminal, Solfoton), 164
Phoenix Biomedical, Diamond™ Valve and shunt system, 92
physician referrals, 58-59
Physicians Who Care advocacy group, 241
pia mater, 5
precocious puberty, 168-169
    causes of, 168
    symptoms of, 168-169
preexisting conditions, insurance and, 223-225
preferred provider organization (PPO), 229
prefrontal cortex, 6
pregnancy, 250-251
proximal catheter, 77
    obstructions, 133-134
PS Medical shunts, 89
PubMed, 264-265

R

radioisotope cisternography, 27-28
radionuclide shuntogram, 130-131
recovery
    follow-up visits, 124
    at home, 123-124
    in hospital, 122-123
referrals
    insurance/HMO, 59-60
    physician, 58-59
    word-of-mouth, 60-61
    See also neurosurgeons, selecting new
researching medical texts, 260
    Internet Grateful Med, 265-266
    Loansome Doc™, 266-267
    medical libraries, 263-264
    online resources, 264-267
    public libraries, 260-263

PubMed, 264-265
responses to diagnosis, 39-45
    anger, 43-44
    confusion, numbness, 40
    denial, 40-41
    fear, 42-43
    friends, 49-50
    hope, 45
    patients, 45-46
    physical, 44-45
    relief, 39-40
    sadness, 41-42
    siblings, 46-48
    spouses, 50-52
    See also diagnosis
rubella, 10

S

schizencephaly, 19
school. *See* learning disabilities
school absences, 198-200
    informing teacher, school regarding, 198-199
    involving teachers, classmates and, 199
    returning after, 200
seizures, 156-160
    antiseizure medication, questions to ask regarding, 160
    causes of, 156-157
    diagnosis of, 159
    first aid for, 166-168
    monitoring, 159-160
    partial, generalized, 158-159
    phases of, 157-158
    surgery for, 166
    treating, 160-168
shunt infections, 137-139
    avoiding, 139
    causes of, 138
    symptoms of, 137-138
    treating, 138-139

shunt revisions
    chronic problems and, 144-145
    complications, signs of and, 126-
        129
    complications and, 140-143
    defined, 126
    infections and, 137-139
    lengthening procedures and, 129-
        130
    obstructions and, 133-135
    silicone allergies and, 140
    subdural hematomas, 135-137
    surgeons, experience of and, 143-
        144
    testing for problems and, 130-133
shunts
    body position changes and, 79-80
    common features of, 85-86
    differences among, 84-86
    how, works, 77-78
    lumboperitoneal (LP), 83
    manufacturers of, 86
    manufacturing, testing, 85
    materials, components of, 85
    parts of, 77
    placement of, 80-84
    placement operations for, 97-101
    valve pressure readings, 79
    ventriculoatrial (VA), 81-83
    ventriculofermoral (VF), 83
    ventriculo-gallbladder (VGB), 84
    ventriculogastric (VG), 84
    ventriculoperitoneal (VP), 81
    ventriculopleural (VPl), 83
    ventriculoureter (VU), 84
    See also specific manufacturers;
        surgery
shunt tap, 131-132
shunt valve, 77
siblings
    diagnosis, impact on, 46-48
    support groups for, 181-182

side effects
    common complaints, 146-147
    diabetes insipidus, 169-171
    eye, visual problems, 152-156
    neuropsychological, testing for,
        147-152
    precocious puberty, 168-169
    seizures, 156-160
    See also neuropsychological
        testing
silicone allergies, 140
16,638 Questionable Doctors, (Public
        Citizen: Health Research
        Group), 66
slit ventricle syndrome (SVS), 143
socialized medicine, 232-233
Social Security Disability Insurance
        (SSDI), 270-272
spina bifida (SB), 16-17
state education agency (SEA), 213
subarachnoid, 5

subdural hematomas (SDH), 135-137
    detecting, 136
    treatment for, 136-137
subdural space, 5
sunsetting eyes, 24, 155
superior sagittal sinus, 2
support
    clergy, 183-184
    conferences on hydrocephalus,
        190-191
    employee assistance programs
        (EAPs), 190
    hospital social workers, 177
    internet and, 192-194
    need for, 172-174
    sources of, 174-176
    starting local group for, 194-196
    See also counseling

ventriculoatrial (VA) shunts, 81-83
    placement of, 99-100
ventriculofemoral (VF) shunts, 83
ventriculo-gallbladder (VGB) shunts,
        84
ventriculogastric (VG) shunts, 84
ventriculoperitoneal (VP) shunts, 81
    placement of, 98-99
ventriculopleural (VPl) shunts, 83
ventriculoureter (VU) shunts, 84
vision problems, 23-24
    sunsetting, 24
    See also eye, visual problems

X
X-linked hydrocephalus, 10

Z
Zarontin (Ethosuximide), 166

About the Authors

Chuck Toporek, originally from the small rural community of Brownstown Township, Michigan, began his career in publishing after four years in the U.S. Navy. He worked at JEMS Publishing Company, where he cut his teeth as a grunt editor and researcher for *JEMS—Journal of Emergency Medical Services*, *Rescue* magazine, the *Journal of Prehospital Disaster Medicine*, and the *Emergency Care Information Center*. After leaving JEMS to move to Vancouver, British Columbia to marry Kellie, Chuck worked for the National Advertising Benevolent Society of Canada (NABS) until 1993, when he and Kellie moved to Bellingham, Washington. There, Chuck worked as a graphic artist and managing editor for The International Society of Photo-Optical Instrumentation Engineers (SPIE). He is currently the managing editor of *Web Review* magazine (*www.webreview.com*). In his spare time, Chuck enjoys riding his mountain bike, digital art design, photography, playing with his cat, Max, watching cartoons, and quoting lines from Monty Python's *The Holy Grail*.

Kellie Robinson, originally from Vancouver, British Columbia, lives in California with her husband and co-author, Chuck Toporek, and their crazy, cool cat, Max. For the past three years, Kellie has been working with young children. She also writes stories for children in her spare time. In addition to writing, Kellie has enjoyed doing voice work and commercials for several years. While living in Bellingham, Washington, she worked as an on-air announcer and board operator for the local National Public Radio station, KZAZ. Ideally, Kellie would like to combine her love of children, writing, and broadcasting to someday host a children's radio show.

You can reach the authors care of O'Reilly & Associates, Inc., by mail or email (*patientguides@oreilly.com*).

Colophon

Patient-Centered Guides are about the experience of illness. They contain personal stories as well as a mixture of practical and medical information. The faces on the covers of our Guides reflect the human side of the information we offer.

The cover of *Hydrocephalus: A Guide for Patients, Families, and Friends* was designed by Edie Freedman using Adobe Photoshop 5.0 and QuarkXPress 3.32 with Onyx BT and Berkeley fonts from Bitstream. The cover photo is from Rubberball Productions, and is used with their permission. The cover mechanical was prepared by Edie Freedman and Kathleen Wilson.

The interior layout for the book was designed by Nancy Priest and Edie Freedman. The interior fonts are Berkeley and Franklin Gothic. The text was prepared by Edie Freedman, Mike Sierra, and Nancy Wolfe Kotary, using QuarkXPress 3.32 and

FrameMaker 5.5. Illustrations were created by Robert Romano using Adobe Photoshop 5.0 and Macromedia FreeHand 8.0. The text was copyedited by Lunaea Hougland and proofread by Gill Kent. Nicole Gipson Arigo, John Files, and Sheryl Avruch provided quality assurance. The index was written by Ruth Rautenberg. Interior composition was done by Claire Cloutier LeBlanc, Sebastian Banker, and Betty Hugh.

Whenever possible, our books use RepKover™ or Otabind™ lay-flat binding. If the page count exceeds the limit for lay-flat binding, perfect binding is used.

Permission to use photographs and illustrations in *Hydrocephalus: A Guide for Patients, Families, and Friends* was provided by the following:

Illustrations of the CSF circulatory pathway, the protective coverings of the brain, the ventricular system, and VP and VA shunt placement have been closely adapted from *About Hydrocephalus: A Book for Parents* © Copyright 1998 Hydrocephalus Association, with permission from the Hydrocephalus Association.

CT images of the brain before and after shunt placement are courtesy of J. Gordon McComb, M.D., and are used with his permission.

Photos of the Codman Hakim™ Precision Valve System, and the Codman Uni-Shunt are courtesy of Johnson & Johnson, and are used with their permission.

Photo of the Delta Valve shunt systems is courtesy of Medtronic PS Medical, and is used with their permission.

Photo of the Novus™ and Novus™ Mini shunt valves is courtesy of NeuroCare Group, and is used with their permission.

Photo of the Diamond™ valve is used by permission of Phoenix Biomedical Corporation, © Copyright Phoenix Biomedical Corporation 1998.

MRI image of the brain, showing bilateral subdural hematomas, is courtesy of Peter M. Black, M.D., and is used with his permission.

Patient-Centered Guides™

Questions Answered
Experiences Shared

We are committed to empowering individuals to evolve into informed consumers armed with the latest information and heartfelt support for their journey.

When your life is turned upside down, your need for information is great. You have to make critical medical decisions, often with what seems little to go on. Plus you have to break the news to family, quiet your own fears, cope with symptoms or treatment side effects, figure out how you're going to pay for things, and sometimes still get to work or get dinner on the table.

Patient-Centered Guides provide authoritative information for intelligent information seekers who want to become advocates of their own health. They cover the whole impact of illness on your life. In each book, there's a mix of:

- **Medical background for treatment decisions**
  We can give you information that can help you to intelligently work with your doctor to come to a decision. We start from the viewpoint that modern medicine has much to offer and also discuss complementary treatments. Where there are treatment controversies we present differing points of view.

- **Practical information**
  Once you've decided what to do about your illness, you still have to deal with treatments and changes to your life. We cover day-to-day practicalities, such as those you'd hear from a good nurse or a knowledgeable support group.

- **Emotional support**
  It's normal to have strong reactions to a condition that threatens your life or changes how you live. It's normal that the whole family is affected. We cover issues like the shock of diagnosis, living with uncertainty, and communicating with loved ones.

Each book also contains stories from both patients and doctors — medical "frequent fliers" who share, in their own words, the lessons and strategies they have learned when maneuvering through the often complicated maze of medical information that's available.

We provide information online, including updated listings of the resources that appear in this book. This is freely available for you to print out and copy to share with others, as long as you retain the copyright notice on the print-outs.

http://www.patientcenters.com

Other Books in the Series

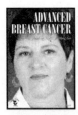

Advanced Breast Cancer
A Guide to Living with Metastatic Disease
By Musa Mayer
ISBN 1-56592-522-X, Paperback 6" x 9", 542 pages, $19.95

"An excellent book...if knowledge is power, this book will be good medicine."
—David Spiegel, M.D.
Stanford University, Author of *Living Beyond Limits*

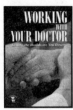

Working with Your Doctor
Getting the Healthcare You Deserve
By Nancy Keene
ISBN 1-56592-273-5, Paperback, 6" x 9", 382 pages, $15.95

"Working with Your Doctor fills a genuine need for patients and their family members caught up in this new and intimidating age of impersonal, economically-driven health care delivery."
—James Dougherty, M.D.
Emeritus Professor of Surgery, Albany Medical College

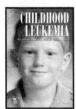

Childhood Leukemia
A Guide for Families, Friends & Caregivers
By Nancy Keene
ISBN 1-56592-191-7, Paperback, 6" x 9", 566 pages, $24.95

"What's so compelling about Childhood Leukemia is the amount of useful medical information and practical advice it contains. Keene avoids jargon and lays out what's needed to deal with the medical system."
—The Washington Post

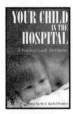

Your Child in the Hospital
A Practical Guide for Parents
By Nancy Keene and Rachel Prentice
ISBN 1-56592-346-4, Paperback, 5" x 8", 136 pages, $9.95

"When your child is ill or injured, the hospital setting can be overwhelming. Here is a terrific 'road map' to help keep families 'on track.'"
—James B. Fahner, M.D., Division Chief
Pediatric Hematology/Oncology
DeVos Children's Hospital, Grand Rapids, Michigan

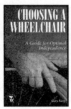

Choosing a Wheelchair
A Guide for Optimal Independence
By Gary Karp
ISBN 1-56592-411-8, Paperback, 5" x 8", 192 pages, $9.95

"I love the idea of putting knowledge often possessed only by professionals into the hands of new consumers. Gary Karp has done it. This book will empower people with disabilities to make informed equipment choices."
—Barry Corbet, Editor
New Mobility Magazine

Patient-Centered Guides
Published by O'Reilly & Associates, Inc.
Our products are available at a bookstore near you.
For information: 800-998-9938 • 707-829-0515 • info@oreilly.com
101 Morris Street • Sebastopol • CA • 95472-9902